Register Now for Online Access to Your Book!

SPRINGER PUBLISHING CONNECT™

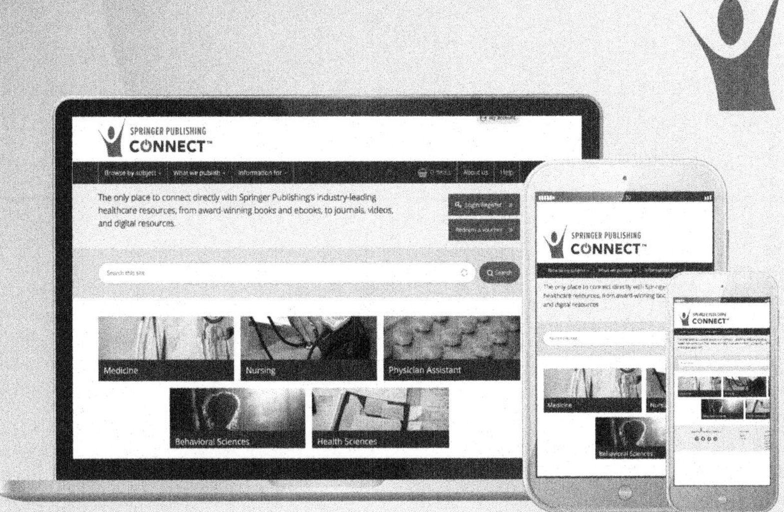

Your print purchase of *A Practical Guide to Child and Adolescent Mental Health Screening, Evidence-Based Assessment, Intervention, and Health Promotion, Third Edition,* **includes online access to the contents of your book**—increasing accessibility, portability, and searchability!

Access today at:
http://connect.springerpub.com/content/book/978-0-8261-6727-9
or scan the QR code at the right with your smartphone. Log in or register, then click "Redeem a voucher" and use the code below.

ESRY8TEL

Scan here for quick access.

Having trouble redeeming a voucher code?
Go to https://connect.springerpub.com/redeeming-voucher-code

If you are experiencing problems accessing the digital component of this product, please contact our customer service department at cs@springerpub.com

The online access with your print purchase is available at the publisher's discretion and may be removed at any time without notice.

Publisher's Note: New and used products purchased from third-party sellers are not guaranteed for quality, authenticity, or access to any included digital components.

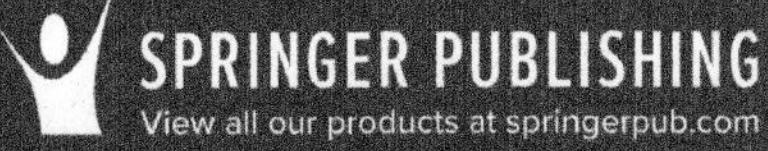

A Practical Guide to Child and Adolescent Mental Health Screening, Evidence-Based Assessment, Intervention, and Health Promotion

Bernadette "Bern" Mazurek Melnyk, PhD, APRN-CNP, FAANP, FNAP, FAAN, is Vice President for Health Promotion, University Chief Wellness Officer, Helene Fuld Health Trust Professor of Evidence-Based Practice, and Dean of the College of Nursing at The Ohio State University, where she also is a Professor of Pediatrics and Psychiatry in the College of Medicine and Executive Director of the Helene Fuld Health Trust National Institute for Evidence-Based Practice. She is recognized nationally and globally for her clinical knowledge and expertise in evidence-based practice, child and adolescent mental health, clinician burnout and resiliency, and intervention research, as well as her innovative approaches to health and wellness. She is sought after as a keynote speaker at national and international conferences and has conducted hundreds of workshops on health and wellness, child and adolescent mental health, and evidence-based practice for healthcare systems, national organizations, and corporations throughout the nation and globe.

Dr. Melnyk is an elected member of the National Academy of Medicine, the American Academy of Nursing, the National Academies of Practice, and the American Association of Nurse Practitioners. She also is a member of the National Academies of Sciences, Engineering and Medicine Expert Panel on Promoting Emotional Well-Being in Children and Adolescents, in collaboration with the Centers for Disease Control and Prevention (CDC), and the National Academy of Medicine's Action Collaborative on Clinician Well-Being and Resilience, as well as a member of the board of directors for the National Forum for Heart Disease and Stroke Prevention. Dr. Melnyk has received over $33 million of sponsored funding from federal agencies, including the National Institutes of Health/National Institute of Nursing Research, and National Institute of Minority Health and Health Disparities, and foundations as a Principal Investigator, is an editor of seven books, and has authored over 450 publications. She is the editor-in-chief of the journal *Worldviews on Evidence-Based Nursing*. Dr. Melnyk has received numerous national and international awards, including induction into Sigma Theta Tau International's Research Hall of Fame and recognition as an Edge Runner three times by the American Academy of Nursing for founding and directing the National Association of Pediatric Nurse Practitioners' KySS child and adolescent mental health campaign, her COPE (Creating Opportunities for Personal Empowerment) program for parents of critically ill children and preterm infants, and her COPE cognitive behavioral skills building program for depressed and anxious children, teens, and young adults, which is being implemented in primary care clinics, schools, universities, community and mental health settings, and private practices throughout the United States and five countries.

Dr. Melnyk earned her Bachelor of Science in Nursing degree from West Virginia University, her Master of Science degree with a specialization in nursing care of children and pediatric nurse practitioner from the University of Pittsburgh, and her PhD in clinical research from the University of Rochester, where she also completed her post-master's certificate as a psychiatric mental health nurse practitioner.

Pamela Lusk, DNP, RN, PMHNP-BC, FAANP, FAAN, is Associate Professor of Clinical Nursing and Director of the KySS Online Child and Adolescent Mental Health Program at The Ohio State University College of Nursing. Dr. Lusk received her BSN from Spalding University in Louisville, Kentucky. She earned her MSN from University of North Carolina, Chapel Hill as a Psychiatric Clinical Nurse Specialist—Child/Adolescent. After years of practice, she returned for a post-master's certificate as a Psychiatric/Mental Health Nurse Practitioner and a Doctor of Nursing Practice degree at Arizona State University. Dr. Lusk has worked in all areas of Child/Adolescent Psychiatric/Mental Health Nursing, including inpatient units, community mental health settings, and most recently as an integrated behavioral health provider (PMHNP) in rural Federally Qualified Health Centers. She currently practices as the integrated PMHNP in a large pediatric practice in Prescott, Arizona.

A Practical Guide to Child and Adolescent Mental Health Screening, Evidence-Based Assessment, Intervention, and Health Promotion

THIRD EDITION

Bernadette Mazurek Melnyk, PhD, APRN-CNP, FAANP, FNAP, FAAN
Pamela Lusk, DNP, RN, PMHNP-BC, FAANP, FAAN

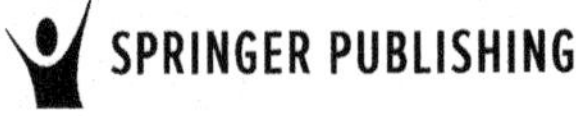

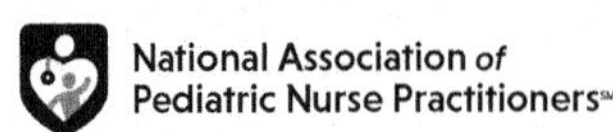

Conflict of Interest Statement: Bernadette Mazurek Melnyk owns a company entitled COPE2Thrive, LLC, that disseminates her evidence-based Creating Opportunities for Personal Empowerment (COPE) programs for children, teens, and young adults that are described in this book.

Springer Publishing Company, LLC
11 West 42nd Street, New York, NY 10036
www.springerpub.com
connect.springerpub.com/

Acquisitions Editor: Elizabeth Nieginski
Compositor: diacriTech

ISBN: 978-0-8261-6726-2
ebook ISBN: 978-0-8261-6727-9
DOI: 10.1891/9780826167279

Printable patient education handouts are available at connect.springerpub.com/content/book/978-0-8261-6727-9
Patient Education Handouts ISBN: 978-0-8261-6033-1

21 22 23 24 / 5 4 3 2 1

Library of Congress Control Number: 2021917662

Printed in the United States of America.

This book is dedicated to all children, teens, and young adults at risk for and suffering with mental health disorders, especially those with severe conditions that require hospitalization and those who have little or no access to evidence-based programs and treatment. I have been blessed to care for so many of these affected children, adolescents, and young adults, including those hospitalized at the Elmira Psychiatric Center Children and Youth In-Patient Unit, who enriched my life for almost two decades. These children and youth taught me that "rainbows follow rain" and that, even with the most severe conditions, there is always hope for a brighter tomorrow.

Bernadette Mazurek Melnyk

I dedicate this book to the incredible first line health professionals who serve our children and adolescents in pediatric and primary care settings. The need for mental health screening, evaluation, and interventions for children, adolescents, and families is great and seems to be ever increasing. With shortages of child psychiatric specialists and wait lists to be seen for initial psychiatric evaluation, primary care and pediatric professionals are tasked with providing the screenings and first-line mental health interventions. I have such admiration for these first-line providers and their dedication to provide the optimal comprehensive care for their patients and families. This text is intended to be a resource for busy practice to help with the mental health aspects of care.

Pamela Lusk

Contents

Printable patient education handouts are available at connect.springerpub.com/content/book/978-0-8261-6727-9 (by clicking on the "Show supplementary" button).

Contributors

Dawn Anderson-Butcher, PhD, LISW-S
Professor
College of Social Work
The Ohio State University
Columbus, Ohio

Annahita Ball, PhD, MSW
Associate Professor
School of Social Work
University at Buffalo, SUNY
Buffalo, New York

Holly Brown, DNP, RN, PMHNP-BC, PMHCS-BC
Associate Professor
Wegmans School of Nursing
Associate Director
Golisano Institute for Developmental Disability Nursing
St. John Fisher College
Rochester, New York

John V. Campo, MD
Professor of Psychiatry and Behavioral Science
Johns Hopkins University School of Medicine
Vice President of Psychiatric Services
Kennedy Krieger Institute
Baltimore, Maryland

Tasha M. Childs, MSW, LSW
Doctoral Candidate
College of Social Work
University of South Carolina
Columbia, South Carolina

Kate Gawlik, DNP, RN, APRN-CNP, FAANP
Associate Professor of Clinical Nursing
College of Nursing
The Ohio State University
Columbus, Ohio

Ann M. Guthery, PhD, RN, PMHNP-BC
Assistant Professor
Specialty Coordinator for Family Psychiatric Mental Health Nurse Practitioner DNP Program
Edson College of Nursing and Health Innovation
Arizona State University
Phoenix, Arizona

Neil E. Herendeen, MD, MS
Professor of Pediatrics
University of Rochester Medical Center
Rochester, New York

Pamela A. Herendeen, DNP, PPCNP-BC
Associate Professor
Wegmans School of Nursing
St. John Fisher College
Pittsford, New York
Senior Nurse Practitioner
Golisano Children's Hospital
Rochester, New York

Jacqueline Hoying, PhD, RN
Assistant Professor
Director MINDSTRONG/MINDBODYSTRONG Program
Director, Helene Fuld Health Trust National Institute for Evidence-Based Practice in Nursing and Healthcare
College of Nursing
The Ohio State University
Columbus, Ohio

Aidyn Iachini, PhD, MSW, LSW
Associate Professor
College of Social Work
University of South Carolina
Columbia, South Carolina

Diana Jacobson, PhD, RN, PPCNP-BC, PMHS, FAANP
Clinical Associate Professor
Pediatric Specialty Coordinator Doctor of Nursing Practice Program
Edson College of Nursing and Health Innovation
Arizona State University
Phoenix, Arizona

Jessica L. Kozlowski, DNP, RN, CPNP-PC
Adjunct Clinical Faculty
Marybelle and S. Paul Musco School of Nursing and Health Professions
umassglobal.edu
Affiliate of University of Massachusetts Global
PNP Palms Medical Group
Chiefland, Florida

Richard E. Kreipe, MD, FAAP, FSAHM, FAED
Professor Emeritus
Division of Adolescent Medicine, Department of Pediatrics
Golisano Children's Hospital, University of Rochester Medical Center
Rochester, New York

Pamela Lusk, DNP, RN, PMHNP-BC, FAANP, FAAN
Associate Professor of Clinical Nursing
Director, KySS Online Child & Adolescent Mental Health Program
College of Nursing
The Ohio State University
Columbus, Ohio

Elizabeth Mellin, PhD, LPC
Associate Professor of Teaching, Learning, and Educational Leadership
College of Community and Public Affairs
Binghamton University—SUNY
Vestal, New York

Bernadette Mazurek Melnyk, PhD, APRN-CNP, FAANP, FNAP, FAAN
Vice President for Health Promotion
University Chief Wellness Officer
Dean and Helene Fuld Health Trust Professor of Evidence-Based Practice, College of Nursing
Professor of Pediatrics and Psychiatry, College of Medicine
Executive Director, the Helene Fuld Health Trust National Institute for Evidence-Based Practice in Nursing and Healthcare
The Ohio State University
Columbus, Ohio

Dianne Morrison-Beedy, PhD, RN, FNAP, FAANP, FAAN
Chief Talent and Global Strategy Officer
The Centennial Professor of Nursing
Martha S. Pitzer Center for Women, Children and Youth
Infectious Disease Institute Faculty
The Ohio State University College of Nursing
Columbus, Ohio

Emily Payton, BA, BS, RN, PhD Candidate
University of Rochester School of Nursing
Rochester, New York

Candra Skrzypek, LMSW
PhD Student
School of Social Work
University at Buffalo
Buffalo, New York

Leigh Small, PhD, RN, CPNPP-PC, FNAP, FAANP, FAAN
Professor and Associate Dean of Academic Affairs
College of Nursing
Michigan State University
East Lansing, Michigan

Alice M. Teall, DNP, APRN-CNP, FAANP
Assistant Professor of Clinical Nursing
College of Nursing
The Ohio State University
Columbus, Ohio

Barbara Jones Warren, PhD, RN, APRN, PMHCNS-BC, FNAP, FAAN
Professor of Clinical Nursing
Director, Psychiatric Mental Health Nurse Practitioner Specialty
The Ohio State University, College of Nursing
Columbus, Ohio

Foreword

I have both a very personal, as well as a professional, connection to the life challenges that affect mental health. I was homeless for the first time when I was 6 years old, and throughout my youth continued to intermittently struggle with hunger and homelessness, in part because my parents both had problems with substance abuse. In addition, I have been a soldier, serving in times of both peace and war and seeing firsthand the emotional devastation that can occur during combat, and even years after combat. As a registered nurse, I have cared for patients with emotional or mental illnesses that interfered with or complicated their physical health. As a law enforcement officer, I have been on the frontlines of rescuing children and teens from abusive situations that left them fearful and emotionally bereft. And, I have focused as a trauma, burns, and critical care surgeon on saving hearts and minds damaged by attempted suicides and other tragedies. I understand on a very deep level what it means to be mentally unhealthy.

When I became the 17th Surgeon General of the United States in 2002, I had the privilege of bringing my training and experience to bear on the largest practice in the world—the 310 million people across our great nation, as well as serving as an advisor to world leaders beyond our own country who often seek the counsel of the U.S. Surgeon General to benefit their own populations. Mental health is a major public health concern for our nation and the world. Daily mental health challenges exist at a magnitude that can only be described as critical. Through the wider lens available to me as the nation's doctor, I practiced with colleagues addressing the multivariate issues that are involved, including a drastic shortage of child and adolescent mental health professionals; increases in mental health problems among youth; the still unrelenting stigma associated with mental illness; and the lack of a comprehensive, coordinated approach to the early diagnosis and treatment of mental illness.

Among children and teens, the need for help can be particularly challenging for health professionals because of acting-out behaviors or the opposite—their silent suffering. The support and treatment our children need may not be readily available due to lack of access to services, the shortage of trained mental health professionals who focus on children and adolescents, as well as the widespread bias against acknowledging mental illness.

An important strategy for addressing these very real and current challenges is to provide information, education, and resources to the health professionals who stand at the gateway of care. Pediatricians, family practice and primary care physicians, physician assistants, nurse practitioners, and other members of the medical community can be even more effective members of the mental health network. This book, edited by my friend and colleague Bernadette Melnyk, is a thorough and relevant first step for health professionals to learn about mental health disorders among children and adolescents, from diagnosis to treatment to resources and prevention. Now is the time to get involved and give our youth the help they so desperately need.

Richard H. Carmona, MD, MPH, FACS
17th Surgeon General of the United States

Preface

Mental health disorders in children and youth were already skyrocketing prior to the historic COVID-19 pandemic. Now, we also have a mental health pandemic. For the millions of children, teens, and young adults at risk for or affected by mental health problems, time is running out to provide them with the evidence-based treatment and programs they need to become healthy adults capable of functioning to their full capacity. We must act NOW to better screen for, identify, manage, and prevent mental health disorders, which are currently affecting one out of every four to five children and adolescents in the United States.

I was 15 years of age and home alone with my mother when she died suddenly right in front of me from a sneeze that precipitated a stroke. Crippled by guilt that I could do nothing to save her and suffering from terrible symptoms of posttraumatic stress disorder, anxiety, and depression, I did not sleep through the night for at least a few years after my mother's death as I continually played the recording of that terrible day over and over again in my head and had continual fears of losing my father, learning that death could come to anyone I loved at any time. After months with these symptoms, I was taken for help to my family physician, who wrote a prescription for valium and told me I would be fine if I took one of those pills to help me sleep every night. There was no psychological evaluation and no mental health counseling for me—just a pill. I took one of those pills that night, which left me feeling groggy in the morning, so I refused to take any more and resigned myself to having to "tough it out" and learn skills on my own to help cope with my tragic loss. In the next 4 years after my mother's death, I lost a cousin following a motor vehicle accident, the only grandparent I ever knew, and my father had his heart attack—tremendous loss and stress in a short period of time during those challenging adolescent years. However, I was fortunate to be blessed with resiliency and a close connection to a much older sister, which helped me through many dark nights and protected me from ongoing mental health issues as an adult. It is this personal experience along with caring for so many children and teens affected by mental health problems who were not identified by their primary care providers or treated until they either attempted suicide or became hospitalized with severe mental illness that fueled my passion to commit much of my career to developing initiatives and programs to promote child and teen mental health, compiling this guide, and developing and implementing evidence-based programs that could help youth who suffer for years without being identified and treated for mental health problems.

Unfortunately, many children today who are suffering with mental health disorders do not have protective factors to buffer them from developing serious mental illness. Further, fewer than 50% of affected children and teens receive any treatment; even fewer receive the best evidence-based treatments. It is unfortunate that, even with all of the accumulated knowledge we have today about evidence-based screening and treatment, primary care practitioners are still not routinely screening for depression and other mental health issues in teens when suicide remains the second leading cause of death in 10- to 34-year-olds. Teens with depression may receive an antidepressant from their primary care provider, but the majority does not receive gold standard cognitive behavioral therapy or skills building, in large part due to the severe shortage of mental health providers in so many areas across the nation.

Primary care providers are ideally suited to screen for, identify, and manage common mental health disorders in children and teens because of established relationships with their families and a practice setting that lessens stigma, which remains alive and well in our country.

Academic programs that prepare healthcare providers also have been slow to integrate in-depth content on the assessment and management of common mental health disorders in children and teens. Thus, primary care providers often report not having the knowledge and skills believed necessary to appropriately and accurately identify and manage common child and adolescent mental health disorders. Further, although there is finally more emphasis nationally on the importance of integrating physical and mental healthcare, the merging of the two remains slow and problematic issues such as reimbursement issues continue. Horrific mass shootings with unnecessary loss of lives often prompt some national action, but too often, the events pass, the momentum once again slows, and our children, teens, and young adults along with their families affected by these problems continue to suffer. Therefore, we must stay consistent and persistent in our efforts to improve the lives of so many families impacted by mental health disorders.

Unfortunately, we still live in a sick care and crisis-oriented healthcare system. We must change that paradigm from sick care to well care and prevention. We must equip our children, teens, and young adults with the coping, cognitive behavioral, and other resiliency skills that we know will protect them from mental health problems. We would not send our children and youth into a deep ocean without an oxygen tank; how can we send them throughout life without equipping them with the knowledge and skills needed to deal with the stressors they are certain to face throughout their lives.

The third edition of this guide has been strengthened with new chapters, evidence-based programs, updated educational materials for families, and resources to assist interprofessional clinicians in being more effective in screening, identifying, managing, and preventing common mental health disorders in children and teens. A major feature of this guide is that it delivers the best "nuts and bolts" evidence-based content in a format that is user friendly and contains screening tools and evidence-based interventions that can be readily used in practice.

In conclusion, I challenge everyone who cares for children, teens and young adults to ACT NOW and enhance their knowledge and skills in screening for, identifying, using evidence-based treatments and programs, and implementing prevention strategies to reverse the alarming epidemic of mental health disorders among our children and youth. The future of our children and youth along with our society depends on it.

Bernadette Mazurek Melnyk, PhD, APRN-CNP, FAANP, FNAP, FAAN
Vice President for Health Promotion
University Chief Wellness Officer
Dean and Helene Fuld Health Trust Professor of Evidence-Based Practice
College of Nursing
Executive Director, the Helene Fuld Health Trust National Institute for Evidence-Based Practice in Nursing and Healthcare
Professor of Pediatrics and Psychiatry, College of Medicine
The Ohio State University

Acknowledgments

The vision and beginnings of this mental health guide began while teaching a pediatric primary care course and recognizing the need for a user-friendly guide on mental health screening, intervention, and health promotion that could be used with nurse practitioner and medical students along with others from the health sciences to enhance their knowledge and skills in caring for the mental health/psychosocial needs of children, youth, and their families. With Dr. Leigh Small, a long-time friend and colleague who was teaching the course with me, and six of our students (Marie Dunn, Christine Emmerson, Kelly Fagan, Kristina Moss, Anita O'Brien, and Nancy Swank), we comprised a rudimentary first draft of this guide that future students said was instrumental in assisting them to be more effective in caring for the mental health needs of children and adolescents. As a result, I would like to acknowledge each of these individuals for their wonderful contributions to a resource that is now widely used by interprofessional healthcare providers and colleges across the nation. I also would like to thank each of the terrific experts who contributed to the first, second, and now third edition of this guide, all who share a deep passion for promoting the mental health of children/teens and their families. I also want to acknowledge my fantastic colleague and friend, Dr. Pamela Lusk, my assistant editor for this guide, who is an expert psychiatric mental health nurses practitioner and terrific teacher who inspires and equips countless numbers of students and practitioners with the knowledge and skills they need to enhance the mental health and well-being of children, teens, and young adults.

In addition, I would like to thank and acknowledge my loving husband, John, and my three wonderful daughters, Angela, Megan, and Kaylin, for their love and support during the writing of this third edition. My two small grandsons, Alexander and Bradley, regularly remind me of the crucial need for mental health prevention and promotion in our children and teens so they can grow up to be resilient adults capable of handling the stressors that are sure to come their way. They provide me with continual inspiration to dream, discover, and deliver a brighter future for our children and youth.

Bernadette Mazurek Melnyk

I discovered as a BSN student that my clinical area of interest is in psychiatric/mental nursing. My first RN position was at a children's psychiatric treatment service, on the adolescent inpatient unit. After a few years as adolescent team nurse, I enrolled at the University of North Carolina, Chapel Hill, and completed the MSN program to become a Psychiatric Clinical Nurse Specialist with a child/adolescent specialty. Since completing that graduate program. I have taught in nursing programs in the psychiatric/mental health or pediatric courses, and I have always continued to practice. Whether my practice was in a rural community mental health center or a university child guidance clinic, I always learned from colleagues and clinical leaders; however, much of the learning that has informed my practice has been from the young patients and their families.

I want to acknowledge all the children, teens, young adults, and their families who have openly shared their stories, struggles, and dreams with me through my years of practice. Their energy, curiosity, honest expression of emotions, and resiliency have inspired me and challenged me. I have also continually learned from the students in psychiatric and pediatric graduate courses and all the professional colleagues participating in the KySS Online Child and Adolescent Mental Health Program. They have shared experiences, keen observations, and perceptive questions as they developed clinical skills and expertise to meet the crucial mental health needs of one our most vulnerable populations.

I want to thank Dr. Bernadette Melnyk for giving me the opportunity to contribute to this book. I have been so fortunate to have Dr. Melnyk as my mentor, colleague, and friend for over 10 years. Dr. Melnyk's determined and sustained devotion to optimizing mental health for all children, adolescents, and young adults has motivated and inspired my work. Her energy and enthusiasm are contagious. Bern envisioned this user-friendly, evidence-based text, used by so many of us in busy everyday practice—now updated in this third edition.

Most importantly, I want to thank my greatest teachers and sources of joy, Sarah, Rachel, Hannah, and Joel, now generous, creative, compassionate young adults. Their young children, my grandchildren Ella, Caleb, Asher, and Millie, continue to teach us all about growth and development and the immense potential and hope of youth.

Pamela Lusk

CHAPTER 1

Bernadette Mazurek Melnyk and Pamela Lusk

Screening for and Assessing Common Mental Health Problems in Children and Adolescents

INTRODUCTION

Mental health/behavioral disorders have been increasing over recent decades and now affect approximately one out of five children and adolescents, creating a major public health epidemic (Kyu et al., 2016). With the COVID-19 pandemic, further increases in mental health problems are occurring. Even with the increased prevalence of these disorders, it is estimated that 50% of affected youth do not receive timely treatment in large part because of insufficient numbers of mental health providers, especially in rural areas of the United States, as well as ongoing issues with mental health stigma that deter families from seeking intervention (Kyu et al., 2016; Reardon et al., 2017; Whitney & Peterson, 2019). The three most common mental health problems in children and adolescents are anxiety disorders, depressive disorders, and attention deficit hyperactivity disorder with depression being the most costly primary mental health diagnosis, accounting for 44.1% of all mental health admissions and costing the U.S. health system $1.33 billion per year (Bardach et al., 2014). Children and teens with one mental health disorder are likely to have another co-occurring mental health problem (Melnyk, 2020). As an example, nearly three in four children aged 3 to 17 years with depression also have anxiety (73.8%) and nearly one in two have behavior problems (47.2%) (Ghandour et al., 2019). Health disparities also exist in that youth in low-income and single parent households are at increased risk for behavior disorders yet youth from disadvantaged ethnic subgroups have been shown to have lower rates of mood disorders (Merikangas, 2018).

Early detection of and evidence-based intervention for mental health/behavioral problems is critical in order to prevent serious ongoing adverse outcomes. Screening for mental health problems can substantially increase the number of children and adolescents identified as possibly having a mental health problem. Screening youth for mental health problems is especially important since half of adults with mental health problems have symptoms by 14 years of age, and 75% have symptoms by 24 years of age (Parekh, 2018).

Significant health disparities also exist in the receipt of mental health services, with a disproportionate number of Hispanic and African American children affected (Ghandour et al., 2019; Marrast et al., 2016). Mental health problems are now surpassing physical health problems in children and youth, including asthma and diabetes. There are many reasons for this increase in incidence, including:

- family instability and malfunctioning,
- stigma of mental health problems,
- access to care and reimbursement issues,
- lack of screening,
- inadequate numbers of mental health professionals,
- genetics,
- and the COVID-19 pandemic.

Every encounter with a child or adolescent, whether for a well-child or illness visit, is an opportunity to screen for and assess a mental health or psychosocial problem. Each healthcare encounter also is an excellent time to provide preventive counseling and educational information on how to recognize these conditions early before the problems become more resistant to early interventions.

Because there is still much stigma associated with mental health/behavior problems and parents often feel guilty about them, use of screening tools can prompt parents to talk about these issues with their healthcare providers. However, it should be remembered that screening tools cannot replace a developmentally sensitive and comprehensive clinical interview. Screening tools are useful in raising "red flags," which can signal underlying mental health disorders. Since less than 50% of children with mental health problems are diagnosed and treated, screening is critical for early recognition and intervention.

RISK FACTORS FOR MENTAL HEALTH DISORDERS IN CHILDREN AND TEENS

Risk factors for mental health disorders in children and teens are important to assess and include:

Screening raises a red flag for a possible mental health disorder, but it cannot replace a developmentally sensitive and comprehensive clinical interview.

- parents who have mental health problems, including use of substances;
- poor self-esteem;
- lack of other developmental assets (e.g., coping skills, optimism);
- altered parenting (e.g., over-protective; controlling, rigid; permissive; lack of supervision and limit setting);
- parental conflict/separation/divorce/re-marriage;
- death of parent, guardian, close family member;
- incarcerated parent (jail or prison);
- chronic illness or handicap of the child or family member;
- hospitalization/life-threatening medical procedures;
- learning disabilities;
- adverse childhood experiences (ACES);
- deteriorating grades;
- the presence of multiple stressors/recent stressful life events;
- peers who engage in risk-taking behaviors;
- social isolation;
- bullying by peers;
- traumatic event(s);
- difficult temperament;
- behavior problems;
- stressful home or school environment;
- gay or bi-sexual orientation;
- overweight/obesity;
- substance use;
- child/teen has been treated badly due to race, sexual orientation, place of birth, or religion;

QUESTIONNAIRES AND TOOLS FOR SCREENING

The following questionnaires in this chapter can be used for the purpose of collecting information on potential mental health/psychosocial problems from families in primary care or other types of pediatric and adolescent clinical settings. Parents can complete the questionnaires while they are waiting for their child's appointment or ahead of the scheduled visits online. It is a good idea to request that parents arrive 15 minutes early if they have not completed the questionnaires so that they have the chance to finish them during their visit. Included also in this chapter are screening tools that can be provided to children and adolescents.

These questionnaires explore issues that parents and teens may be thinking about or may reveal areas of concern. The items on the KySS mental health assessment questionnaires were developed by pediatric and mental health experts through a consensus-building process. Once completed, the questionnaires provide healthcare providers with a quick overview of potential or actual mental health/psychosocial issues that need to be more fully assessed during the clinical interview.

A commonly used valid and reliable general mental health screening tool for use in primary care that is in the public domain and that can be downloaded free of charge is the Pediatric Symptom Checklist (both the 35-item checklist and shorter 17-item version) (Jellinek, 2002). Information about this screening tool and others are contained in this chapter.

The U.S. Preventive Services Task Force recommends screening all adolescents (12–18 years of age) for major depressive disorder (MDD). Adequate systems should be in place to ensure accurate diagnosis, effective treatment (cognitive behavioral or interpersonal therapy), and appropriate follow-up. See www.uspreventiveservicestaskforce.org/uspstf/document/RecommendationStatementFinal/depression-in-children-and-adolescents-screening.

If the response from the parents is affirmative, assessment of the concern should include:

- degree of impairment;
- distress (by patient and caregiver);
- severity of symptoms;
- frequency;
- intensity;
- duration, and
- actions being taken to deal with the concern, and degree to which they are helpful.

> At every well and ill child visit, it is important to pose the following question to parents:
>
> **Do you have any concerns or worry about your child's mental/emotional health or their behaviors, or has there been a change in how they usually are at home or at school?**

If problems are occurring at home *and* at school, the problem is more serious. Additional questions for assessing mental health/behavior concerns are included in this chapter. See Foy et al., 2019, for mental health competencies for pediatric practice.

PERFORMING A MENTAL STATUS EXAM

If a child is suspected of having a mental health problem after screening and clinical interview, it is important to perform a mental status exam along with a thorough physical exam to rule out potential physical causes of mental health problems. For example, children or teens with depression could have underlying iron deficiency or hypothyroidism.

Components of the mental status exam include the following:

- appearance (e.g., how is the child dressed and groomed?);
- attitude and interaction (e.g., is the child cooperative, guarded, or avoidant?);

- activity level/behavior (e.g., is the child calm, active, or restless; are psychomotor activity, abnormal movements, and/or tics present?);
- speech (e.g., is the child's speech loud or quiet, flat in tone or full of intonation, slow or rushed? How are words formed? Does the child understand what is being said to them? Does the child express themselves appropriately?);
- thought processes (e.g., coherent, disorganized, flight of ideas [rapid skipping from topic to topic], blocking [inability to fill memory gaps], loosening associations [the shifting of topics quickly even though unrelated; echolalia [mocking repetition of another person's words]; perseveration: [repetition of verbal or motor response]);
- thought content (including delusions [false, irrational beliefs, such as "I am superman"]; obsessions [persistent thoughts or impulses]; perceptual disorders [including hallucinations (altered sensory perceptions, such as hearing voices inside or outside their head that others are unaware of)]; phobias [irrational fears]; hypochondriasis [excessive worry about personal health without an actual reason);
- impulse control (e.g., is the child able to control aggressive, hostile, and sexual impulses);
- mood/affect (e.g., depressed, anxious, flat, ambivalent, fearful, irritable, elated, euphoric, and inappropriate);
- suicidal and/or homicidal behavior/ideation;
- cognitive functioning (e.g., orientation to surroundings, attention span/concentration, memory [recent and remote]; ability to abstract; insight/judgment);
- parent-child interaction (e.g., warm, nurturing, conflicted, rejecting, appropriate use of limit setting, in tune with child's feeling/needs, affectionate, eye contact, and other body language);
- engagement with interviewer (e.g., friendly, initiates conversation, initiates/maintains eye contact, oppositional, withdrawn, hostile, disinterested, unable to attend to interview) (Cepeda & Gotanco, 2017);

EXAMPLE OF A MENTAL STATUS ASSESSMENT WRITE-UP

Shannon is a well-groomed, healthy-appearing, overweight adolescent who is cooperative and pleasant in her conversation. She sits calmly without making abnormal movements and makes good eye contact. Her rate and quality of speech are normal. Her thought processes are generally well organized and free of delusions. Shannon states that she can go quickly from a 0 to 10 in terms of anger. It is evident that she has a pattern of depressive cognitive thinking as she degrades herself frequently.

On a scale of 0 to 10, Shannon rates her depression as 6 to 7 on average and talks about the fact that she sometimes worries, especially about how other people view her. She denies hallucinations or any sleep problems. Shannon states that she needs help with anger management. She has poor impulse control as evidenced by frequent anger outbursts in her home. Shannon denies suicidal or homicidal ideations. She has some insight into her problems and talks about her desire to be a landscape designer. Short- and long-term memories are intact.

RULE OUT PHYSICAL HEALTH CONDITIONS

When a child has a suspected mental health disorder, it is important to rule out physical conditions as etiological factors, although remember that **many children with mental health problems present with somatic symptoms that can lead to unnecessary medical testing and interventions.**

Obtain a general health history:

- Conduct a thorough review of all systems (e.g., has your child ever had or do they now have problems with their head (e.g., headaches, head injuries), eyes (e.g., difficulty seeing, blurry vision); ears (e.g., ear infections, hearing), and so forth.

- Has your child ever been hospitalized or had any surgeries?
- Does your child have any type of chronic illness, such as diabetes, asthma, seizures?
- What medications does your child take along with the dosage? Do they experience any side effects from the medications?
- Assess prenatal, natal, and developmental history, including whether the child attained developmental milestones on time.

Conduct a thorough physical exam and laboratory testing as indicated by the history.

- *Rule out:*
  - vision or hearing problems;
  - anemia;
  - hypothyroidism;
  - mononucleosis and chronic fatigue syndrome;
  - eating disorders;
  - substance abuse;
  - premenstrual syndrome;
  - diabetes mellitus;
  - head trauma;
  - CNS lesions;
  - seizures;
  - cushing syndrome;
  - HIV and AIDS;
  - mitral valve prolapse;
  - systemic lupus erythematosus;
  - chronic conditions;
  - developmental delays, and
  - failure to thrive.

SPECIAL CONSIDERATIONS WHEN INTERVIEWING ADOLESCENTS ABOUT MENTAL HEALTH ISSUES

It is very important to assure teens about confidentiality before the clinical interview begins. Not informing teens of confidentiality is the main reason that they do not confide in their healthcare providers. However, it also is critical to inform them that you cannot hold their information confidential if they tell you that they want to hurt themselves or that someone else has hurt them.

If time for the interview is limited, the HEADSS (Home, Education, Activities, Drugs, Sexuality, and Suicide/Depression) Assessment, developed by J. M. Goldenring and E. Cohen, can be very helpful in identifying potential mental health problems.

- **H**ome (e.g., where is the teen living; who lives in the home; how is the teen getting along with people in the home; has the teen ever run away or been incarcerated?);
- **E**ducation (e.g., how is the teen functioning in school in terms of grades, teacher and peer relations, suspensions, missed school days, and so forth?);

- **A**ctivities (e.g., what extracurricular and sports activities is the teen involved in; what do they do with their friends; and so forth);
- **D**rugs (e.g., which drugs, including IV drugs, alcohol, cigarettes, vaping, and caffeine, have been and are used by the teen, their family, and friends?);
- **S**exuality (e.g., when was the first time the teen had sex; what is the teen's sexual preference; does the teen use contraceptives—and, specifically, does the teen use condoms; how many partners have they had; what is the teen's past history of sexually transmitted infections, pregnancy, and abortion, sexual or physical abuse?); and
- **S**uicide (e.g., has the teen had any suicidal ideations or past history of suicidal attempts; if there have been suicidal ideations, does the teen have a plan and access to means to commit suicide?).

GUIDELINES FOR ADOLESCENT PREVENTIVE SERVICES (GAPS)

The American Medical Association has a set of Guidelines for Adolescent Preventive Services (GAPS) materials with tools that provide a framework, an assessment system, and resources for preventive health services in adolescents. The GAPS recommendations were created to be delivered as a preventive services package during health visits between the ages of 11 and 21 (see www.ncbi.nlm.nih.gov/books/NBK232700/).

The GAPS questionnaires are available in this chapter.

Remember, if you do not screen for or ask questions regarding the mental/behavioral health of the children and adolescents for whom you care, you will not discover and have the opportunity to provide evidence-based preventive information and treatment for potential disorders that can have serious adverse outcomes for the children themselves, their families and society.

Bottom Line: Screen, Ask, and Assess!

REFERENCES

American Medical Association. (1994). *Guidelines for adolescent preventive services.* https://www.uptodate.com/contents/guidelines-for-adolescent-preventive-services

Bardach, N. S., Coker, T. R., Zima, B. T., Mangione-Smith, R. (2014). Common and costly hospitalizations for pediatric mental health disorders. *Pediatrics, 133*(4), 602–609. https://doi.org/10.1542/peds.2013-3165.

Cepeda, C., & Gotanco, L. (2017). *Psychiatric interview of children and adolescents.* American Psychiatric Association Publishing. ISBN-13: 978-1615370481, ISBN-10: 9781615370481

Foy, J. M., Green, C., Earls, M., & Committee on Psychosocial Aspects of Child and Family Health, Mental Health Leadership Work Group. (2019). Mental health competencies for pediatric practice. *Pediatrics, 144*(5), e20192757. https://doi.org/10.1542/peds.2019-2757

Gardner, W., Lucas, A., Kolko D. J., & Campo, J. V. (2007). Comparison of the PSC-17 and alternative mental health screens in an at-risk primary care sample. *Journal of the American Academy of Child & Adolescent Psychiatry, 46*(5), 611–618.

Ghandour, R. M., Sherman, L. J., Vladutiu, C. J., Ali, M. M., Lynch, S. E., Bitsko, R. H., & Blumberg, S. J. (2019). Prevalence and treatment of depression, anxiety, and conduct problems in U.S. children. *The Journal of Pediatrics, 206*, 256–267. https://doi.org/10.1016/j.jpeds.2018.09.021.

Jellinek, M. S., & Murphy, J. M. (1988). Screening for psychosocial disorders in pediatric practice. *American Journal of Diseases of Children, 145*(11), 1153–1157.

Jellinek, M., Patel, B. P., & Froehle, M. (2002). *Bright futures in practice: Mental health-Vol I. Practice guide.* National Center for Education in Maternal and Child Health.

Jellinek, M., & Patel, B. P., & Froehle, M. (2002). *Bright futures in practice: Mental health-Vol II. Tool kit.* National Center for Education in Maternal and Child Health.

Kessler, R. C., Berglund, P., Demier, O., Jin, R., Merikangas, K. R., Walters, E. E. (2005). Lifetime prevalence and age of onset distributions of DSM-IV disorders in the National Co-morbidity Survey Replication. *Archives of General Psychiatry, 62*(6), 593–602.

Kyu, H. H., Pinho, C., Wagner, J. A., Brown, J. C., Bertozzi-Villa, A., Charlson, F. J., Coffeng, L. C., Dandona, L., Erskine, H. E., Ferrari, A. J., Fitzmaurice, C., Fleming, T. D., Forouzanfar, M. H., Graetz, N., Guinovart, C., Haagsma, J., Higashi, H., Kassebaum, N. J., Larson, H. J., Global Burden of Disease Pediatrics Collaboration, . . . Vos, T. (2016). Global and national burden of diseases and injuries among children and adolescents between 1990 and 2013: Findings from the Global Burden of Disease 2013 Study. *JAMA Pediatrics, 170*(3), 267–287. https://doi.org/10.1001/jamapediatrics.2015.4276

Marrast, L., Himmelstein, D., & Woolhandler, S. (2016). Racial and ethnic disparities in mental health care for children and young adults: A national study. *International Journal of Health Services, 46*, 1–15. https://doi.org/10.1177/0020731416662736

Melnyk, B. M. (2020). Reducing healthcare costs for mental health hospitalizations with the evidence-based COPE program for child and adolescent depression and anxiety: A cost analysis. *Journal of Pediatric Health Care, 34*(2), 117–121. https://doi.org/10.1016/j.pedhc.2019.08.002

Merikangas K. R. (2018). Time trends in the global prevalence of mental disorders in children and adolescents: Gap in data on U.S. youth. *Journal of the American Academy of Child and Adolescent Psychiatry, 57*(5), 306–307. https://doi.org/10.1016/j.jaac.2018.03.002. PMID:29706158

Murphy, J. M., Arnett, H. L., Bishop, S. J., Jellinek, M. S., & Reede, J. Y. (1992). Screening for psychosocial dysfunction in pediatric practice. A naturalistic study of the Pediatric Symptom Checklist. *Clinical Pediatrics, 31*(11), 660–667.

Murphy, J. M., Ichinose, C., Hicks, R. C., Kingdon, D., Crist-Whitzel, J., Jordan, P., Feldman, G., & Jellinek, M. S. (1996). Screening for psychosocial dysfunction in pediatric practice. A naturalistic study of the Pediatric Symptom Checklist. *Journal of Pediatrics, 129*(6), 864–869.

Murphy, J., & Jellinek, M. S. (1985). *Development of a brief psychosocial screening instrument for pediatric practice: Final report. NIMH Contract No. 84M0213612*. National Institute of Mental Health.

Pagano, M., Murphy, J. M., Pederson, M., Mosbacher, D., Crist-Whitzel, J., Jordan, P., Rodas, C., & Jellinek, M. S. (1996). Screening for psychosocial problems in four- and five-year-olds during routine EPSDT examinations; validity and reliability in a Mexican American sample. *Clinical Pediatrics, 35*, 139–146.

Parekh, R. (2018). *Warning signs of mental illness*. American Psychiatric Association. https://www.psychiatry.org/patients-families/warning-signs-of-mental-illness.

Reardon, T., Harvey, K., Baranowska, M., O'Brien, D., Smith, L., & Creswell, C. (2017). What do parents perceive are the barriers and facilitators to accessing psychological treatment for mental health problems in children and adolescents? A systematic review of qualitative and quantitative studies. *European Child & Adolescent Psychiatry, 26*(6), 623–47. https://doi.org/10.1007/s00787-016-0930-6.

Sheldrick, R. C., Henson, B. S., Merchant, S., Neger, E. N., Murphy, J. M., & Perrin, E. C. (2012a). The preschool pediatric symptom checklist (PPSC): Development and initial validation of a new social/emotional screening instrument. *Academic Pediatrics, 12*(5), 456–467.

Sheldrick, R. C., Hensen, B. S., Neger, E. N., Merchant, S., Murphy, J. M., & Perrin, E. C. (2012b). The baby pediatric symptom checklist: Development and initial validation of a new social/emotional screening instrument for very young children. *Academic Pediatrics, 13*, 72–80. https://doi.org/10.1016/j.acap.2012.08.003. [Epub ahead of print].

Stoppelbein, L., Greening, L., Moll, G., Jordan, S., & Suozzi, A. (2012). Factor analysis of the Pediatric Symptom Checklist-17 with African American and Caucasian pediatric populations. *Journal of Pediatric Psychology, 37*(3), 348–357.

Whitney, D. G., & Peterson, M. D. (2019). Children. *JAMA Pediatrics, 173*(4), 389–391. https://doi.org/10.1001/jamapediatrics.2018.5399.

KySS Assessment Questions for Parents of Older Infants and Toddlers

Child's Name________________________________ DOB________________ Age_________

Parent's/Guardian's Name____________________ Relationship to Child ____________

Because your child's physical as well as mental/emotional health are very important, please complete each of the following questions. We will have the opportunity to talk about some of these issues during your visit. Please indicate which items are most important to talk about today by placing a check mark in front of those items.

1. What worries or concerns you most about your child's emotions and/or behaviors at this time? _______
2. Have there been changes in your family in the past year, such as marital separation, remarriage, move, family illness or death)? If yes, what: No ☐ Yes ☐
3. Are you afraid of anyone in your home? If yes, who: No ☐ Yes ☐
4. Do you ever feel so frustrated that you may hit or hurt your child? No ☐ Yes ☐
5. On a scale of 0 (not at all) to 10 (a lot), how stressed is your child on a day-to-day basis? _______
6. Have you been worried about your child being angry, irritable, sad, fearful, or having a change in behavior in the last month? If yes, what is worrying you: No ☐ Yes ☐
7. Do you have any worries about your child being sad? No ☐ Yes ☐
8. Are you concerned about your child's weight? If yes, what concerns you: No ☐ Yes ☐
9. Who usually watches your child when you are not with them? _______
10. What is the easiest part about being your child's parent? _______
11. What is the hardest part about being your child's parent? _______
12. What worries you most about your child? _______
13. On a scale of 0 (not at all) to 10 (a lot), how stressed are you on a day-to-day basis? _______
14. On a scale of 0 (not at all) to 10 (a lot), how depressed are you from day-to-day? _______
15. How do you discipline your child? _______
16. Do you think that the way that you discipline your child is effective? No ☐ Yes ☐
17. Do you think that your child has ever been abused? If yes, when: No ☐ Yes ☐
18. Has your child ever been through a traumatic or very frightening experience (e.g., a motor vehicle accident, hospitalization, death of a loved one, watching arguments)? If yes, when and what was the trauma? No ☐ Yes ☐

This handout may be distributed to families.

From Melnyk, B. M., & Lusk, P. (2022). *A Practical Guide to Child and Adolescent Mental Health Screening, Evidence-Based Assessment, Intervention, and Health Promotion* (3rd ed.).

National Association of Pediatric Nurse Practitioners℠

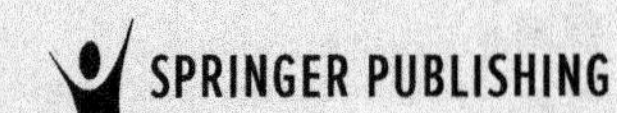

19. Has your child ever been diagnosed with an emotional, behavioral, or mental health problem? If yes, what and when: No ☐ Yes ☐
20. Has your child ever been on medication for an emotional, behavioral, or mental health problem? If yes, what medication and when: No ☐ Yes ☐
21. Do you have guns in your home? No ☐ Yes ☐
22. Are there stressful things that your family has been dealing with recently? If yes, what? No ☐ Yes ☐
23. On a scale of 0 (not at all) to 10 (very), how emotionally connected do you feel with your child? ______
24. On a scale of 0 (very easy) to 10 (very difficult), how is your child's temperament? ______
25. Does your child have difficulty sleeping? If yes, what specifically (e.g., difficulty falling asleep; waking up with nightmares): No ☐ Yes ☐
26. Does anyone in your home smoke? If yes, who: No ☐ Yes ☐
27. Does anyone in your home use alcohol or drugs to the point that you wish they would stop? No ☐ Yes ☐
28. On a scale of 0 (none) to 10 (a lot), how much arguing goes on in your home? ______
29. On a scale of 0 (not at all) to 10 (a lot), do you overprotect your child? ______
30. On a scale of 0 (not at all) to 10 (very much so), how satisfied are you with being a parent to your child? ______
31. On a scale of 0 (not at all) to 10 (very much so), how consistent are you in setting limits with your child? ______
32. Have you or any other of your child's blood relatives ever been diagnosed with a mental health disorder? If yes, who and what: No ☐ Yes ☐

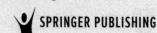

This handout may be distributed to families.
From Melnyk, B. M., & Lusk, P. (2022). *A Practical Guide to Child and Adolescent Mental Health Screening, Evidence-Based Assessment, Intervention, and Health Promotion* (3rd ed.).

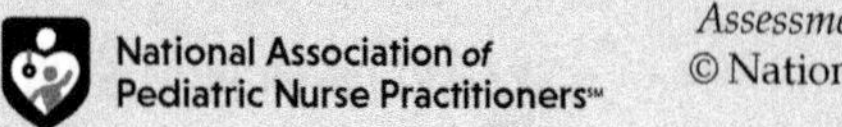

SPRINGER PUBLISHING

KySS Assessment Questions for Parents of Preschool Children

Child's Name________________________________ DOB________________ Age________

Parent's/Guardian's Name____________________ Relationship to Child ____________

Because your child's physical as well as mental/emotional health are very important, please complete each of the following questions. We will have the opportunity to talk about some of these issues during your visit. Please indicate which items are most important to talk about today by placing a check mark in front of those items.

1. What worries or concerns you most about your child's emotions and/or behaviors at this time? _______
2. Have there been changes in your family in the past year, such as marital separation, remarriage, move, family illness or death? If yes, what: No ☐ Yes ☐
3. Are you afraid of anyone in your home? If yes, who: No ☐ Yes ☐
4. Do you ever feel so frustrated that you may hit or hurt your child? No ☐ Yes ☐
5. On a scale of 0 (not at all) to 10 (a lot), how much does your child worry on a day-to-day basis? _______
6. What does your child worry most about? _______
7. On a scale of 0 (not at all) to 10 (a lot), how stressed is your child on a day-to-day basis? _______
8. Have you been worried about your child being angry, irritable, sad, fearful, or having a change in behavior in the last month? If yes, what is worrying you? No ☐ Yes ☐
9. How often does your child complain of headaches or stomachaches?

   a. never, b. 1×/month, c. 2×/month, d. 1×/week, e. more that 1x/week _______
10. Do you have any worries about your child being sad or depressed? No ☐ Yes ☐
11. Are you concerned about your child's weight? If yes, what concerns you: No ☐ Yes ☐
12. Who usually watches your child when you are not with him or her? _______
13. Do you talk about safety with your child? No ☐ Yes ☐
14. What is the easiest part about being your child's parent?
15. What is the hardest part about being your child's parent?
16. What worries you most about your relationship with your child?
17. On a scale of 0 (not at all) to 10 (a lot), how stressed are you on a day-to-day basis? _______

This handout may be distributed to families.

From Melnyk, B. M., & Lusk, P. (2022). *A Practical Guide to Child and Adolescent Mental Health Screening, Evidence-Based Assessment, Intervention, and Health Promotion* (3rd ed.).

National Association *of* Pediatric Nurse Practitioners℠

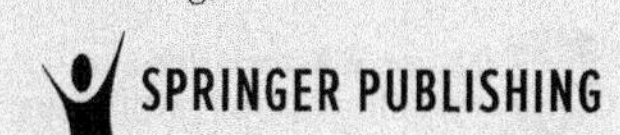

18. On a scale of 0 (not at all) to 10 (a lot), how depressed are you on a day-to day basis? ______

19. On a scale of 0 (not good at all) to 10 (excellent), how does your child cope with stress? ______

20. How do you discipline your child?

21. Do you think that the way that you discipline your child is effective? No ☐ Yes ☐

22. Do you think that your child has ever been abused? If yes, when: No ☐ Yes ☐

23. Has your child ever been through a traumatic or very frightening experience (e.g., a motor vehicle accident, hospitalization, death of a loved one, watching arguments)? If yes, when and what was the trauma? No ☐ Yes ☐

24. Has your child ever been diagnosed with an emotional, behavioral, or mental health problem? If yes, what and when? No ☐ Yes ☐

25. Has your child ever been on medication for an emotional, behavioral, or mental health problem? If yes, what medication and when? No ☐ Yes ☐

26. Do you have guns in your home? No ☐ Yes ☐

27. Are there stressful things that your family has been dealing with recently? If yes, what? No ☐ Yes ☐

28. On a scale of 0 (poor) to 10 (excellent), how is your child's self-esteem? ______

29. On a scale of 0 (not at all) to 10 (very), how emotionally connected do you feel with your child? ______

30. On a scale of 0 (very difficult) to 10 (very easy), how is your child's temperament? ______

31. Does your child have difficulty sleeping? If yes, what specifically (e.g., difficulty falling asleep; waking up with nightmares): No ☐ Yes ☐

32. Does anyone in your home smoke? If yes, who? No ☐ Yes ☐

33. Does anyone in your home use alcohol or drugs to the point that you wish they would stop? No ☐ Yes ☐

34. On a scale of 0 (none) to 10 (a lot), how much arguing goes on in your home? ______

35. On a scale of 0 (not good) to 10 (very good), how well does your child get along with their peers or friends? ______

36. On a scale of 0 (not at all) to 10 (a lot), do you overprotect your child? ______

37. On a scale of 0 (not at all) to 10 (very much so), how satisfied are you with being a parent to your child? ______

38. On a scale of 0 (not at all) to 10 (very much so), are you consistent in setting limits with your child? ______

39. Is your child ever cruel to animals? No ☐ Yes ☐

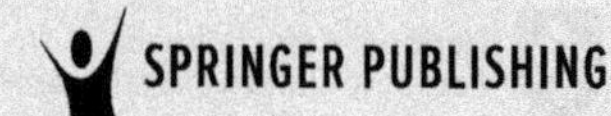

KySS Assessment Questions For Parents of School-Age Children and Teens

Child's/Teen's Name______________________________ DOB________________ Age_________

Parent's/Guardian's Name____________________ Relationship to Child ____________

Because your child's physical as well as mental/emotional health are very important, please complete each of the following questions. We will have the opportunity to talk about some of these issues during your visit. Please indicate which items are most important to talk about today by placing a check mark before those items.

1. What worries or concerns you most about your child's emotions and/or behaviors at this time? ________
2. Have there been changes in your family in the past year, such as marital separation, remarriage, move, family illness or death? If yes, what: No ☐ Yes ☐
3. Are you afraid of anyone in your home? If yes, who: No ☐ Yes ☐
4. Do you ever feel so frustrated that you may hit or hurt your child? No ☐ Yes ☐
5. On a scale of 0 (not at all) to 10 (a lot), how much does your child worry on a day-to-day basis? ________
6. What does your child worry most about?
7. On a scale of 0 (not at all) to 10 (a lot), how stressed is your child on a day-to-day basis. ________
8. Have you been worried about your child being angry, irritable, sad, fearful, or having a change in behavior in the last month? If yes, what is worrying you: No ☐ Yes ☐
9. How often does your child complain of headaches or stomachaches?

   a. Never, b. 1×/month, c. 2×/month, d. 1×/week, e. more that 1×/week ________
10. Do you have any worries about your child being depressed? No ☐ Yes ☐
11. If yes, do you ever think that your child thinks about hurting themselves? No ☐ Yes ☐
12. Are you concerned about your child's weight? If yes, what concerns you? No ☐ Yes ☐
13. Does your child make negative comments about their body or weight? No ☐ Yes ☐
14. Where does your child spend their free time?
15. Who usually watches your child when you are not with them?
16. Do you talk about safety with your child? No ☐ Yes ☐
17. What is the easiest part about being your child's parent?
18. What is the hardest part about being your child's parent?

This handout may be distributed to families.

From Melnyk, B. M., & Lusk, P. (2022). *A Practical Guide to Child and Adolescent Mental Health Screening, Evidence-Based Assessment, Intervention, and Health Promotion* (3rd ed.).

National Association of Pediatric Nurse Practitioners℠

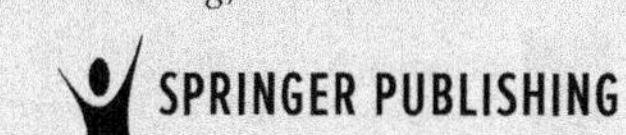

19. What worries you most about your relationship with your child?
20. On a scale of 0 (not at all) to 10 (a lot), how stressed are you on a day-to-day basis? ______
21. On a scale of 0 (not at all) to 10 (a lot), how depressed are you on a day-to-day basis? ______
22. On a scale of 0 (not good at all) to 10 (excellent), how does your child cope with stress? ______
23. How do you discipline your child?
24. Do you think that the way that you discipline your child is effective? No ☐ Yes ☐
25. Has your child ever been through a traumatic or very frightening experience (e.g., a motor vehicle accident, hospitalization, death of a loved one, rape)? If yes, when and what was the trauma? No ☐ Yes ☐
26. On a scale of 0 (not at all) to 10 (a lot), how comfortable do you feel in talking with your child about sexuality? ______
27. Are you worried about your child becoming sexually active? No ☐ Yes ☐
28. Are you worried about your child and drug or alcohol use? No ☐ Yes ☐
29. Are you worried about your child and cigarette smoking tobacco use, or vaping? No ☐ Yes ☐
30. Does your child ever get bullied? No ☐ Yes ☐
31. Has your child ever been diagnosed with an emotional, behavioral, or mental health problem? If yes, what and when? No ☐ Yes ☐
32. Has your child ever been on medication for an emotional, behavioral, or mental health problem? If yes, what medication and when? No ☐ Yes ☐
33. Do you have guns in your home? No ☐ Yes ☐
34. Are there stressful things that your family has been dealing with recently? If yes, what? No ☐ Yes ☐
35. On a scale of 0 (poor) to 10 (excellent), how is your child's self-esteem? ______
36. On a scale of 0 (not at all) to 10 (very), how emotionally connected do you feel with your child? ______
37. On a scale of 0 (very difficult) to 10 (very easy), how is your child's temperament? ______
38. Has your child had a recent decline in their school performance/grades? If yes, when and what? No ☐ Yes ☐
39. Does your child have difficulty sleeping? If yes, what specifically (e.g., difficulty falling asleep; waking up with nightmares): No ☐ Yes ☐
40. Does anyone in your home smoke? If yes, who? No ☐ Yes ☐

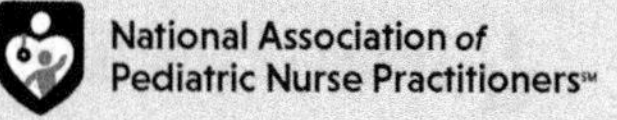

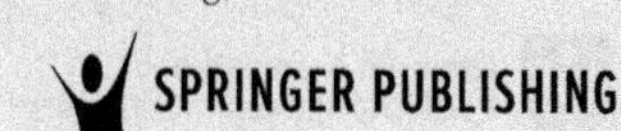

41. Does anyone in your home use alcohol or drugs to the point that you wish they would stop? No ☐ Yes ☐

42. On a scale of 0 (none) to 10 (a lot), how much arguing goes on in your home? _______

43. On a scale of 0 (not good) to 10 (very good), how well does your child get along with their peers or friends? _______

44. On a scale of 0 (not at all) to 10 (a lot), do you overprotect your child? _______

45. On a scale of 0 (not at all) to 10 (very much so), how satisfied are you with being a parent to your child? _______

46. On a scale of 0 (not at all) to 10 (very much so), are you consistent in setting limits with your child? _______

47. Is your child ever cruel to animals? No ☐ Yes ☐

48. Have you or any other of your child's blood relatives ever been diagnosed with a mental health disorder? If yes, who and what? No ☐ Yes ☐

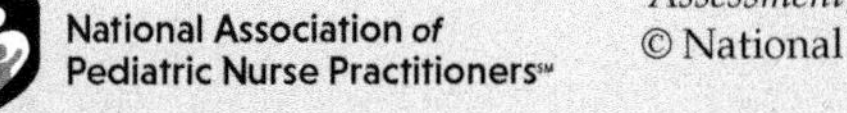

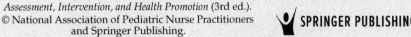

Assessment Questions for a Specific Emotional or Behavioral Problem

When parents report that they have a specific concern or worry about their child's mental/emotional health or behaviors or that there has been a change in the way the child is functioning at home or school, proceed with the following questions regarding history or background to shed more light on the parents' concern:

1. **What?**
   a. What specifically occurs?
   b. What precipitates it?
   c. What are the associated symptoms (e.g., headaches, stomachaches)?
2. **Where?**
   a. At home and/or school/day care?
3. **When?**
   a. Time of day? During a transition?
4. **Who?**
   a. Who is with the child when it occurs and who is involved?
5. **How?**
   a. How do the parent and others involved react?
   b. How long has it been going on?
6. **Why?**
   a. What makes the parent and child think that this is occurring?

Refer to a mental health specialist if the problem has been persistent, increasing in severity, and/or interfering with functioning at home or in school.

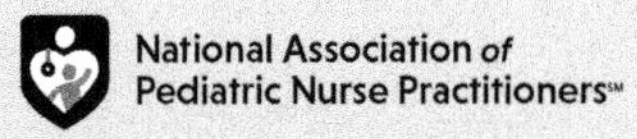

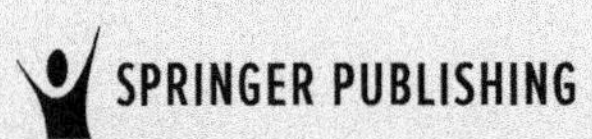

The Pediatric Symptom Checklist (PSC)
(M. S. Jellinek and J. M. Murphy)

DESCRIPTION OF THE PSC

The Pediatric Symptom Checklist (PSC) is a one-page questionnaire that lists a range of children's emotional and behavioral concerns as perceived by parents; it is available in several different languages. There is also a youth self-reported version of the scale. The PSC can be easily administered in a pediatric or family practice clinic's waiting room or online and scored by a receptionist or healthcare provider. A high score indicates likelihood of significant psychosocial dysfunction. All versions of the PSC are freely downloadable from used in www.massgeneral.org/psychiatry/treatments-and-services/pediatric-symptom-checklist

Age Range: 4 to 18 years

Psychometric Properties of the PSC

Instructions for Scoring: The PSC consists of 35 items that are rated as "never," "sometimes," or "often" present and scored as 0, 1, and 2, respectively. Item scores are summed, and the total score is recoded into a dichotomous variable indicating psychosocial impairment. For children aged 6 through 16 years, the cut-off score is 28 or higher. For 4- and 5-year-old children, the PSC cut-off is 24 or higher (Pagano et al., 1996). Items that are left blank by parents are simply ignored (score = 0). If 4 or more items are left blank, the questionnaire is considered invalid.

How to Interpret the PSC: A positive score on the PSC suggests the need for further evaluation by a qualified health professional (MD, NP, RN) or mental health professional (PhD, LICSW, Nurse Practitioner of Psychiatry). Both false positives and false negatives occur, and only an experienced clinician should interpret a positive PSC score as anything other than a suggestion that further evaluation may be helpful. Data from past studies using the PSC indicate that two out of three children who screen positive on the PSC will be correctly identified as having moderate to serious impairment in psychosocial functioning. The one child "incorrectly" identified usually has at least mild impairment, although a small percentage of children turn out to have very little actually wrong with them (e.g., an adequately functioning child of an overly anxious parent). Data on PSC-negative screens indicate 95% accuracy, which still suggest that 1 out of 20 children rated as functioning adequately may actually be impaired. The inevitability of both false-positive and false-negative screens underscores the importance of experienced clinical judgment in interpreting PSC scores. Therefore, it is especially important for parents or other lay persons who administer the form to consult with a licensed professional if their child receives a PSC-positive score.

Validity: Using a receiver operating characteristic curve, Jellinek, Murphy, Robinson, et al. (1988) found that a PSC cut-off score of 28 has a specificity of 0.68 and a sensitivity of 0.95 when compared with clinicians' ratings of children's psychosocial dysfunction.

Reliability: Test-retest reliability of the PSC ranges from $r = 0.84$-0.91. Over time, case/not case classification ranges from 83% to 87%. (Jellinek & Murphy, 1988; Murphy et al., 1992).

Inter-item Analysis: Studies (Murphy & Jellinek, 1985; Murphy et al., 1996) also indicate strong internal consistency reliability (Cronbach's alpha = 0.91) of the PSC items and highly significant ($p < 0.0001$) correlations between individual PSC items and positive PSC screening scores.

Qualifications for Use of the PSC: The training required may differ according to the ways in which the data are to be used. Professional school (e.g., medicine or nursing) or graduate training in psychology of at least the master's degree level would ordinarily be expected. However, no amount of prior training can substitute for professional maturity, a thorough knowledge of clinical research methodology, and supervised training in working with parents and children. There are no special qualifications for scoring.

Source: Jellinek, M. S., Murphy, J. M., Robinson, J., et al. (1988). Pediatric Symptom Checklist: Screening school age children for psychosocial dysfunction. *Journal of Pediatrics, 112*, 201–209. The PSC is one of only a few public domain measures and can be downloaded in English or Spanish at: psc.partners.org/, free of charge.

***From:** Pediatric Development and Behavior Online, available at http://www.dbpeds.org*

The PSC is in the public domain, available in several languages and can be downloaded for use at www.massgeneral.org/psychiatry/services/psc_home.aspx

Please Note: It is suggested that the Child Behavior Checklist (CBCL) be administered if a positive score is found on the PSC (see information on the CBCL that follows the PSC in this guide).

OTHER VERSIONS OF THE PEDIATRIC SYMPTOM CHECKLIST

The PSC also is available in a 17-item short form (free and downloadable at www.massgeneral.org/psychiatry/treatments-and-services/pediatric-symptom-checklist. A total cut off score of 15 has been recommended (Gardner et al., 2007). Although the shorter version of the PSC-17 has similar properties to the PSC-35, research suggests a greater degree of accuracy with the longer 35-item version. As a result, the PSC-35 remains the recommended instrument unless time limitations call for the 17-item version.

The Pediatric Symptom Checklist has recently been adapted for young children, 18–60 months (Sheldrick et al., 2012a) and children less than 18 months (Sheldrick et al., 2012b). It also has been psychometrically evaluated with diverse populations of children (Stoppelbein et al., 2012).

Pediatric Symptom Checklist

Child's Name____________________ Record Number____________________

Today's Date____________________ Filled out by____________________

Date of Birth____________________

Please mark under the heading that best fits your child:

	Never (0)	**Sometimes (1)**	**Often (2)**
1. Complains of aches/pains	☐	☐	☐
2. Spends more time alone	☐	☐	☐
3. Tires easily, has little energy	☐	☐	☐
4. Fidgety, unable to sit still	☐	☐	☐
5. Has trouble with a teacher	☐	☐	☐
6. Less interested in school	☐	☐	☐
7. Acts as if driven by a motor	☐	☐	☐
8. Daydreams too much	☐	☐	☐
9. Distracted easily	☐	☐	☐
10. Is afraid of new situations	☐	☐	☐
11. Feels sad, unhappy	☐	☐	☐
12. Is irritable, angry	☐	☐	☐
13. Feels hopeless	☐	☐	☐
14. Has trouble concentrating	☐	☐	☐
15. Has less interest in friends	☐	☐	☐
16. Fights with others	☐	☐	☐
17. Absent from school	☐	☐	☐
18. School grades dropping	☐	☐	☐
19. Is down on him or herself	☐	☐	☐
20. Visits doctor with doctor finding nothing wrong	☐	☐	☐
21. Has trouble sleeping	☐	☐	☐
22. Worries a lot	☐	☐	☐
23. Wants to be with you more than before	☐	☐	☐
24. Feels he or she is bad	☐	☐	☐
25. Takes unnecessary risks	☐	☐	☐
26. Gets hurt frequently	☐	☐	☐
27. Seems to be having less fun	☐	☐	☐

Reproduced with permission from Jellinek, M., & Murphy, M. (1986).
Massachusetts General Hospital.
https://www.massgeneral.org/psychiatry/treatments-and-services/pediatric-symptom-checklist.

National Association of Pediatric Nurse Practitioners℠

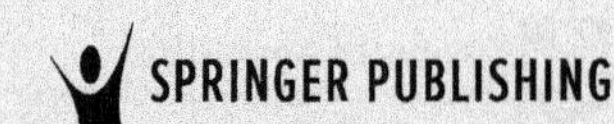

	Never (0)	Sometimes (1)	Often (2)
28. Acts younger than children his or her age	☐	☐	☐
29. Does not listen to rules	☐	☐	☐
30. Does not show feelings	☐	☐	☐
31. Does not understand other people's feelings	☐	☐	☐
32. Teases others	☐	☐	☐
33. Blames others for his or her troubles	☐	☐	☐
34. Takes things that do not belong to him or her	☐	☐	☐
35. Refuses to share	☐	☐	☐
Totals:	_____	_____	_____

Other comments:

Does your child have any emotional or behavioral problems for which they need help?

( ) N ( ) Y

Are there any services that you would like your child to receive for these problems?

( ) N ( ) Y

If yes, what services? ____

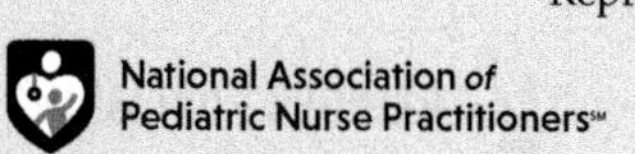

Reproduced with permission from Jellinek, M., & Murphy, M. (1986). *Massachusetts General Hospital.* https://www.massgeneral.org/psychiatry/treatments-and-services/pediatric-symptom-checklist.

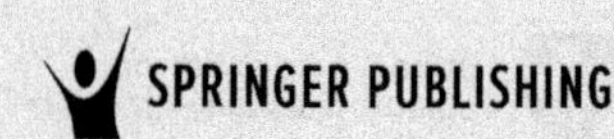

Estudio Sobre Adaptacion Social Y Emocional De Los Ninos

La salud fisica y emocional son importantes para cada niño. Los padres son los primeros que notan un problema de la conducta emocional o de aprendizaje. Ud puede ayudar a su hijo a obtener el mejor cuidado del doctor por medio de contestar estas preguntas. Favor de indicar cual frase describe a su niño/a.

Indique cual síntoma mejor describe a su niño/a:

	NUNCA (0)	ALGUNAS (1)	SEGUIDO (2)
1. Se queja de dolores y malestares...................	☐	☐	☐
2. Pasa mucho tiempo solo(a)	☐	☐	☐
3. Se cansa fácilmente, tiene poca energiá......	☐	☐	☐
4. Nervioso, incapaz de estarse quieto...........	☐	☐	☐
5. Tiene problemas con un maestro................	☐	☐	☐
6. Menos interesado en la escuela.................	☐	☐	☐
7. Es incansable..	☐	☐	☐
8. Esta muy un sonador....................................	☐	☐	☐
9. Se distrae facilmente.....................................	☐	☐	☐
10. Temeroso/a a nuevas situaciónes...............	☐	☐	☐
11. Se siete triste, infelix.......................................	☐	☐	☐
12. Es irritable, enojon...	☐	☐	☐
13. Se siente sin esperanzas................................	☐	☐	☐
14. Tiene problemas para concentrarse.............	☐	☐	☐
15. Menos interesado en amistades...................	☐	☐	☐
16. Pelea con otros niños.....................................	☐	☐	☐
17. Se ausenta de la escuela a menudo..............	☐	☐	☐
18. Se critica a si mismo/a..................................	☐	☐	☐
19. Visita al doctor sin que le encuentren nada.	☐	☐	☐
20. Tiene problemas para dormer.......................	☐	☐	☐
21. Se preocupa mucho..	☐	☐	☐
22. Quiere estar con usted mas que antes.........	☐	☐	☐
23. Cree que el/ella es malo/a	☐	☐	☐
24. Toma riezgos innecesarios.............................	☐	☐	☐
25. Se lastima frecuentemente.............................	☐	☐	☐

National Association *of* Pediatric Nurse Practitioners℠

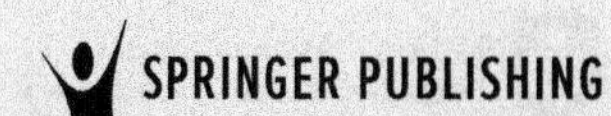

	NUNCA (0)	ALGUNAS (1)	SEGUIDO (2)
26. Parece divertirse menos................................	☐	☐	☐
27. Actua mas chico que niños de su propia edad	☐	☐	☐
28. No obedece las reglas..	☐	☐	☐
29. No demuestra sus sentimientos........................	☐	☐	☐
30. No comprende los sentimientos de otros.........	☐	☐	☐
31. Molesta o se burla de otros..............................	☐	☐	☐
32. Culpa a otros por sus problemas.....................	☐	☐	☐
33. Toma cosas que no le pertenecen.....................	☐	☐	☐
34. Se rehusa a compartir...	☐	☐	☐
Totals:	____	____	____

Necesita su nino(a) ayuda con problemas en el comportamiento con problemas emocionales? .... ___Si ____No

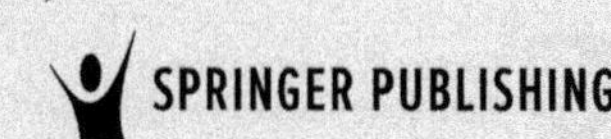

Pediatric Symptom Checklist—Youth Report (Y-PSC)

Child's Name____________________________ Record Number____________________________

Today's Date____________________________ Filled out by____________________________

Date of Birth____________________________

The questionnaire that follows can be used to see if you are having emotional, attentional, or behavioral difficulties. For each item, please mark how often you:

	Never (0)	Sometimes (1)	Often (2)
1. Complain of aches or pains	☐	☐	☐
2. Spend more time alone	☐	☐	☐
3. Tire easily, have little energy	☐	☐	☐
4. Are fidgety, unable to sit still	☐	☐	☐
5. Have trouble with teacher	☐	☐	☐
6. Are less interested in school	☐	☐	☐
7. Act as if driven by motor	☐	☐	☐
8. Daydream too much	☐	☐	☐
9. Distract easily	☐	☐	☐
10. Are afraid of new situations	☐	☐	☐
11. Feel sad, unhappy	☐	☐	☐
12. Are irritable, angry	☐	☐	☐
13. Feel hopeless	☐	☐	☐
14. Have trouble concentrating	☐	☐	☐
15. Are less interested in friends	☐	☐	☐
16. Fight with other children	☐	☐	☐
17. Are absent from school	☐	☐	☐
18. School grades dropping	☐	☐	☐
19. Are down on yourself	☐	☐	☐
20. Visit the doctor who finds nothing wrong	☐	☐	☐
21. Have trouble sleeping	☐	☐	☐
22. Worry a lot	☐	☐	☐
23. Want to be with parent more than before	☐	☐	☐
24. Feel that you are bad	☐	☐	☐

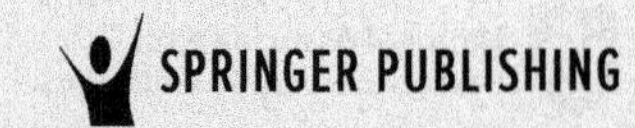

	Never (0)	Sometimes (1)	Often (2)
25. Take unnecessary risks	☐	☐	☐
26. Get hurt frequently	☐	☐	☐
27. Seem to be having less fun	☐	☐	☐
28. Act younger than children your age	☐	☐	☐
29. Do not listen to rules	☐	☐	☐
30. Do not show feelings	☐	☐	☐
31. Do not understand other people's feelings	☐	☐	☐
32. Tease others	☐	☐	☐
33. Blame others for your troubles	☐	☐	☐
34. Take things that do not belong to you	☐	☐	☐
35. Refuse to share	☐	☐	☐
Totals:	_____	_____	_____

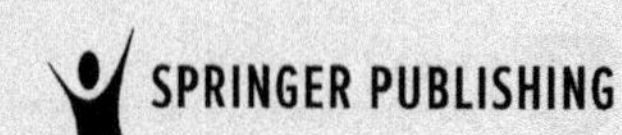

Cuestionario (PSC-Y)

La salud fisica y emocional van juntas. Usted pueda ayudar al doctor/a obtener el mejor servicio posible, contestando unas pocas preguntas acerca de usted. La informacion que nos de es parte de la visita de hov.

Indique cual síntoma mejor describe a su niño/a:

	NUNCA (0)	ALGUNAS (1)	SEGUIDO (2)
1. Se queja de dolores y malestares	☐	☐	☐
2. Pasa mucho tiempo solo(a)	☐	☐	☐
3. Es inquieto(a)	☐	☐	☐
4. Problemas con un maestro(a)	☐	☐	☐
5. Menos interesado en la escuela	☐	☐	☐
6. Es incansable	☐	☐	☐
7. Es muy sonador	☐	☐	☐
8. Se distrae facilmente	☐	☐	☐
9. Temeroso(a) a nuevas situaciónes	☐	☐	☐
10. Se siete triste, infeliz	☐	☐	☐
11. Es irritable, enojon	☐	☐	☐
12. Se siente sin esperanzas	☐	☐	☐
13. Tiene problemas para concentrandose	☐	☐	☐
14. Menos interesado(a) en amigos(as)	☐	☐	☐
15. Pelea con otros niños(as)	☐	☐	☐
16. Falta a la escuela a menudo	☐	☐	☐
17. Estan bejando sus calificaciones	☐	☐	☐
18. Se critica a si mismo(a)	☐	☐	☐
19. Va al doctor y no encuentren nada	☐	☐	☐
20. Tiene problemas para dormir	☐	☐	☐
21. Se preocupa mucho	☐	☐	☐
22. Cree que eres malo(a)	☐	☐	☐
23. Se pone en peligro sin necesidad	☐	☐	☐
24. Se lastima facilmente	☐	☐	☐
25. Parece divertise menos	☐	☐	☐
26. Actua como un nino a su edad	☐	☐	☐

National Association *of* Pediatric Nurse Practitioners℠

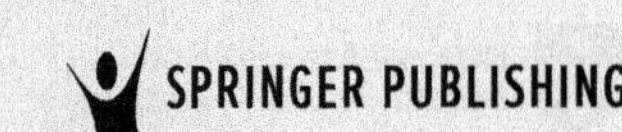

	NUNCA (0)	ALGUNAS (1)	SEGUIDO (2)
27. No obedece reglas..	☐	☐	☐
28. No demuestra sus sentimientos....................	☐	☐	☐
29. No comprende el sentir de otros..................	☐	☐	☐
30. Molesta a otros..	☐	☐	☐
31. Culpa a otros de sus problemas...................	☐	☐	☐
32. Toma cosas que no le pertenecen.................	☐	☐	☐
33. Se rehusa a compartir....................................	☐	☐	☐
Totals:	_____	_____	_____

Necesita usted ayuda con problemas de comportamiento, emocionales o aprendizaje? .... ____Si ____ No

National Association *of* Pediatric Nurse Practitioners℠

Reproduced with permission from Jellinek, M., & Murphy, M. (1986). *Massachusetts General Hospital.* https://www.massgeneral.org/psychiatry/treatments-and-services/pediatric-symptom-checklist

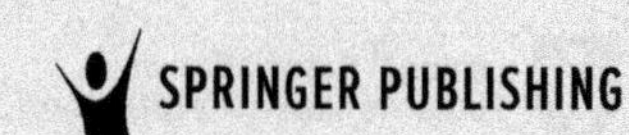

Pediatric Symptom Checklist (PSC-17) for Parents

Please mark under the heading that best describes your child:

	NEVER (0)	SOMETIMES (1)	OFTEN (2)
1. Feels sad, unhappy	☐	☐	☐
2. Feels hopeless	☐	☐	☐
3. Is down on self	☐	☐	☐
4. Worries a lot	☐	☐	☐
5. Seems to be having less fun	☐	☐	☐
6. Fidgety, unable to sit still	☐	☐	☐
7. Daydreams too much	☐	☐	☐
8. Distracted easily	☐	☐	☐
9. Has trouble concentrating	☐	☐	☐
10. Acts as if driven by a motor	☐	☐	☐
11. Fights with other children	☐	☐	☐
12. Does not listen to rules	☐	☐	☐
13. Does not understand other people's feelings	☐	☐	☐
14. Teases others	☐	☐	☐
15. Blames others for their troubles	☐	☐	☐
16. Refuses to share	☐	☐	☐
17. Takes things that do not belong to them	☐	☐	☐

Does your child have any emotional or behavioral problems for which they need help? __No __Yes

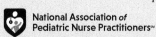

Reproduced with permission from Jellinek, M., & Murphy, M. (1986). *Massachusetts General Hospital.* https://www.massgeneral.org/psychiatry/treatments-and-services/pediatric-symptom-checklist

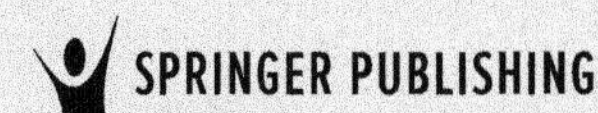

Lista De Síntomas Pediátricos (Pediatric Symptom Checklist—PSC)

La salud física y emocional son importantes para cada niño. Los padres son los primeros que notan un problema de la conducta emocional o del aprendizaje de su hijo(a). Ud. puede ayudar a su hijo(a) a obtener el mejor cuidado de su doctor por medio de contestar estas preguntas. Favor de indicar cual frase describe a su hijo(a)

Indique cual síntoma mejor describe a su hijo/a:

	NUNCA (0)	ALGUNAS VECES (1)	FRECUENTEMENTE (2)
1. Se siente triste, infeliz	_____	_____	_____
2. Se siente sin esperanzas	_____	_____	_____
3. Se siente mal de sí mismo(a)	_____	_____	_____
4. Se preocupa mucho	_____	_____	_____
5. Parece divertirse menos	_____	_____	_____
6. Es inquieto(a), incapaz de sentarse tranquilo(a)	_____	_____	_____
7. Sueña despierto demasiado	_____	_____	_____
8. Se distrae fácilmente	_____	_____	_____
9. Tiene problemas para concentrarse	_____	_____	_____
10. Es muy activo(a), tiene mucha energía	_____	_____	_____
11. Pelea con otros niños	_____	_____	_____
12. No obedece las reglas	_____	_____	_____
13. No comprende los sentimientos de otros	_____	_____	_____
14. Molesta o se burla de otros	_____	_____	_____
15. Culpa a otros por sus problemas	_____	_____	_____
16. Se niega a compartir	_____	_____	_____
17. Toma cosas que no le pertenecen	_____	_____	_____

Total____________________

¿Tiene su hijo(a) algún problema emocional o del comportamiento para el cual necesita ayuda?............ __☐ No __☐ Sí

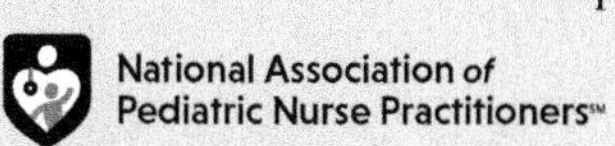

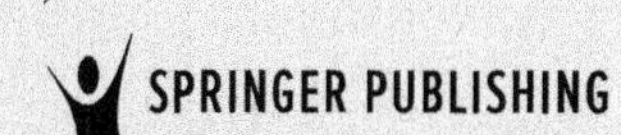

The Child Behavior Checklist (CBCL)
(T. Achenbach and C. S. Edelbrock)

DESCRIPTION

The Child Behavior Checklist (CBCL) is a tool on which parents or other individuals rate a child's problem behaviors and competencies. This Likert scale tool can either be self-administered or administered through an interview and now includes *DSM*-oriented scales. The CBCL also can be used to measure a child's change in behavior over time or following a treatment. The first section of the CBCL consists of 20 competence items and the second section consists of 120 items on behavior or emotional problems during the past 6 months (e.g., aggression, hyperactivity, bullying, conduct problems, defiance, violence). Parents rate their child for how true each item is now or within the past 6 months using the following scale: 0 = not true (as far as you know); 1 = somewhat or sometimes true; and 2 = very true or often true. Teacher Report Forms (TRF), Youth Report Forms (YRF), and Direct Observation Forms are also available. It is suggested that the CBCL be used for further evaluation if a positive score is found on the Pediatric Symptom Checklist (PSC).

Age Range: Two versions of the tool exist: one for children 1½ to 5 years of age and another for ages 6 to 18. The Youth Self Report tool is targeted for teens 11 to 18 years of age.

PSYCHOMETRIC PROPERTIES OF THE CBCL

The CBCL has been extensively studied and supported by multiple studies to be a valid and highly reliable tool for use with African American, Caucasian, and Hispanic/Latino children across all socioeconomic levels. The range of internal consistency reliability is reported as 0.78–0.97.

Manual and computer scoring is available.

Examiner Qualifications: Master's degree

Permission Required to Use Instrument: Yes

Contact Information for Ordering the CBCL

Achenbach System of Empirically Based Assessment

1 South Prospect Street, Room 6436

Burlington, Vermont 05401-3456

Phone: 802-656-8313

Fax: 802-656-2608

Email: mail@aseba.org

Website: www.ASEBA.org

Sources: Achenbach, T. (1991). *Integrative guide to the 1991 CBCL/4-18, YSR, and TRF Profiles.* University of Vermont, Department of Psychology.

Achenbach, T., & Edelbrock, C. S. (1983). *Manual for the child behavior checklist and revised child behavior profile.* University of Vermont.

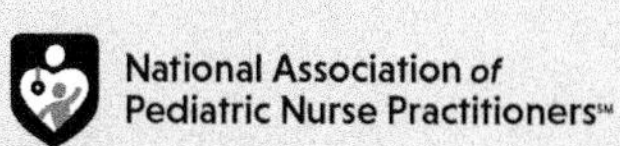

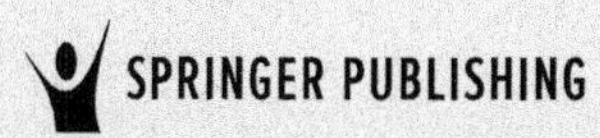

Guidelines for Adolescent Preventive Services

Several tools have been designed to support implementing the American Medical Association's (AMA, 1994) Guidelines for Adolescent Preventive Services (GAPS) program in your clinical setting. The six forms that follow include the Younger Adolescent Questionnaire in English and Spanish, Middle-Older Adolescent Questionnaire in English and Spanish, and the Parent/Guardian Questionnaire in English and Spanish. The questionnaires are considered master copies that you can reproduce but not alter, modify, or revise without the expressed written consent of the Child and Adolescent Health Program at the American Medical Association.

Pediatric Nurse Practitioners® — National Association of

Guidelines for Adolescent Preventive Services
Younger Adolescent Questionnaire
Confidential (Your answers will not be given out.)

Chart # ________________

Name ______________________________ Today's Date ______________
Last First Middle Initial month day year

Birthdate ______________ Grade in School __________ **Boy** or **Girl** (*circle one*) Age ________
month day year

Address ______________________________ City __________ State __________ Zip __________

Phone Number ______________________ Pager/Beeper Number ______________________
area code

What languages are spoken where you live? ______________________________

Are you: ☐ White ☐ African American ☐ Asian/Pacific Islander
☐ Latino/Hispanic ☐ Native American ☐ Other ______________

MEDICAL HISTORY

1. What languages are spoken where you live? ______________________________
____
2. Are you allergic to any medicines?
☐ No ☐ Yes, name of medicine(s): ______________________ ☐ Not Sure
3. Do you have any health problems?
☐ No ☐ Yes, problem(s): ______________________ ☐ Not Sure
4. Are you taking any medicine now?
☐ No ☐ Yes, name of medicine(s): ______________________ ☐ Not Sure

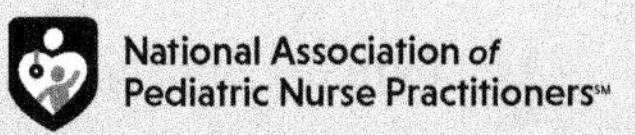

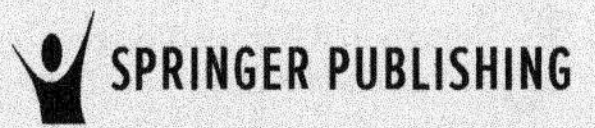

5. Have you been to the dentist in the last year? .... ☐ No ☐ Yes ☐ Not Sure
6. Have you stayed overnight in a hospital in the last year? .... ☐ No ☐ Yes ☐ Not Sure
7. Have you ever had any of the problems below?

	Yes	No	Not Sure		Yes	No	Not Sure
Allergies or hay fever	☐	☐	☐	Seizures	☐	☐	☐
Asthma	☐	☐	☐	Cancer	☐	☐	☐
Tuberculosis (TB)	☐	☐	☐	Diabetes	☐	☐	☐

FOR GIRLS ONLY

8. Have you started having periods? .... ☐ No ☐ Yes
   a. *If yes*, are your periods regular (once a month) ? .... ☐ No ☐ Yes
   b. *If yes*, what was the 1st day of your last period? Month _________ Day _______
9. Have you ever been pregnant? .... ☐ Yes ☐ No

FAMILY INFORMATION

10. Who do you live with? (Check all that apply).

☐ Mother ☐ Stepmother ☐ Brother(s)/ages________________

☐ Father ☐ Stepfather ☐ Sister(s)/ages__________________

☐ Guardian ☐ Other adult relative ☐ Other/(explain)________________

11. Do you have older brothers or sisters who live away from home? ...... ☐ Yes ☐ No ☐ Not Sure
12. During the past year, have there been any changes in your family such as: (Check all that apply)

☐ Marriage ☐ Loss of job ☐ Births ☐ Other changes _______

☐ Separation ☐ Moved to a new neighborhood ☐ Serious Illness/Injury _____________________

☐ Divorce ☐ A new school ☐ Deaths _____________________

SPECIFIC HEALTH ISSUES

13. Please check whether you have questions or are worried about any of the following:

☐ Height ☐ Neck or back ☐ Muscle or pain in arms/legs ☐ Anger or temper

☐ Weight ☐ Breasts ☐ Menstruation or periods ☐ Feeling tired

☐ Eyes or vision ☐ Heart ☐ Wetting the bed ☐ Trouble sleeping

☐ Hearing or earaches ☐ Coughing or wheezing ☐ Trouble urinating or peeing ☐ Fitting in/belonging

☐ Colds/runny or stuffy nose ☐ Chest pain or trouble breathing ☐ Drip from penis or vagina ☐ Cancer

National Association of Pediatric Nurse Practitioners℠

SPRINGER PUBLISHING

☐ Mouth or teeth or breath ☐ Stomachache ☐ Wet dreams ☐ HIV/AIDS

☐ Headaches ☐ Vomiting or throwing up ☐ Skin (rash/acne) ☐ Dying

Other ________________________________

These questions will help us get to know you better. Choose the answer that best describes what you feel or do. Your answers will be seen only by your health care provider and their assistant.

HEALTH PROFILE

Eating/Weight/Body

14. Do you eat fruits and vegetables every day? ☐ No ☐ Yes
15. Do you drink milk and/or eat milk products every day? ☐ No ☐ Yes
16. Do you spend a lot of time thinking about ways to be skinny? ☐ Yes ☐ No
17. Do you do things to lose weight (skip meals, take pills, starve yourself, vomit, etc.) ☐ Yes ☐ No
18. Do you work, play, or exercise enough to make you sweat or breathe hard at least 3 times a week? ☐ No ☐ Yes
19. Have you pierced your body (not including ears) or gotten a tattoo? ☐ Yes ☐ No

School

20. Is doing well in school important to you? ☐ No ☐ Yes
21. Is doing well in school important to your family and friends? ☐ No ☐ Yes
22. Are your grades this year worse than last year? ☐ Yes ☐ No ☐ Not Sure
23. Are you getting failing grades in any subjects this year? ☐ Yes ☐ No ☐ Not Sure
24. Have you been told that you have a learning problem? ☐ Yes ☐ No
25. Have you been suspended from school this year? ☐ Yes ☐ No

Friends and Family

26. Do you know at least one person who you can talk to about problems? ☐ No ☐ Yes
27. Do you think that your parent(s) or guardian(s) usually listen to you and take your feelings seriously? ☐ No ☐ Yes
28. Have your parents talked with you about things like alcohol, drugs, and sex? ☐ No ☐ Yes ☐ Not Sure
29. Are you worried about problems at home or in your family? ☐ Yes ☐ No ☐ Not Sure
30. Have you ever thought seriously about running away from home? ☐ Yes ☐ No

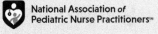

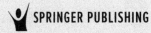

Weapons/Violence/Safety

31. Is there a gun, rifle, or other firearm where you live? .... ☐ Yes ☐ No ☐ Not Sure
32. Have you ever carried a gun, knife, club, or other weapon to protect yourself? .... ☐ Yes ☐ No
33. Have you ever been in a physical fight where you or someone else got hurt?... ☐ Yes ☐ No
34. Have you ever been in trouble with the police? .... ☐ Yes ☐ No
35. Have you ever seen a violent act take place at home, school, or in your neighborhood? .... ☐ Yes ☐ No
36. Are you worried about violence or your safety? .... ☐ Yes ☐ No ☐ Not Sure
37. Do you usually wear a helmet and/or protective gear when you rollerblade, skateboard, or ride a bike? .... ☐ No ☐ Yes
38. Do you always wear a seat belt when you ride in a car, truck, or van? .... ☐ Yes ☐ No

Tobacco

39. Have you ever tried cigarettes or chewing tobacco? .... ☐ Yes ☐ No
40. Have any of your close friends ever tried cigarettes or chewing tobacco? .... ☐ Yes ☐ No
41. Does anyone you live with smoke cigarettes/cigars or chew tobacco? .... ☐ Yes ☐ No

Alcohol

42. Have you ever tried beer, wine, or other liquor (except for religious purposes)? .... ☐ Yes ☐ No
43. Have any of your close friends ever tried beer, wine, or other liquor (except for religious purposes)? .... ☐ Yes ☐ No
44. Have you ever been in a car when the driver has been using drugs or drinking beer, wine, or other liquor? .... ☐ Yes ☐ No
45. Does anyone in your family drink so much that it worries you? .... ☐ Yes ☐ No ☐ Not Sure

Drugs

46. Have you ever taken things to get high, stay awake, calm down, or go to sleep? .... ☐ Yes ☐ No ☐ Not Sure
47. Have you ever used marijuana (pot, grass, weed, reefer, or blunt)? .... ☐ Yes ☐ No ☐ Not Sure
48. Have you ever used other drugs such as cocaine, speed, LSD, mushrooms, etc.? .... ☐ Yes ☐ No ☐ Not Sure
49. Have you ever sniffed or huffed things like paint, White-Out, glue, gasoline, etc.? .... ☐ Yes ☐ No ☐ Not Sure

50. Have any of your close friends ever used marijuana, other drugs, or done other things to get high? ☐ Yes ☐ No ☐ Not Sure

51. Does anyone in your family use drugs so much that it worries you? ☐ Yes ☐ No ☐ Not Sure

Development/Relationships

52. Are you dating someone or going steady? ☐ Yes ☐ No ☐ Not Sure

53. Are you thinking about having sex ("going all the way "or "doing it")? ☐ Yes ☐ No ☐ Not Sure

54. Have you ever had sex? ☐ Yes ☐ No ☐ Not Sure

55. Have any of your friends ever had sex? ☐ Yes ☐ No ☐ Not Sure

56. Have you ever felt pressured by anyone to have sex or had sex when you did not want to? ☐ Yes ☐ No ☐ Not Sure

57. Have you ever been told by a doctor or a nurse that you had a sexually transmitted disease like herpes, gonorrhea, or chlamydia? ☐ Yes ☐ No ☐ Not Sure

58. Would you like to receive information on abstinence ("how to say no to sex")? ☐ Yes ☐ No ☐ Not Sure

59. Would you like to know how to avoid getting pregnant, getting HIV/AIDS, or getting sexually transmitted diseases? ☐ Yes ☐ No ☐ Not Sure

Emotions

60. Have you done something fun during the past 2 weeks? ☐ No ☐ Yes

61. When you get angry, do you do violent things? ☐ Yes ☐ No

62. During the past few weeks, have you felt very sad or down as though you have nothing to look forward to? ☐ Yes ☐ No

63. Have you ever seriously thought about killing yourself, made a plan, or tried to kill yourself? ☐ Yes ☐ No

64. Is there something you often worry about or fear? ☐ Yes ☐ No

65. Have you ever been physically, emotionally, or sexually abused? ☐ Yes ☐ No ☐ Not Sure

66. Would you like to get counseling about something that is bothering you? ☐ Yes ☐ No ☐ Not Sure

Special Circumstances

67. In the past year have you been around someone with tuberculosis (TB)? ☐ Yes ☐ No ☐ Not Sure

68. In the past year, have you stayed overnight in a homeless shelter, jail, or detention center? ☐ Yes ☐ No

69. Have you ever lived in foster care or a group home? ☐ Yes ☐ No

Self

70. What two words best describe you?

    1) ______________________ 2) ______________________

71. What would you like to be when you grow up?

    ____

72. If you could have three wishes come true, what would they be?

    1) ____

    2) ____

    3) ____

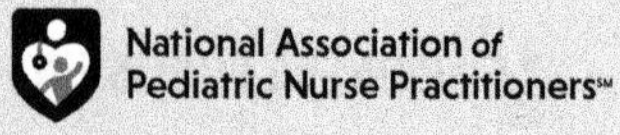

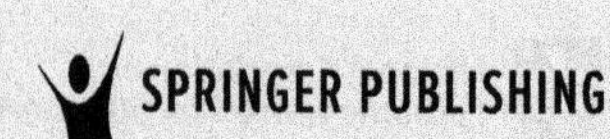

Guía de Servicios Preventivos Para los Adolescentes

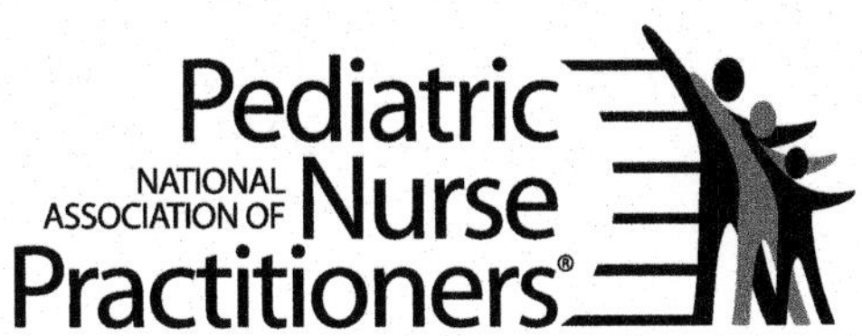

Guía de Servicios Preventivos Para los Adolescentes
Cuestionario para Adolescentes Jóvenes
Confidencial (No le diremos a nadie lo que nos diga)

Archivo # ______________________________

Nombre ______________________________ (Apellido) (Nombre) (Inicial) Fecha de Hoy ______________ mes/dia/año

Fecha de Nacimiento______ Añp/Curso Escoloar ______ Niño o Niña (*marque con círculo*) Edad ______

Direción______________________Ciudad_____________CódigoPostal/Zip________________

Teléfono ( ) ____________ (Código) Anunciador/Pager/Beeper ( )______________________

¿ Cuales idiomas se hablan donde vive Ud.? ______________________________

¿ ES Ud.?: ☐ Blanco ☐ Afro-Aericano ☐ Asiático/Isleño del Pacifico
☐ Latino/Hispano ☐ Indígena Norteamericano ☐ Otro

HISTORIA MÉDICA

1. ¿Porqué vino all consultorio hoy?______________________________
____
2. ¿Tiene alergias a cualqier medicina?
☐ No ☐ Sí, (nombre(s) de la (s) medicina (s): __________) ☐ No estoy seguro
3. ¿Tiene cualquier problema con la salud?
☐ No ☐ Sí, (nombre(s) de la (s) medicina (s): __________) ☐ No estoy seguro
4. ¿Esta tomando medicinas actualmente?
☐ No ☐ Sí, (nombre(s) de la (s) medicina (s): __________) ☐ No estoy seguro
5. ¿En el ú;tomp año ha consultado al dentist? .... ☐ No ☐ Sí ☐ No estoy seguro
6. En el ultimo año Ha pasado la noche en el hospital? ☐ No ☐ Sí ☐ No estoy seguro
7. ¿Alguna vez padeció cualqiera de los siguientes prolemes de salud?

	Sí	No	No estoy seguro		Sí	No	No estoy seguro
Alergias o "hay fever"	☐	☐	☐	Convulsiones/ Ataques	☐	☐	☐
Asma	☐	☐	☐	Cáncer	☐	☐	☐
Tuberculosis (TB)	☐	☐	☐	Diabetes	☐	☐	☐

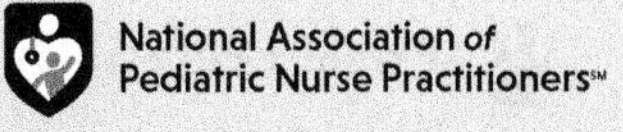

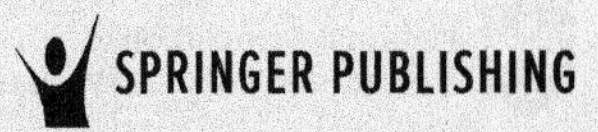

UNICAMETE PARA NIÑUS

8. Ha comenzado a tener su período/la regla? .... ☐ No ☐ Sí
   a. Si ya comenzó Le viene regularmente (una vez al mes)? .... ☐ No ☐ Sí
   b. Si es el caso, ¿Cual fue el primer día de la última regla? .... Mes____ Día____
9. ¿Alguna vez ha estado embarazada?... ☐ No ☐ Sí

INFORMATION FAMILIAR

10. ¿Con quién vive? (Marque todas que sean ciertas).

☐ Madre	☐ Madrastra	☐ Hermanos/edades
☐ Padre	☐ Padrastro	☐ Heranas/edades
☐ Guardián Legal	☐ Otro pariente adulto	☐ Otra/(explique)

11. ¿Tiene hermanos mayors que no viven en casa?............ ☐ Sí ☐ No ☐ No estoy seguro
12. En el ultimo año Han habido cambios importantes en su familia? (Marque todas que sean ciertas),

☐ Matrimonios	☐ Alguien perdi su empleo	☐ Nacimientos	☐ Otros cambios
☐ Separaciones	☐ Mudanzas a otros vecindarios	☐ Enfermedades graves	
☐ Divorcios	☐ Cambio de escuela	☐ Muertes	

PROBLEMAS ESPECÍFICOS DE LA SALUD

13. Por favor, marque a continuación si tiene preguntas o alguna preocupación sobre:

☐ Estatura/desarrollo físico	☐ Cuello o espalda	☐ Músculos o dolor en los brazos/piernas	☐ Enojo o mal genio
☐ Peso	☐ Pechos/senos	☐ Menstruación o la regla	☐ Cansancio
☐ Ojos/la vista	☐ Corazón	☐ Mojarse la cama	☐ Difficultad al dormer
☐ Dificultad para oir o dolor del oído	☐ Tos o le chilla el pecho hacer pipí	☐ Difficultad para orinar o	☐ Su relación con los compañeros
☐ Catarro/moquillo o las narices tapadas	☐ Dolor del pecho o difficultad en respirar	☐ Gota del pene o la vagina	☐ Cáncer
☐ Boca o dientes o aliento	☐ Dolor del estómago	☐ Sueño mojado	☐ VIH/SIDA
☐ Dolores de cabeza	☐ Vómito o náuseas	☐ Piel (salpullido/espinillas)	☐ La muerte

Estas preguntas nos ayudarán a conocerle mejor. Escoja la respuesta que mejor indica lo que siente o hace.

Sus respuestas ser n vistas nicamente por su medico/enfermera y su asistente.

National Association of Pediatric Nurse Practitioners℠

SPRINGER PUBLISHING

SU SALUD

Comer/Peso/Cuerpo

14. ¿Come Ud. frutas y vegetales cada día? ☐ No ☐ Sí
15. ¿Toma Ud. leche y/o come productos lácteos cada día? ☐ No ☐ Sí
16. ¿Gasta mucho tiempo pensando en como adelgazar? ☐ No ☐ Sí
17. ¿Trata de bajar de peso (evita comidas, toma pastillas, ayuna, vomita, eta) ☐ No ☐ Sí
18. ¿Trabaja Ud, juega, o hace suficiente ejercicio como para sudar orespirar fuerte por lo menos 3 veces por semana? ☐ No ☐ Sí
19. Ha perforado su cuerpo (sin incluir las orejas) o ha puesto un tatuaje? ☐ Sí ☐ No

La Escuela

20. ¿Salir bien en sus estudios es importante para Ud.? ☐ No ☐ Sí
21. ¿Salir bien en sus estudios es importante para su familia y sus amigos? ☐ No ☐ Sí
22. ¿Sus notas (calificaciones) son peores este año ? ☐ Sí ☐ No ☐ No estoy seguro
23. ¿Está saliendo mal en alguna materia ? ☐ Sí ☐ No ☐ No estoy seguro
24. ¿Le han dicho que tiene dificultad en aprender? ☐ Sí ☐ No
25. ¿Le han suspendido de clases este año? ☐ Sí ☐ No

Los Amigos y la Familia

26. ¿Conoce al menos una persona con quien puede hablar si tiene un problema? ☐ No ☐ Sí
27. ¿ Cree Ud. que sus padres o su guardián le escuchan y toman en seriosus sentimientos? ☐ No ☐ Sí
28. ¿Sus padres han hablado con Ud. sobre alcohol, drogas, y sexo ? ☐ No ☐ Sí ☐ No estoy seguro
29. ¿Está preocupado por problemas en su casa o en su familia ? ☐ No ☐ Sí ☐ No estoy seguro
30. ¿Alguna vez ha contemplado seriamente fugarse de la casa? ☐ No ☐ Sí

Las Armas/la Violencia/la Seguridad

31. ¿Hay una pistola, rifle u otra arma de fuego en la casa donde vive ? ☐ No ☐ Sí ☐ No estoy seguro
32. ¿Alguna vez ha portado una pistola, cuchillo, palo u otra arma para protegerse? ☐ No ☐ Sí
33. ¿Alguna vez ha estado en una pelea donde Ud. u otra persona fue lesionado? ☐ No ☐ Sí
34. ¿Alguna vez ha tenido problemas con la policía? ☐ No ☐ Sí
35. ¿Alguna vez ha visto un acto de violencia en la casa, la escuela,o en el vecindario? ☐ No ☐ Sí

National Association of Pediatric Nurse Practitioners™

SPRINGER PUBLISHING

36. ¿Está Ud. preocupado por la violencia o por su seguridad? .... ☐ Sí ☐ No ☐ No estoy seguro

37. ¿Normalmente usa Ud. un casco y/o equipo protectivo cuando patina ("roller blade," "skateboard", o monta a bicicleta? .... ☐ No ☐ Sí

38. ¿Siempre usa Ud. el cinturón de seguridad cuando monta en un auto, vehículo de carga, o camioneta? .... ☐ No ☐ Sí

El Tabaco

39. Ha probado Ud. cigarrillos o tabaco de mascar (rapé)? .... ☐ Sí ☐ No

40. ¿Alguno de sus mejores amigos ha probado cigarrillos o tabaco de mascar? .... ☐ Sí ☐ No

41. ¿Alguien con quien vive Ud. fuma cigarrillos/puros o usa tabaco de mascar? .... ☐ Sí ☐ No

El Alcohol

42. ¿Alguna vez ha probado Ud. cerveza, vino, u otro licor (fuera de propósitos religiosos)? .... ☐ Sí ☐ No

43. ¿Alguno de sus mejores amigos ha probado cerveza, vino, u otro licor (fuera de propósitos religiosos)? .... ☐ Sí ☐ No

44. ¿Alguna vez ha estado en un veh culo cuando el motorista ha estado tomando drogas, cerveza, vino, u otro licor? .... ☐ Sí ☐ No

45. ¿Hay alguien en su familia que toma tanto que le preocupa? .... ☐ Sí ☐ No ☐ No estoy seguro

Las Drogas

46. ¿Alguna vez ha tomado sustancias para elevarse, para mantenerse despierto, calmarse, o para dormir? .... ☐ Sí ☐ No ☐ No estoy seguro

47. ¿Alguna vez ha usado marijuana (hierba, pasto, maría, mota, "refer, o pot")? .... ☐ Sí ☐ No ☐ No estoy seguro

48. ¿Alguna vez ha usado otras drogas como la coca na, la metanfetamina "speed", LSD, hongos.? .... ☐ Sí ☐ No ☐ No estoy seguro

49. ¿Alguna vez ha inhalado sustancias: pintura, "white-out", gases de los pegantes o gomas, gasolina? .... ☐ Sí ☐ No ☐ No estoy seguro

50. ¿Alguno de sus mejores amigos ha usado la marijuana, otras drogas o hecho otras cosas para elevarse o sentirse "bien"? .... ☐ Sí ☐ No ☐ No estoy seguro

51. ¿Hay alguien en su familia que usa tanta droga que le preocupa? .... ☐ Sí ☐ No ☐ No estoy seguro

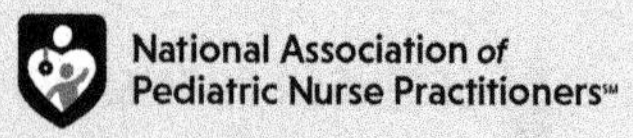

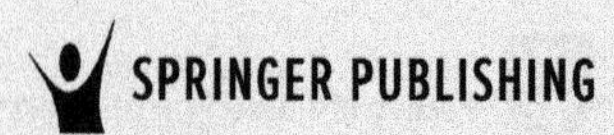

El Desarrollo/Relaciones Personales

52. ¿Tiene novio(a) o esta saliendo con alguien? .... ☐ Sí ☐ No ☐ No estoy seguro
53. ¿Está pensando en tener relaciones sexuales (en hacerlo, tener sexo)?.. ☐ Sí ☐ No ☐ No estoy seguro
54. ¿Quisiera recibir información sobre como abstenerse (como decir que "no" a tener sexo)?. .... ☐ Sí ☐ No ☐ No estoy seguro
55. ¿Alguna vez ha tenido relaciones sexuales? .... ☐ Sí ☐ No ☐ No estoy seguro
56. ¿Alguno de sus amigos ha tenido relaciones sexuales ya? .... ☐ Sí ☐ No ☐ No estoy seguro
57. ¿Alguna vez ha sido presionado por alguien a tener relaciones o ha tenido relaciones cuando no quería? .... ☐ Sí ☐ No ☐ No estoy seguro
58. ¿Alguna vez un médico le ha dicho que tuvo una enfermedad transmitida sexualmente como el herpes, la gonorrea, o la sífilis? .... ☐ Sí ☐ No ☐ No estoy seguro
59. ¿Quisiera saber como evitar el embarazo, el VIH/SIDA, o una enfermedad "venérea"? .... ☐ Sí ☐ No ☐ No estoy seguro

Las Emociones

60. ¿ Ha hecho algo divertido en las últimas dos semanas? ....☐ No ☐ Sí
61. ¿Cuando se pone enojado, se hace cosas violentas? .... ☐ No ☐ Sí
62. ¿Durante las últimas semanas ha sentido muy triste, desanimado, desalentado? ....☐ No ☐ Sí
63. ¿Alguna vez ha pensado seriamente en matarse, ha hecho un plan, o ha intentado matarse? .... ☐ No ☐ Sí
64. ¿Hay algo que le preocupa o teme con frecuencia? ....☐ No ☐ Sí
65. ¿Alguna vez ha sido abusado físicamente, emocionalmente, o sexualmente? .... ☐ No ☐ Sí ☐ No estoy seguro
66. ¿Quisiera hablar con un(a) consejero(a) de algo que le preocupa? .... ☐ No ☐ Sí ☐ No estoy seguro

Circunstancias Especiales

67. En este año pasado, ¿Ha pasado tiempo con alguien que tiene la tuberculosis? .... ☐ Sí ☐ No ☐ No estoy seguro
68. En este año pasado, ¿Ha pasado la noche en un albergue, la cárcel, o un centro detención juvenil? .... ☐ Sí ☐ No
69. ¿Alguna vez ha vivido con padres de crianza, o en una casa juvenil? .... ☐ Sí ☐ No

National Association of Pediatric Nurse Practitioners™

SPRINGER PUBLISHING

Sí Mismo

70. ¿Cuales dos palabras describen mejor a Ud.? 1) ________________ 2) ________________

71. ¿Que quiere hacer cuando sea adulto? ____

72. Si podrían concederle tres deseos, cuales serían?

1) ____

2) ____

3) ____

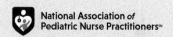

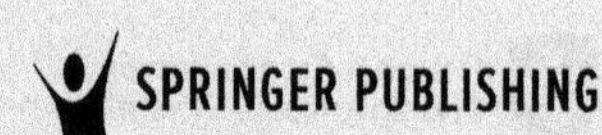

Guidelines for Adolescent Preventive Services

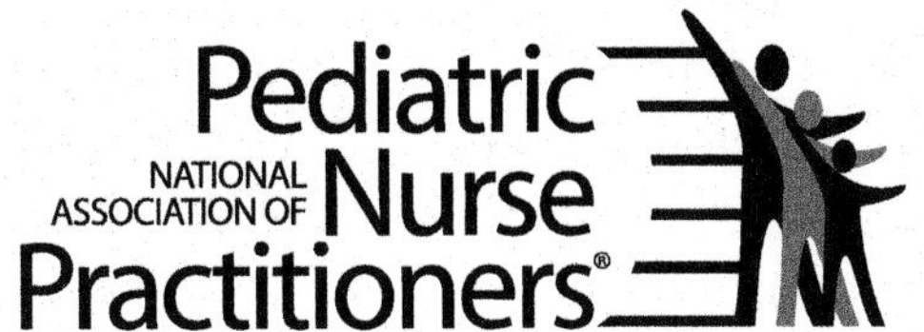

Guidelines for Adolescent Preventive Services
Middle-Older Adolescent Questionnaire
Confidential (Your answers will not be given out.)

Chart # __________

Name ______________________________ Date __________
Last First Middle Initial

Date of Birth ________ Grade in School ______ Year in college ________ Sex: Male Female Age ______

Address ____________________ City ____________________ Zip __________

Phone number where you can be reached ______________ Pager/beeper number ______________

What languages are spoken where you live? ____________________ Race ______________

MEDICAL HISTORY

1. Why did you come to the clinic/office today? ____________________
2. Do you have any health problems? ☐ Yes ☐ No Problem(s) ______________
3. Did you have any health problems in the past 12 months? ☐ Yes ☐ No Problem(s) ____
4. Are you taking any medicine now? ☐ Yes ☐ No Name of medicine ______________

For Girls

5. Date when last period started _______ Are your periods regular (monthly)? ☐ No ☐ Yes
Month Date
6. Have you had a miscarriage, an abortion, or live birth in the past 12 months? ☐ Yes ☐ No

SPECIFIC HEALTH ISSUES

7. Please check whether you have questions or are worried about any of the following:

☐ Height/weight ☐ Mouth/teeth/breath ☐ Frequent or painful urination ☐ Trouble sleeping
☐ Blood pressure ☐ Neck/back ☐ Feeling tired a lot
☐ Diet/food/appetite ☐ Chest pain/trouble breathing ☐ Discharge from penis or vagina ☐ Cancer
☐ Future plans/job ☐ Wetting the bed ☐ Dying
☐ Skin (rash, acne) ☐ Coughing/wheezing

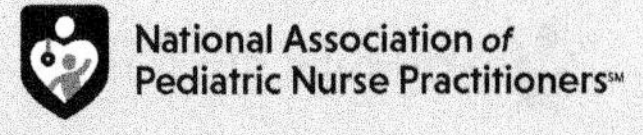

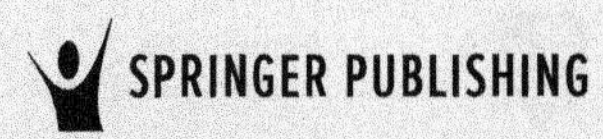

☐ Headaches/migraines	☐ Breasts	☐ Sexual organs/genitals	☐ Sad or crying a lot
☐ Dizziness/fainting	☐ Heart	☐ Menstruation/periods	☐ Stress
☐ Eyes/vision	☐ Stomachache	☐ Wet dreams	☐ Anger/temper
☐ Ears/hearing/ear aches	☐ Nausea/vomiting	☐ Physical or sexual abuse	☐ Violence/personal safety
☐ Nose	☐ Diarrhea/constipation	☐ Masturbation	☐ Other (explain)
☐ Lots of colds	☐ Muscle or joint pain in arms/legs	☐ HIV/AIDS	____________________ ____________________

HEALTH PROFILE

These questions will help us get to know you better. Choose the answer that best describes what you feel or do. Your answers will be seen only by your health care provider and their assistant.

Eating/Weight

8. Are you satisfied with your eating habits? .... ☐ No ☐ Yes
9. Do you ever eat in secret? .... ☐ Yes ☐ No
10. Do you spend a lot of time thinking about ways to be thin? .... ☐ Yes ☐ No
11. In the past year, have you tried to lose weight or control your weight by vomiting, taking diet pills or laxatives, or starving yourself? .... ☐ Yes ☐ No
12. Do you exercise or participate in sport activities that make you sweat and breathe hard for 20 minutes or more at a time at least three or more times during the week? .... ☐ No ☐ Yes

School

13. Are your grades this year worse than last year? .... ☐ Yes ☐ No ☐ Not in school
14. Have you either been told you have a learning problem or do you think you have a learning problem? .... ☐ Yes ☐ No
15. Have you been suspended from school this year? .... ☐ Yes ☐ No ☐ Not in school

Friends & Family

16. Do you have at least one friend who you really like and feel you can talk to? .... ☐ No ☐ Yes
17. Do you think that your parent(s) or guardian(s) *usually* listen to you and take your feelings seriously? .... ☐ No ☐ Yes
18. Have you ever thought seriously about running away from home? .... ☐ Yes ☐ No ☐ Not sure

National Association *of* Pediatric Nurse Practitioners™ SPRINGER PUBLISHING

Weapons/Violence/Safety

19. Do you or anyone you live with have a gun, rifle, or other firearm? .... ☐ Yes ☐ No ☐ Not sure
20. In the past year, have you carried a gun, knife, club, or other weapon for protection? .... ☐ Yes ☐ No
21. Have you been in a physical fight during the *past 3 months*? .... ☐ Yes ☐ No
22. Have you ever been in trouble with the law? .... ☐ Yes ☐ No
23. Are you worried about violence or your safety? .... ☐ Yes ☐ No ☐ Not sure
24. Do you usually wear a helmet when you rollerblade, skateboard, ride a bicycle, motorcycle, minibike, or ride in an all-terrain vehicle (ATV)? .... ☐ No ☐ Yes
25. Do you usually wear a seat belt when you ride in or drive a car, truck, or van? .... ☐ No ☐ Yes

Tobacco

26. Do you ever smoke cigarettes/cigars, use snuff or chew tobacco? .... ☐ Yes ☐ No
27. Do any of your close friends ever smoke cigarettes/cigars, use snuff or chew tobacco? .... ☐ Yes ☐ No
28. Does anyone you live with smoke cigarettes/cigars, use snuff or chew tobacco? .... ☐ Yes ☐ No

Alcohol

29. In the past month, did you get drunk or very high on beer, wine, or other alcohol? .... ☐ Yes ☐ No
30. In the past month, did any of your close friends get drunk or very high on beer, wine, or other alcohol? .... ☐ Yes ☐ No
31. Have you ever been criticized or gotten into trouble because of drinking? .... ☐ Yes ☐ No ☐ Not sure
32. In the past year have you used alcohol and then driven a car/truck/van/motorcycle? .... ☐ Yes ☐ No ☐ Does not apply
33. In the past year, have you been in a car or other motor vehicle when the driver has been drinking alcohol or using drugs? .... ☐ Yes ☐ No
34. Does anyone in your family drink or take drugs so much that it worries you? .... ☐ Yes ☐ No

Drugs

35. Do you ever use marijuana or other drugs, or sniff inhalants? .... ☐ Yes ☐ No ☐ Not sure
36. Do any of your close friends ever use marijuana or other drugs, or sniff inhalants? .... ☐ Yes ☐ No ☐ Not sure

37. Do you ever use non prescription drugs to get to sleep, stay awake, calm down, or get high?
(These drugs can be bought at a store without a doctor's prescription.) .... ☐ Yes ☐ No

38. Have you ever used steroid pills or shots without a doctor telling you to? .... ☐ Yes ☐ No ☐ Not sure

Development

39. Do you have any concerns or questions about the size or shape of your body, or your physical appearance?.......... ☐ Yes ☐ No ☐ Not sure

40. Do you think you may be gay, lesbian, or bisexual? .... ☐ Yes ☐ No ☐ Not sure

41. Have you ever had sexual intercourse?
(How old were you the first time?________________) .... ☐ Yes ☐ No ☐ Not sure

42. Are you using a method to prevent pregnancy?
(Which:______________________________) .... ☐ No ☐ Yes ☐ Not active

43. Do you and your partner(s) *always* use condoms when you have sex? .... ☐ No ☐ Yes ☐ Not active

44. Have any of your close friends ever had sexual intercourse? ...... ☐ Yes ☐ No ☐ Not sure

45. Have you ever been told by a doctor or nurse that you had a sexually transmitted infection or disease? .... ☐ Yes ☐ No ☐ Not sure

46. Have you ever been pregnant or gotten someone pregnant? .... ☐ Yes ☐ No ☐ Not sure

47. Would you like to receive information or supplies to prevent pregnancy or sexually transmitted infections? .... ☐ Yes ☐ No ☐ Not sure

48. Would you like to know how to avoid getting HIV/AIDS? .... ☐ Yes ☐ No ☐ Not sure

49. Have you pierced your body (not including ears) or gotten a tattoo? .... ☐ Yes ☐ No ☐ Thinking about it

Emotions

50. Have you had fun during the past 2 weeks? .... ☐ No ☐ Yes

51. During the past few weeks, have you *often* felt sad or down or as though you have nothing to look forward to? .... ☐ Yes ☐ No

52. Have you ever *seriously* thought about killing yourself, made a plan or actually tried to kill yourself? .... ☐ Yes ☐ No

53. Have you ever been physically, sexually, or emotionally abused? .... ☐ Yes ☐ No ☐ Not sure

54. When you get angry, do you do violent things? .... ☐ Yes ☐ No

55. Would you like to get counseling about something you have on your mind? .... ☐ Yes ☐ No ☐ Not sure

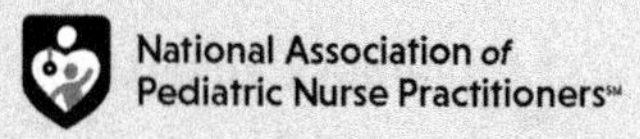

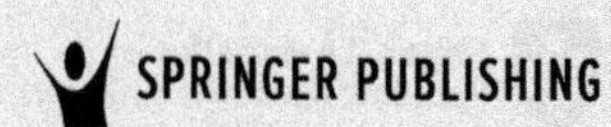

SPECIAL CIRCUMSTANCES

56. In the past year, have you been around someone with tuberculosis (TB)? .... ☐ Yes ☐ No ☐ Not sure

57. In the past year, have you stayed overnight in a homeless shelter, jail, or detention center? .... ☐ Yes ☐ No

58. Have you ever lived in foster care or a group home? .... ☐ Yes ☐ No

SELF

59. What four words best describe you? ____________________

60. If you could change one thing about your life or yourself, what would it be? ____________________

____

61. What do you want to talk about today? ____________________

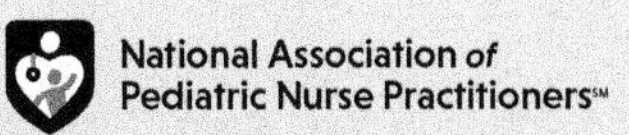

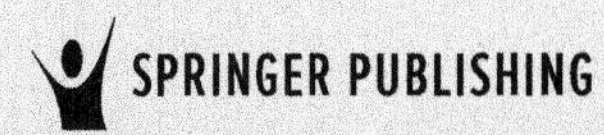

Guía de Servicios Preventivos Para los Adolescentes

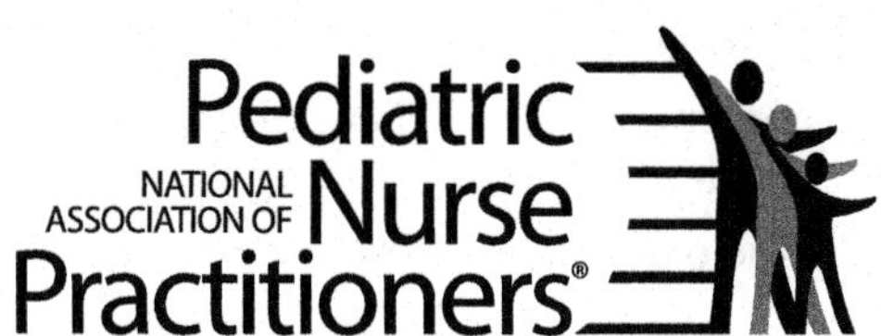

Guía de Servicios Preventivos Para los Adolescentes
Cuestionario Mayores Para Adolescentes
Confidencial (No le diremos a nadie lo que tú nos digas)

Expediente # ____________________

Nombre ____ Fecha ____________
(apellido) (nombre) (inicial del Segundo nombre)

Fecha de Nacimiento____ Año Escolar ___ Año Universitario ____ Sexo: ☐ Hombre ☐ Mujer Edad ___

Direción______________________________Ciudad___________AreaPostal__________________

Teléfono donde te podemos Ilamar ____________________________ Beeper ___________________

¿Qué idiomas se hablan en tu hogar? ____________________________ Raza ___________________

HISTORIAL MÉDICO

1. ¿Por qué viniste hoy a clinical/oficina? ____
2. ¿Tienes algún problema de salud? ☐ Sí ☐ No Problem(s) ____________________
3. ¿Hastenido algún problema de salud en el año pasado? ☐ Sí ☐ No
4. ¿Estás tomando alguna medicina abora? ☐ Sí ☐ No Nombre de la medicina _______

Para Mujeres Jóvenes

5. ¿Cuál fue el primer dia de u última regla? _________ ¿ Te viene la regla regularmente cada mes? .... ☐ No ☐ Sí
6. ¿Has tenido un aborto (natural o provocado) o has tenido un hijo en los ultimos 12 meses? .... ☐ No ☐ Sí

SOBRE LA SALUD

7. Si tienes alguna pregunta o preocupación sobre alguno de los siguientes temas, márcalos.

☐ Estatura/peso	☐ Tos/te silba el pecho	☐ Eyaculas cuando sueñas (el despertar mojado)
☐ LR o baja presión	☐ Senos (el busto)	☐ Abuso fisico o sexual
☐ Dieta/comida/apetito	☐ Corazón	☐ Masturbación
☐ Planes para el futuro/ trabajo	☐ Dolores de estómago	☐ VIH/SIDA
☐ Piel (sarpullido, acne)	☐ Náusea/vómitos	☐ No dueres bien
☐ Dolores de cabeza/ migrañas	☐ Diarrea/estreñimiento	☐ Cansancio todo el tiempo

National Association of Pediatric Nurse Practitioners℠ SPRINGER PUBLISHING

☐ Mareos/desmayos	☐ Dolor muscular o en las articulaciones	☐ Cáncer
☐ Ojos/vision	☐ Orinas frecuentamente o tienes dolor al orinar	☐ La muerte
☐ Oídos/dolor de oídos	☐ Orinas frecuentamente o tienes dolor al orinar	☐ Triste o lloras mucho
☐ Nariz	☐ Secreción del pene o de la vagina	☐ Estrés
☐ Muchos catarros	☐ Te orinas en la cama	☐ Enojo/mal humor
☐ Cuello/espalda	☐ Organos sexuales/genitals	☐ Violencia/seguridad personal
☐ Dolor de pecho/ dificultad al respirar	☐ Menstruación/regla	

☐ Otros (explica) ____

____

TU SALUD

Estas preguntas os ayudarán a conocerte mejor. Escoge la respuesta que mejor describe lo que sientes o haces. Tus respuestas solo las repasan el doctor y su asistente.

Dieta/Peso

8. ¿Estás satisfecho con tus hábitos alimenticios? .... ☐ No ☐ Sí
9. ¿Coes a escondidas o en secreto de vez en cuando? .... ☐ Sí ☐ No
10. ¿ Te pasas horas pensando en cómo bajar de peso? .... ☐ Sí ☐ No
11. Eb ek año pasado. ¿trataste de bajar o controlar tu peso haciédote vomitar, usando pastillas, axantes o purgantes, o dejando de comer? .... ☐ xSí ☐ No
12. ¿ Haces ejercicios o participas en actividades deportivas tres veces o más durante la semana que te hacen sudar y respirar fuerte y que duran 20 minutos? .... ☐ No ☐ Sí

Escuela

13. ¿Tus notas de este año son peores que las del año pasado? .... ☐ Sí ☐ No ☐ No estoy en la escuela
14. ¿Te han dicho o piensas que tienes problemas para aprender? .... ☐ Sí ☐ No
15. ¿Te han suspendido de clases en la escuela este año .... ☐ Sí ☐ No ☐ No estoy en la escuela

National Association of Pediatric Nurse Practitioners℠ SPRINGER PUBLISHING

Amistades y Familia

16. ¿Tienes un amigo a quien estimas mucho y quien puedes hablar de todo? .... ☐ No ☐ Sí
17. ¿ Piensas que tus padres o tus guardians te escuchan usualmente y te toman tus sentamientos en serio? .... ☐ No ☐ Sí
18. ¿Alguna vez has pensado seriamente en escaparte de tu casa? .... ☐ No ☐ Sí ☐ No estoy en la seguro(a)

Armas/Violencia/Seguridad

19. ¿Alguna de las personas con quien vives tú mismo tiene una pistol, rifle, o alguna otra arma de fuego? .... ☐ Sí ☐ No ☐ No estoy en la seguro(a)
20. ¿Has portado una pistol, navaja, garrote o alguna otra arma para protegerte en los últimos 12 meses? .... ☐ Sí ☐ No
21. ¿Has tenido alguna pelea fiscia en los últimos 3 meses? .... ☐ Sí ☐ No
22. ¿Has tenido problemas con la key? .... ☐ Sí ☐ No
23. ¿Te preocupa la violencia o tu seguridad? .... ☐ Sí ☐ No ☐ No estoy en la seguro(a)
24. ¿Usas un casco cuando montas en patines, patineta, bicicleta, motocicleta, miniciclo, trimoto o arenero? .... ☐ No ☐ Sí
25. ¿Usas el cinturón de seguridad cuando viajas en carro, camion, o camioneta? .... ☐ No ☐ Sí

Tabaco

26. ¿Fumas cigarrillos/puros, masticas tabaco, o "snuff?" .... ☐ Sí ☐ No
27. ¿Alguno de tus amigos fuma cigarrillos/ puros, mastica tabaco, o usa "snuff?" .... ☐ Sí ☐ No
28. ¿Alguna de las personas con quien vives fuma cigarrillos/puros, mastica tabaco, o usa "snuff?" .... ☐ Sí ☐ No

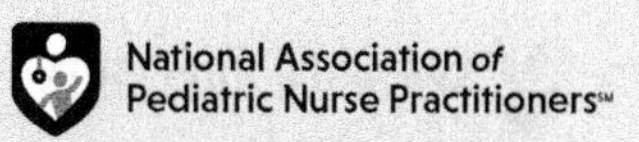

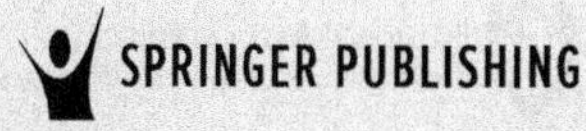

Alcohol

29. El mes pasado, ¿tuviste una borrachera con cerveza, vino, o alguna otra bebida alcohólica? .... ☐ Sí ☐ No
30. El mes pasado, ¿alguno de tus mejores amigos tuvo una borrachera con cerveza, vino, o alguma otra bebida alcohólica? ..... ☐ Sí ☐ No
31. ¿Alguna vez te han criticado o has tenido problemas porque tomas? .... ☐ Sí ☐ No ☐ No estoy seguro(a)
32. ¿Bebiste alcohol este año pasado, y después manejaste un carro, camion, camioneta o motocicleta? .... ☐ Sí ☐ No ☐ No aplica
33. ¿Estuviste en un carro o algún otro vehículo este año pasado, en el cual el chofer estaba bebido o había usado drogas? .... ☐ Sí ☐ No
34. ¿Te preocupas por alguno de tu familia que torma mucho o usa drogas? .... ☐ Sí ☐ No

Drogas

35. ¿A veces usas arihuana u otras drogas, o inhalas goma o cosas parecidas? .... ☐ Sí ☐ No ☐ No estoy seguro(a)
36. ¿Alguno de tus mejores amigos usa marihuana u otras drogas, o inhala goma o cosas parecidas? .... ☐ Sí ☐ No ☐ No estoy seguro(a)
37. ¿Alguna vez has usado medicinas sin receta medica para poder domir, estar despierto, calmarte, o ponerte en onda? .... (Medicinas que se pueden comprar en cualquier farmacia, sin receta médica) ☐ Sí ☐ No
38. ¿Has usado esteroides en pastille o como inyección sin receta medica? .... ☐ Sí ☐ No ☐ No estoy seguro(a)

Desarrollo

39. ¿Te preocupa o quileres más información sobre la forma o tamaño de tu cuerpo, o tu apariencia física? .... ☐ Sí ☐ No ☐ No estoy seguro(a)
40. ¿Crees ser hormosexual, lesbian, o bisexual? .... ☐ Sí ☐ No ☐ No estoy seguro(a)

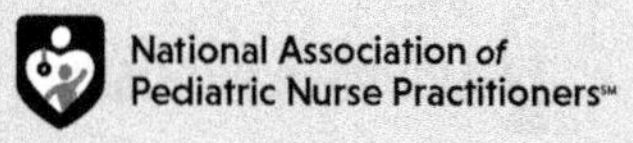

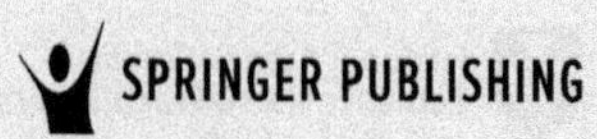

41. ¿Has tenido relaciones sexuales? .... ☐ Sí ☐ No ☐ No estoy seguro(a)
¿Cuántos años tenías la primera vez?
____

42. ¿Estás usando algún metodo para prewenir el embarao?.................................. ☐ Sí ☐ No ☐ No estoy seguro(a)
¿Cuál? ______________________________

43. ¿Usas condones cuando slempre tienes relaciones sexuals con tus pareja(s)? .... ☐ Sí ☐ No ☐ No tengo relaciones

44. ¿Alguno de tus mejores amigos ha tenido relaciones sexuales? .... ☐ Sí ☐ No ☐ No estoy seguro(a)

45. ¿Te ha dicho alguna vez algún doctor o enfermera que tienes una enfermedad o infeción que se transmite sexualmente? .... ☐ Sí ☐ No ☐ No estoy seguro(a)

46. ¿Has estado ernbarazada alguna vez, o has sido tú el que embarazó alguna jowen? .... ☐ Sí ☐ No ☐ No estoy seguro(a)

47. ¿Quieres información o cosas que te ayuden a evitar ebarazos, o infeciones transmitidas sexualmente? .... ☐ Sí ☐ No ☐ No estoy seguro(a)

48. ¿Quieres saber cómo evitar contraer el virus del VIH/SIDA? ☐ Sí ☐ No ☐ No estoy seguro(a)

49. ¿Te has perforaste (excluyendo las orejas) o recibiste algún tatuaje en el cuerpo? .... ☐ Sí ☐ No ☐ Lo estoy seguro(a)

Emociones

50. ¿Te has divertido en las últimas dos semanas? .... ☐ No ☐ Sí

51. Durante las últimas dos semanas, ¿te has sentido triste con frecuencia, o desganado, o como si no tuvieras nada que buscar en la mañana? .... ☐ Sí ☐ No

52. ¿Alguna vez has seriamente pensado en el suicidio, hecho planes para hacerlo, o tratado de matarte? .... ☐ Sí ☐ No

53. ¿Alguna vez te han abusado fisicamente, sexualmente, o emocionalmente? .... ☐ Sí ☐ No ☐ No estoy seguro(a)

54. ¿Haces cosas violentas cuando te enojas? . ☐ Sí ☐ No

55. ¿Deseas tener una consulta professional sobre algo que te está molestando? .... ☐ Sí ☐ No ☐ No estoy seguro (a)

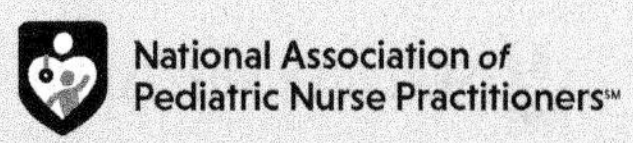

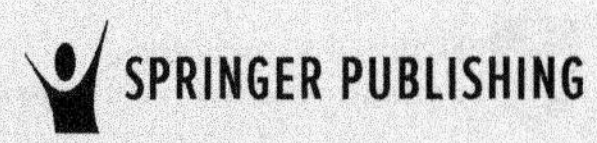

CIRCUNSTANCIAS ESPECIALES

56. En los últimos 12 meses, ¿estuviste con alguien que tiene tuberculosis? .... ☐ Sí ☐ No ☐ No estoy seguro (a)

57. ¿Te has quedado alguma noche en un refugio para desamparados, cárcel, o prisión juvenile? .... ☐ Sí ☐ No

58. ¿Has vivido en un hogar adoptive o una casa para grupos de jóvenes? .... ☐ Sí ☐ No

SOBRE TU PERSONA

59. ¿Cuáles son las cuatro palabras que mejor describen cómo eres? ________________________

60. Si pudieras cambiar algo en tu vida, o en tu persona, ¿qué cosa cambiarias? ______________
____

61. ¿De qué cosas quieres hablar hoy? ____

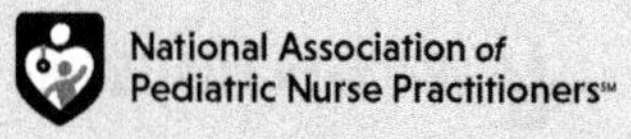

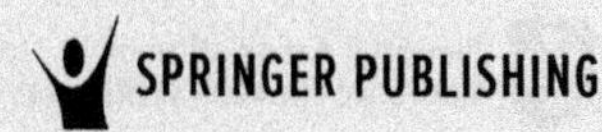

Guidelines for Adolescent Preventive Services

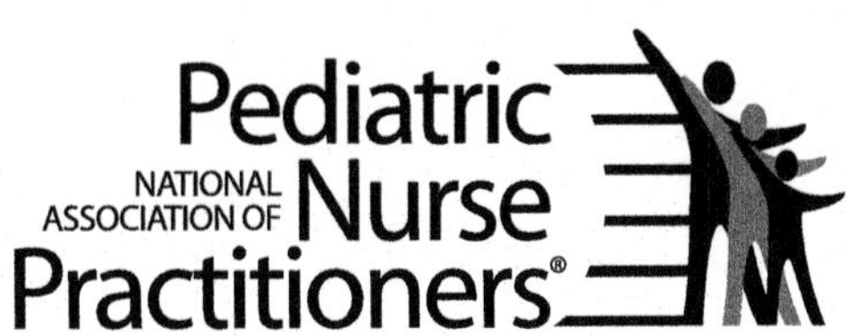

Guidelines for Adolescent Preventive Services
Parent/Guardian Questionnaire
Confidential (Your answers will not be given out.)

Date ____________________

Adolescent's name ____________________ Adolescent's birthday ____________ Age ___________

Parent/Guardian name ________________ Relationship to adolescent ________________________

Your phone number: Home ___________ Work ______________________________________

ADOLESCENT HEALTH HISTORY

1. Is your adolescent allergic to any medicines?

   ☐ Yes ☐ No If yes, what medicines? ________________________________

2. Please provide the following information about medicines your adolescent is taking.

Name of medicine	Reason taken	How long taken

3. Has your adolescent ever been hospitalized overnight?

   ☐ Yes ☐ No If yes, give the age at time of hospitalization and describe the problem.

Age	Problem

4. Has your adolescent ever had any serious injuries?

   ☐ Yes ☐ No If yes, please explain. ______________________________

5. Have there been any changes in your adolescent's health during the past 12 months?

   ☐ Yes ☐ No If yes, please explain. ______________________________

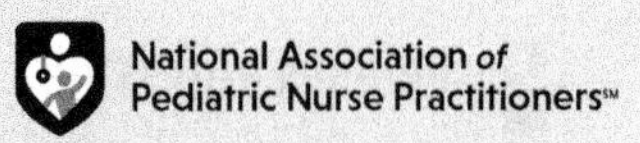

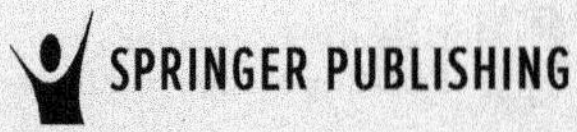

6. Please check (✓) whether your adolescent ever had any of the following health problems: If yes, at what age did the problem start?

	Yes	No	Age
ADHD/learning disability	☐	☐	________
Allergies/hayfever	☐	☐	________
Asthma	☐	☐	________
Bladder or kidney infections	☐	☐	________
Blood disorders/sickle cell anemia	☐	☐	________
Cancer	☐	☐	________
Chicken pox	☐	☐	________
Depression	☐	☐	________
Diabetes	☐	☐	________
Eating disorder	☐	☐	________
Emotional disorder	☐	☐	________
Hepatitis (liver disease)	☐	☐	________
Headaches/migraines	☐	☐	________
Low iron in blood (anemia)	☐	☐	________
Mononucleosis (mono)	☐	☐	________
Rheumatic fever or heart disease	☐	☐	________
Scoliosis (curved spine)	☐	☐	________
Seizures/epilepsy	☐	☐	________
Severe acne	☐	☐	________
Stomach problems	☐	☐	________
Tuberculosis (TB)/lung disease	☐	☐	________
Pneumonia	☐	☐	________
Other: ____________________	☐	☐	________

7. Does this office or clinic have an up-to-date record of your adolescent's immunizations (record of "shots")?

☐ Yes ☐ No ☐ Not sure

FAMILY HISTORY

8. Some health problems are passed from one generation to the next. Have you or any of your adolescent's *blood* relatives (parents, grandparents, aunts, uncles, brothers, or sisters), living or deceased, had any of the following problems? If the answer is "yes," please state the age of the person when the problem occurred and his or her relationship to your adolescent.

	Yes	**No**	**Unsure**	**Age at Onset**	**Relationship**
Allergies/asthma	☐	☐	☐	________	____________

National Association of Pediatric Nurse Practitioners℠

SPRINGER PUBLISHING

	Yes	No	Unsure	Age at Onset	Relationship
Arthritis	☐	☐	☐	____________	________________
Birth defects	☐	☐	☐	____________	________________
Blood disorders/sickle cell anemia	☐	☐	☐	____________	________________
Cancer (type________________)	☐	☐	☐	____________	________________
Depression	☐	☐	☐	____________	________________
Diabetes	☐	☐	☐	____________	________________
Drinking problem/alcoholism	☐	☐	☐	____________	________________
Drug addiction	☐	☐	☐	____________	________________
Endocrine/gland disease	☐	☐	☐	____________	________________
Heart attack or stroke *before* age 55	☐	☐	☐	____________	________________
Heart attack or stroke *after* age 55	☐	☐	☐	____________	________________
High blood pressure	☐	☐	☐	____________	________________
High cholesterol	☐	☐	☐	____________	________________
Kidney disease	☐	☐	☐	____________	________________
Learning disability	☐	☐	☐	____________	________________
Liver disease	☐	☐	☐	____________	________________
Mental health	☐	☐	☐	____________	________________
Mental retardation	☐	☐	☐	____________	________________
Migraine headaches	☐	☐	☐	____________	________________
Obesity	☐	☐	☐	____________	________________
Seizures/epilepsy	☐	☐	☐	____________	________________
Smoking	☐	☐	☐	____________	________________
Tuberculosis/lung disease	☐	☐	☐	____________	________________

9. With whom does the adolescent live most of the time? *(Check all that apply.)*

☐ Both parents in same household
☐ Mother
☐ Father
☐ Other adult relative
☐ Stepmother
☐ Stepfather
☐ Guardian
☐ Brother(s)/ages ________
☐ Sister(s)/ages ________________
☐ Other ________________________
☐ Alone

10. In the past year, have there been any changes in your family? *(Check all that apply.)*

☐ Marriage
☐ Separation
☐ Divorce
☐ Loss of job
☐ Move to a new neighborhood
☐ A new school or college
☐ Births
☐ Serious illness
☐ Deaths
☐ Other ________________

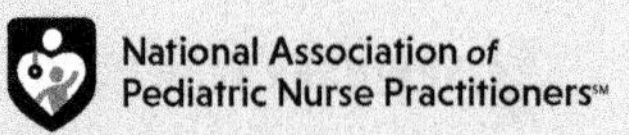

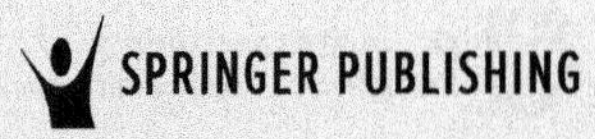

PARENTAL/GUARDIAN CONCERNS

11. Please review the topics listed below. Check (✓) if you have a concern about your adolescent.

	Concern About My Adolescent
Physical problems	☐
Physical development	☐
Weight	☐
Change of appetite	☐
Sleep patterns	☐
Diet/nutrition	☐
Amount of physical activity	☐
Emotional development	☐
Relationships with parents and family	☐
Choice of friends	☐
Self-image or self-worth	☐
Excessive moodiness or rebellion	☐
Depression	☐
Lying, stealing, or vandalism	☐
Violence/gangs	☐
Guns/weapons	☐
School grades/absences/dropout	☐
Smoking cigarettes/chewing tobacco	☐
Drug use	☐
Alcohol use	☐
Dating/parties	☐
Sexual behavior	☐
Unprotected sex	☐
HIV/AIDS	☐
Sexual transmitted diseases (STDs)	☐
Pregnancy	☐
Sexual identity (heterosexual/homosexual/bisexual)	☐
Work or job	☐
Other: ______________________________	☐

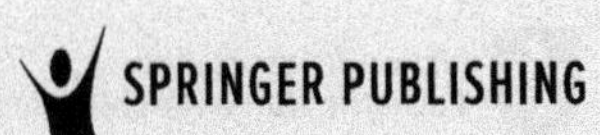

12. What seems to be the greatest challenge for your teen? ______________________

13. What is it about your teen that makes you proud of them? ______________________

14. Is there something on your mind that you would like to talk about today?
    What is it? ______________________

15. Can we share your answers to Question 13 with your teen? ☐ Yes ☐ No

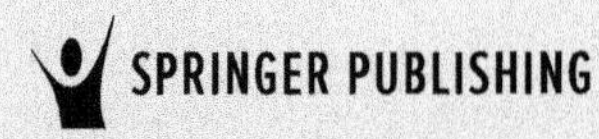

Guía de Servicios Preventivos Para Los Adolescentes

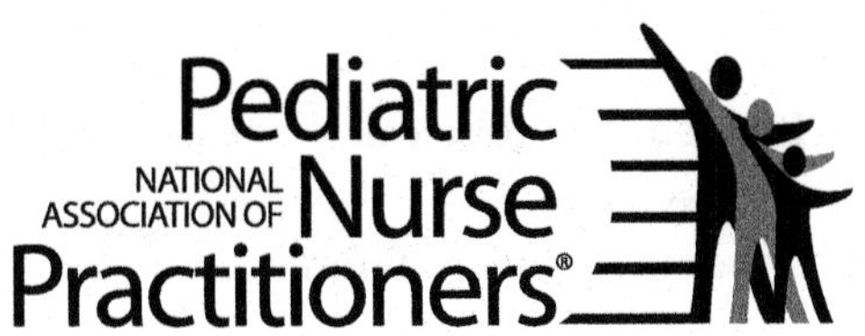

Guía de Servicios Preventivos Para Los Adolescentes
Cuestionario Para Padres o Guardianes
Confidencial (No le diremos a nadie lo que nos diga)

Fecha ______________

Nombre del adolescente ____________ Fecha de nacimiento _____________ Edad ____________

Nombre del Padre o Guardián _______ Su re:acoón el adolescene____________________________

Su número de teléfono: de casa ( ) del trabajo ( )

HISTORIAL MÉDICO DEL ADOLESCENTE

1. ¿Es su adolescente alérgico a alguna medicina?

   ¿ Sí ¿ No Si la respuesta es ***Sí***, ¿a cuál medicina? ______________________

2. Por favor, diganos qué medicinas está tomando su adolescente.

Nombre de la medicina	Razón para tomada	Cuánto tiempo tiene tomándola
______________	______________	______________
______________	______________	______________

3. ¿Su adolescente alguna ve se ha lastimado seriamente?

   ☐ Sí ☐ No Si su respuesta es. ***Sí***/por favor esplique. ______________

4. ¿Ha notado cambios en la salud de su adolescente en los últimos 12 meses?

   ☐ Sí ☐ No Si su respuesta es. ***Sí***/por favor esplique. ______________

5. Por favor, marque (✓) si su adolescente alguna vez padeció de alguno de los siguientes problemas de salud. Sí su respuesta es ***Sí***/, marque cuántos años tenía cuando coenzó el problema.

	Sí	No	Edad		Sí	No	Edad
Problemas de aprendizaje/ADHD	☐	☐	____	Doloes de Cabeza/ Migrañas	☐	☐	____
Alerias	☐	☐	____	Falta de Hierro en la Sangre (anemia)	☐	☐	____
Asma	☐	☐	____	Pulmonia	☐	☐	____
Infeción de la vejiga o de los riñones	☐	☐	____	Fiebre reumática o enfermed del corazón	☐	☐	____

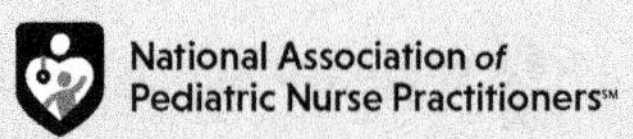

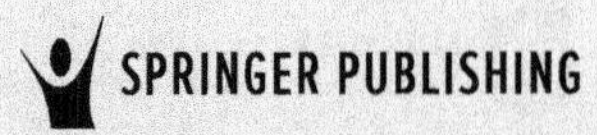

Enfermedad de la Sangre	☐	☐	____	Escoliosis (columna vertebral curva)	☐	☐	____
Cáncer	☐	☐	____	Convulsiones/Epilepsia	☐	☐	____
Varicela	☐	☐	____	Aené	☐	☐	____
Depresión	☐	☐	____	Problemas Estomacales	☐	☐	____
Diabetes	☐	☐	____	Tuberculosis/ enfermedad del pulmón	☐	☐	____
Problemas Alimenticios	☐	☐	____	Mononucleois	☐	☐	____
Problmas Emocionales	☐	☐	____	Otra(s): ____________	☐	☐	____
Hepatitis (enfermedad del higado)	☐	☐	____				

6. ¿Tiene esta clinica toda la información sobre las bacunas de su adolescente?

☐ Sí ☐ No ☐ No estoy seguro

HISTORIAL FAMILIAR

7. Algunos problemas de salud se pasan de generación a generación. ¿Hay alún pariente biológico, de su adolescente (padres, abuelos, tíos, o hermanos), que haya tenido alguna de las siguientes enfermedades? Incluyua parientes vivos y difuntos. Sí la respueta es. ***Sí*** marque cuántos años tenia la persona cuando empezó el problema y su relación con su adolescene.

	Sí	No	No estoy seguro	Edad cuando empezó	Relación con el adolescente
Alergias/Asma	☐	☐	☐	____	____________
Artritis	☐	☐	☐	____	____________
Defectos de Nacimiento	☐	☐	☐	____	____________
Enfermedad de sangre	☐	☐	☐	____	____________
Cáncer (de qué tipo ____________)	☐	☐	☐	____	____________
Depresión	☐	☐	☐	____	____________
Diabetes	☐	☐	☐	____	____________
Problema con la bebida/ Alcoholismo	☐	☐	☐	____	____________
Adicción a drogas	☐	☐	☐	____	____________
Enfermedad del sistema endocrino	☐	☐	☐	____	____________
Ataques al Corazón o Embolias antes de los 55 años	☐	☐	☐	____	____________
Ataques al Corazón o Embolias después de los 55 años	☐	☐	☐	____	____________

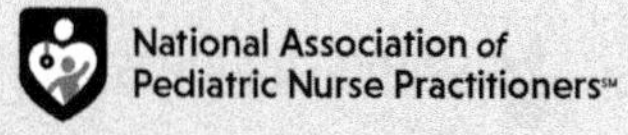

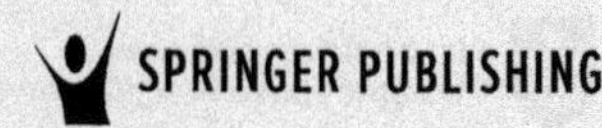

Presión Alta	☐	☐	☐	_____	______________
Alto Nivel de Colesterol	☐	☐	☐	_____	______________
Enfermedad de los Riñones	☐	☐	☐	_____	______________
Problemas de Aprendizaje	☐	☐	☐	_____	______________
Enfermedad del Hígado	☐	☐	☐	_____	______________
Salud Mental	☐	☐	☐	_____	______________
Retardo Mental	☐	☐	☐	_____	______________
Migrañas	☐	☐	☐	_____	______________
Obesidad	☐	☐	☐	_____	______________
Convulsiones/Epilepsia	☐	☐	☐	_____	______________
Fumar	☐	☐	☐	_____	______________
Tuberculosis/enfermedad del pulmón	☐	☐	☐	_____	______________

8. ¿Con quién vive el adolescente la mayor parte del año? (Marque todas las que sean ciertas)

   ☐ Ambos padres en la misma casa ☐ Madrastra ☐ Hermanas/edades _________

   ☐ Madre ☐ Padrastro ☐ Otra persona _________

   ☐ Padre ☐ Guardián Legal ☐ Solo

   ☐ Otro pariente adulto ☐ Hermanos/edades _________

9. En estos últimos 12 meses, ¿han habido cambios importantes en su familia? (Marque todos los que sean ciertos.)

   ☐ Matrimonios ☐ Alguien perdió el trabajo ☐ Nacimientos ☐ Otros _______

   ☐ Separaciones ☐ Mudanzas a otros vecindarios ☐ Enfermedades graves

   ☐ Divorcios ☐ Cambio de escuela o universidad ☐ Muertes

PREOCUPACIONES DE LOS PADRES O GUARDIÁN

10. ¿Cuáles son los retos personales más difíciles para su adolescente?
11. ¿Qué lo enorgullece de su adolescente?
12. Hoy, ¿Quisiera hablarnos sobre algo en especial? ¿Que?
13. ¿Nos permite mostrarle a su adolescente su respuesta a la Pregunta #13? ☐ Sí ☐ No

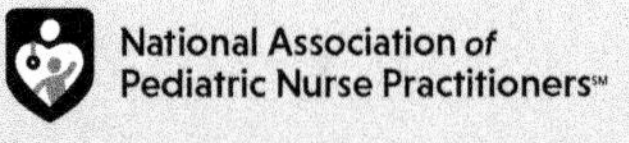

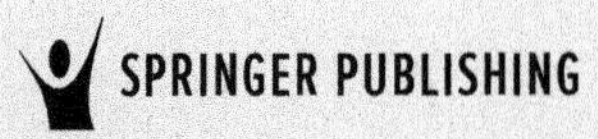

Important Information About Well-Child Visits for Parents

UNDERSTANDING THE WELL-CHILD VISIT

Every day, "healthy" children are brought to doctors and nurse practitioners for well-child visits. Leading pediatric authorities recommend routine visits, ideally beginning with a prenatal visit and continuing throughout infancy, childhood, and adolescence. The purpose of these visits is to help families keep children healthy as well as to pick up early signs of potential problems. These visits are so important to a child's health that both private and public insurance companies pay for them. This is because childhood is a unique period of time to lay the foundation for a person's health throughout life.

Yet a funny thing sometimes happens during these visits. The most important part of the visit gets overlooked. Many parents don't even realize that both they and their healthcare provider are forgetting to talk about the biggest threats to their child's well-being.

Many things happen during these visits. Many of the activities are very visible, like weighing a child and providing the child with necessary immunizations. But sometimes, the most important part of the visit, the part that is not so easy to see, gets forgotten. That is the part of the visit that should be spent talking to your doctor or nurse practitioner about how your child is growing emotionally and mentally and the important role that behavior plays in keeping your child healthy.

Unlike 100 years ago, the greatest threats faced by children in this country today are not infection and physical illnesses. The Surgeon General and others have often called attention to the real risks to children's health today. **Children's health today is threatened most by behaviors**—their own behaviors, the behaviors of their families and friends, or sometimes the behavior of strangers. Many children and adolescents die from accidents and injuries, from homicide, and suicide. One in five has a mental health disorder and many more have behavior problems that interfere with their family relationships, their friendships, and their performance in school. Mental health problems appear in families of all social classes and backgrounds. Child mental health problems often continue into adulthood and worsen if untreated. Yet, more is known today than ever before about how to recognize early mental health problems in children and how to help them during the critical childhood years. It is most important that you talk to your healthcare provider about your child's emotions and behaviors on a regular basis and share your concerns.

There is nothing to be ashamed of if your child has an emotional or behavior problem. The sooner you share your concerns with your child's doctor or nurse practitioner, the faster your child can be helped.

Parents: Did you remember to talk to your doctor/nurse practitioner today about your child's behavior and emotions?

Remember:

Both parents and healthcare providers have a role to play in keeping children mentally and physically healthy.

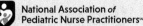

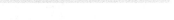

SPRINGER PUBLISHING

HOW CAN PARENTS ENSURE THIS HAPPENS?

1. Expect your pediatric healthcare provider to talk to you routinely about your child's behavior and emotions. Many doctors and nurse practitioners will use screening tools at every visit to help recognize when children are having more difficulties than usual.
2. Call or make an appointment to talk to your healthcare provider when you have concerns or worries about your child's behavior or emotions.
3. Some concerns can be dealt with in a single visit, but most will require follow-up calls or appointments. **Following up is most important.**
4. Some pediatric healthcare providers have more experience in behavior/mental health management than others. After taking a careful history, some providers may suggest that you be referred to a mental health clinician. Yet others will talk to you about some short-term interventions they may be able to provide, such as:
    a. formal screening for mental health problems and strengths,
    b. discussions to help you and your child better understand the problem,
    c. brief solution-focused counseling sessions that help you and your child manage the problem, and
    d. participation in group sessions with other parents or children.
5. If the problem is not getting better or seems to be getting worse, do not hesitate to ask your healthcare provider for a referral to someone with expertise in the mental healthcare of children.
6. When your healthcare provider suggests certain treatments to deal with the problem, ask the provider for the evidence behind what is being recommended.
7. Keep your pediatric provider informed about your child's progress even after referral to a specialist. Your pediatric primary care provider has an important role to play in helping you to advocate for your child's continued mental and physical health.

Internet Resources and Professional Development Programs in Child and Adolescent Mental Health

American Academy of Child and Adolescent Psychiatry

www.aacap.org

This website provides excellent information on the assessment and treatment of child and adolescent mental health disorders. Handouts addressing a multitude of problems (i.e., *Facts for Families*) are available.

American Academy of Pediatrics (AAP): Development And Behavior

https://services.aap.org/en/community/aap-sections/developmental-and-behavioral-pediatrics/about-us/ **https://www.healthychildren.org/English/Pages/default.aspx**

This website, sponsored by the AAP Section on Developmental and Behavioral Pediatrics (SODBP), is targeted to professionals interested in child development and behavior, especially in the clinical setting. It houses a variety of screening tools as well as educational handouts on developmental and behavioral problems that are downloadable for use in practice. There is a learning section that features "the toolbox," which is a link to special articles, features, keywords, and evidence. There also is a practice section that emphasizes practical information and tools to support primary care and specialty practice.

AAP Mental Health Competencies for Pediatric Practice 2019

https://pediatrics.aappublications.org/content/144/5/e20192757

Kidshealth

www.kidshealth.org

This is an outstanding website that contains health information for healthcare providers, parents, teens, and children. Many of the topics relate to emotions and behaviors (e.g., anxiety, fears, depression) and are developmentally sensitive to specific age groups. Physicians and other healthcare providers review all material before it is posted on this website.

National Association of Pediatric Nurse Practitioners (NAPNAP)

www.napnap.org

http://www.dbmhresource.org/

This site can be accessed to keep abreast of all ongoing and new initiatives of NAPNAP. Mental health resources for providers are housed at the site in addition to fact sheets on a variety of mental health issues, which can be downloaded and printed for distribution.

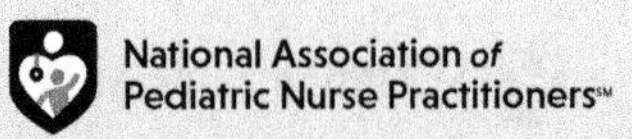

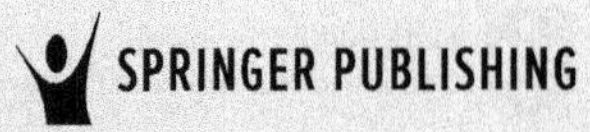

National Institute of Mental Health

www.nimh.nih.gov

This is a website that contains outstanding evidence-based educational resources and publications on a variety of mental health disorders. Health information is arranged by age/gender and treatment across the life span. Fact sheets on a variety of disorders are available for downloading and distribution.

The Ohio State University's KySS℠ Child and Adolescent Mental Health Online Fellowship Program

https://nursing.osu.edu/offices-and-initiatives/office-continuing-education/kyss-mental-health-fellowship-child-and

The KySS (Keep your children/yourself Safe and Secure) program prepares pediatric and family nurse practitioners, family physicians, pediatricians, social workers, and other health professionals who care for children to accurately screen for, identify and deliver early evidence-based interventions for affected children and teens. It is a collaborative among the Ohio State Colleges of Nursing, Medicine and Social Work. Uniqueness of the KySS℠ program includes: 12 on-line modules that are self-paced to fit busy schedules, complemented by clinical learning activities, and guided by a faculty mentor with expertise in child and adolescent health. For more information, see: https://nursing.osu.edu/offices-and-initiatives/office-continuing-education/kyss-mental-health-fellowship-child-and. Upon satisfactory completion of the entire fellowship program, the participants receive 50.1 Nursing Contact hours, 3.6 Psychopharmacology CE with KySS Fellowship Certificate from The Ohio State University and are well prepared to take the Pediatric Nursing Certification Board's pediatric primary care mental health specialist certification exam. https://www.pncb.org/pmhs—KySS is listed as a recommended clinical resource—online preparation program https://www.pncb.org/pmhs-clinical-resources

The REACH Institute

https://www.thereachinstitute.org/

The REACH Institute is dedicated to improving the mental health of American children and adolescents with emotional and behavioral challenges. It provides workshops for healthcare providers that teach the best evidence-based therapies, from psychotherapy to pharmacology, to improve the mental health of children and teens. Excellent resources at the website are available for healthcare providers, agencies, and families.

U.S. Preventive Services Task Force

http://www.ahrq.gov/clinic/uspstfix.htm

The U.S. Preventive Services Task Force (USPSTF) is an independent group of national experts in prevention and evidence-based practice that works to improve the health of all Americans by making evidence-based recommendations about clinical preventive services such as screenings, counseling services, or preventive medications. The USPSTF is made up of 16 volunteer members from the fields of preventive medicine and primary care, including internal medicine, family medicine, pediatrics, behavioral health, obstetrics/gynecology, and nursing.

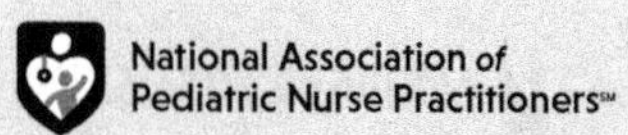

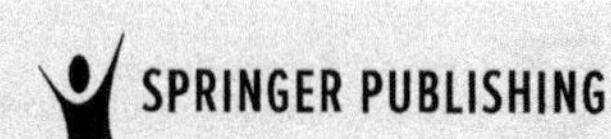

CHAPTER 2

Bernadette Mazurek Melnyk and Pamela Lusk

Diagnosing, Managing, and Preventing Mental Health Disorders in Children and Adolescents

DIAGNOSING MENTAL HEALTH DISORDERS

The reliable diagnosis of mental health disorders is essential for guiding appropriate evidence-based treatment along with identifying prevalence rates for the planning of mental health services and accurately documenting important public health information, such as morbidity and mortality rates. Mental health disorders are diagnosed according to criteria in the *Diagnostic and Statistical Manual of Mental Disorders* (*Fifth Edition*) (*DSM-5*™) by the American Psychiatric Association. Diagnostic criteria include symptoms, behaviors, cognitive functions, personality traits, physical signs, syndrome combinations, and durations requiring clinical expertize to differentiate from normal life variation and treatment responses to stress (*DSM-5*).

The *International Classification of Diseases (ICD)* is updated yearly (at the time of the writing of this book, the current version is ICD-10 [2021]; the ICD-11 codes will be released in 2022) and has thousands of diagnoses from which to choose. In Chapter 17, there is a list of ICD codes for the more common diagnoses for the psychosocial and mental health needs of children, adolescents, and young adults. The list includes:

ICD-10 Codes

F41.9	Anxiety state: unspecified
F41.1	Generalized anxiety disorder
F48.9	Suicide ideation
F34.1	Dysthymic disorder
F43.21	Brief depressive reaction
F33.0	Major depressive disorder, recurrent mild
F31	Bipolar disorder, unspecified
F34.8	Disruptive mood dysregulation disorder
F91.3	Oppositional defiant disorder
F43.22	Adjustment disorder with anxious mood
F43.25	Adjustment disorder with mixed emotions and conduct
F43.24	Adjustment disorder with conduct disturbance
F43.21	Adjustment disorder with depressed mood
F43.29	Adjustment disorder with physical symptoms
F43.10	Post-traumatic stress disorder, unspecified
G47.9	Sleep disturbance, unspecified

Z55.3	Academic underachiever disorder
F90.0	Attention deficit hyperactivity disorder, inattentive
F90.2	Attention deficit hyperactivity disorder, combined type
E66.01	Obesity, morbid
E66.9	Obesity, unspecified
Z71.3	Dietary counseling
R62.0	Delayed developmental milestones
F84.0	Autism
Z62.820	Counseling for parent/child problem
Z71.1	Feared condition, not present
F99	Other unknown and unspecified cause (still trying to figure it out)
T43.95XA	Adverse effects of psychoactive medication
F99	Mental disorder, not otherwise specified

It is important to exercise much caution when assigning *DSM-5* diagnoses to children and adolescents as stigma and labeling can place additional burdens upon an already stressed family system, especially if the diagnosis is not accurate. However, correctly identifying a diagnosis and beginning early intervention as well as providing comprehensive psychoeducation can be of enormous relief and assist the child and family in obtaining positive outcomes. An example of exercising care and caution in diagnosing is to consider using the DSM-5 diagnosis of disruptive mood dysregulation disorder for a child or teen, ages 6 to 18 years, initially; then, if the symptoms over time meet full criteria for bipolar disorder, updating the diagnosis.

Before a diagnosis is made, it is necessary to gain collateral information from multiple sources (e.g., the child's parents, day care, workers, and schoolteachers) and to conduct a comprehensive interview with the child and family. If the diagnosis is in doubt and/or the disorder is complex or not responsive to early intervention strategies, it is critical to have the child seen and concurrently managed by a mental health provider (e.g., psychiatrist, psychiatric mental health nurse practitioner, or psychologist).

A template for a comprehensive mental health interview with a child or adolescent is included in Chapter 1. This is a strength-based format for interviewing youth that has been used for the past decade in the KySS Online Child and Adolescent Mental Health Program at The Ohio State University College of Nursing. The data obtained will lead to formulation of a diagnosis. See https://nursing.osu.edu/offices-and-initiatives/office-continuing-education/kyss-mental-health-fellowship-child-and.

GENERAL APPROACH TO THE EVIDENCE-BASED MANAGEMENT OF MENTAL HEALTH DISORDERS IN CHILDREN AND ADOLESCENTS

Based upon the mental health assessment, a decision must be made to:

- Triage the child or adolescent immediately.
- Intervene.
- Consult with a mental health professional.
- Refer to a mental health professional (it is important to know the mental health specialists in your area and preferably to send the family to someone in close proximity; follow-up is critical to ensure that the family has adhered to the referral).
    - A good referral form template can be accessed at www.brightfutures.org/mentalhealth/pdf/index.html

- Good referral rule of thumb: Always refer when a child is exhibiting behaviors that are dangerous to self or others, including vandalism, fire setting, cruelty to animals, and self-harm.
- Possible referrals include:
  - psychiatrists, psychiatric mental health nurse practitioners, psychologists
  - outpatient services
  - partial hospital services
  - inpatient services
  - emergency and urgent care services
  - youth emergency services, lifeline, preventive services of the department of social services
- Barriers to referral include:
  - lack of mental health providers/services
  - family reluctance to accept a mental health diagnosis
  - reluctance to "label" the child

In making a decision about management, consider severity, persistence, and resistance to change. Once a mental health problem is identified, support of and therapeutic communications with the family are critical. Treating a child/teen for a mental health problem typically requires more than one person or system. Many early interventions, especially with young children, are parent-focused. School-age and teen interventions need to be skills oriented, and it is best to teach the skills to both children and parents. Conduct therapeutic communication with the child and family (active listening and acknowledgment of the challenge). Promote optimism and hope about the process and outcomes: ***Emphasize that there are excellent evidence-based interventions and that mental health problems are treatable!*** Engage parents and child in an active role. Focus on one achievable goal—what can be changed? Children and parents need to learn where to turn for help and information, so it is important to know your community resources. Encourage families to use multiple resources (reliable internet resources, books, TV, school staff, healthcare professionals, clergy, friends, extended family, and mental health professionals).

FOUR GOAL MODEL FOR THE BRIEF MENTAL HEALTH VISIT

Begin treatment while the diagnostic process is underway:

- Understand the concern-active listening.
- Rule out an emergency.
- Make a diagnosis and start treatment.
- Agree on a plan (engage the child/teen/parents and do something!).

PSYCHOEDUCATION

Counseling parents and children/teens about what to expect in dealing with a particular condition is critical as it will assist them in coping with the condition and adhering to treatment. The most effective way to address this problem is by achieving positive and effective communication with families about mental health issues. The American Academy of Pediatrics contends that there is an urgent need for improvement in how mental health issues are communicated between pediatric providers and families. Engaging families to identify mental health needs, giving effective advice, and having therapeutic encounters with angry or discouraged patients and families require skill and practice. Leveraging the techniques of motivational interviewing and implementation of brief psychosocial interventions in pediatric practice facilitates development of a strong therapeutic relationship and improved collaboration with families in addressing mental health concerns (see American Academy of Pediatrics Mental Health Initiatives at www.aap.org/en-us/advocacy-and-policy/aap-health-initiatives/Mental-Health/Pages/introduction.aspx).

PSYCHOSOCIAL/COGNITIVE BEHAVIORAL INTERVENTIONS

A large body of evidence exists for psychosocial interventions (e.g., cognitive behavior therapy/cognitive behavioral skills building) than for any other type of intervention in support of their efficacy for treating mood (e.g., depression), anxiety, and behavior disorders. Examples of evidence-based programs readily available include:

- The COPE (Creating Opportunities for Personal Empowerment) Program developed by Dr. Bernadette Melnyk is a seven-session structured manualized cognitive behavioral skills building program for children, teens, and young adults that is available at www.cope2thrive.com. A digitalized online interactive version of the manualized program also is available for teens. Findings from several studies support the positive effects of COPE in decreasing depression, anxiety, stress and suicidal ideation along with improving healthy lifestyle behaviors in children, teens, and college students (Hart Abney et al., 2019; Hoying & Melnyk, 2016; Hoying, Melnyk, & Arcoleo, 2016; Lusk & Melnyk, 2011; Melnyk et al., 2009; Melnyk, Kelly, & Lusk, 2014; Erlich et al., 2018; Kozlowski, Lusk, & Melnyk, 2015; Melnyk et al., 2014; Melnyk et al., 2013; Lusk & Melnyk, 2011; Melnyk, Amaya, Szalacha et al., 2015). A 15-session COPE Healthy Lifestyles TEEN (Thinking, Emotions, Exercise, and Nutrition) program that contains the seven-session cognitive behavioral skills building program with eight additional sessions on nutrition and physical activity also is available and, through a large clinical trial funded by National Institutes of Health (NIH)/the National Institute for Nursing Research, has been shown to improve healthy lifestyle behaviors, physical and mental health, social skills, and academic competence in adolescents as well as decrease overweight and obesity (Melnyk, Jacobson, Kelly et al., 2015; Melnyk, Jacobson, Kelly et al., 2013). The COPE Healthy Lifestyles TEEN program is recognized as a research tested intervention program for adolescents by the NIH with the highest score for dissemination capability (see www.ebccp.cancercontrol.cancer.gov/programDetails.do?programId=22686590).

  The COPE programs are currently being delivered by nurse practitioners and physicians in primary care and community mental health practices and being reimbursed with the 99214 CPT code (Melnyk, 2020). Teachers, nurses, nurse practitioners, counselors, psychologists, and social workers also are delivering the COPE programs in individual, small group, and classroom formats in schools, universities, and community health settings across the United States. Health professionals are able to deliver COPE after completing a 4-hour online training program. The COPE programs are used for prevention as well as for evidence-based intervention with children, teens, and college students who are experiencing mild to moderate anxiety, stress, and depression.
- Lewinsohn and Clark's group cognitive behavioral "Adolescent Coping with Stress and Coping with Depression" courses are evidence-based and downloadable for use by mental health professionals without permission at www.kpchr.org/public/acwd/acwd.html. There is a group treatment intervention for actively depressed adolescents, a group prevention intervention for youth at risk for future depression, and a brief individual treatment for depressed youth receiving a selective serotonin reuptake inhibitor (SSRI). These courses are not self-help materials.

PSYCHOPHARMACOLOGY

Medications supported as the most effective on the basis of clinical trials with children and teens include stimulant medications for attention deficit hyperactivity disorder (ADHD) and SSRIs for obsessive-compulsive disorder and moderate to severe major depressive disorder. However, medication alone is usually not fully effective in treating a mental health disorder. A combination of medication with therapy/counseling typically leads to the best outcomes. Risperidone and aripiprazole also have been empirically supported as an effective treatment for irritability associated with autism.

- General rule of thumb when starting medication in children and teens: **Start Low, Go Slow!**

Providers without in-depth psychopharmacology education and skills training should be extremely cautious about prescribing medications for mental health disorders in children and teens without consultation from a child psychiatrist or psychiatric mental health nurse practitioner.

Evidence-based management guidelines for some mental health disorders in children and adolescents can be found at www.ecri.org/solutions/ecri-guidelines-trust. ECRI Guidelines Trust® is an interactive guideline portal that puts current evidence-based clinical practice guideline summaries directly into the hands of clinicians, researchers, medical librarians, and patients. This publicly available guideline repository was created by the same team that developed and maintained the Agency for Healthcare Research and Quality's National Guideline Clearinghouse™ (NGC) for more than 20 years. For information about how to critically appraise evidence-based guidelines, see Melnyk and Fineout-Overholt (2019). Two excellent psychopharmacology books specifically for children and adolescent prescribing are:

- Riddle, M. (2019). *Pediatric psychopharmacology for primary care* (2nd ed.). American Academy of Pediatrics. This is a concise, portable paperback that has very helpful charts of starting and maximum doses of medications used in pediatric mental health. Charts are helpful in daily practice to share with patients and families.
- Stahl, S. M. (2019). *The prescriber's guide: Children and adolescents. Stahl's essential psychopharmacology.* Cambridge University Press. This publication is an excellent psychopharmacology handbook.

EXCELLENT MENTAL HEALTH RESOURCES FOR HEALTHCARE PROVIDERS

- The NAPNAP Position Statement on the integration of mental health care in pediatric primary care settings by Frye, L., Lusk, P., Van Cleve, S., Heighway, S., & Johnson-Smith, A. (2020). *Journal of Pediatric Health Care, 34*(5), 514–517.
- *Bright Futures in Practice: Mental Health*-Volume I (Practice Guide) and Volume II (Tool kit) (2002) can be downloaded with no charge at: www.brightfutures.org/mentalhealth/. *Bright Futures* is a national health promotion initiative dedicated to the principle that every child deserves to be healthy; it is now housed at the Bright Futures Educational Center at the American Academy of Pediatrics. Although nearly two decades since publication, it still contains relevant resources and tools.
- The American Academy of Pediatrics' Task Force on Mental Health has created resources and a chapter action tool kit to assist pediatric primary care providers in dealing with child and adolescent mental health problems, which can be downloaded at www.aap.org/mentalhealth.
- Foy, J. M., Green, C. M., & Earls, M. F. (2019). American Academy of Pediatrics. AAP Committee on Psychosocial Aspects of Child and Family Health, Mental Health Leadership Work Group on Mental Health Competencies for Pediatric Practice. *Pediatrics, 144*(5): e20192757 (see www.aappublications.org/cgi/collection/development:behavior).
- The National Institute of Mental Health has a website that contains outstanding evidence-based educational resources and publications on a variety of mental health disorders for healthcare providers (see www.nimh.nih.gov).
- The REACH Institute (The *RE*source for *A*dvancing *C*hildren's *H*ealth) is committed to accelerating the acceptance and use of evidence-based interventions that foster children's emotional and behavioral health. REACH's website contains helpful resources for health professionals and families at www.thereachinstitute.org/.

> **"Knowing is not enough; we must apply.**
> **Willing is not enough; we must do."**—*Goethe*

PREVENTION OF MENTAL HEALTH/PSYCHOSOCIAL MORBIDITIES IN CHILDREN AND TEENS

Prevention of mental health disorders should occur at the primary, secondary, and tertiary levels. Interventions should target the family, school, and community. Primary prevention must start during pregnancy or at birth with parenting education and support (e.g., anticipatory guidance about normal developmental milestones and characteristics, temperament, discipline, and positive parenting strategies to facilitate self-esteem and close relationships). Remember that it is much easier to prevent behaviors that have never started than to curtail negative patterns. It is never too early to begin parent effectiveness training.

Parent Effectiveness Training as a Preventive and Early Intervention Strategy

Important tips to provide to parents:

- Provide positive reinforcement/praise: "Catch children being good!"
- Provide specific praise (e.g., "I like the way you brushed your teeth without me telling you to today" instead of "You are a good girl").
- Promote independence and age-appropriate control.
- Set age-appropriate limits.
- Reward cooperative behavior (e.g., special time together, stickers).
- Provide age-appropriate independence and competencies.
- Give gradual increases in work responsibilities with increasing age.
- Allow children to make choices.
- Allow children to struggle some with challenges to build their coping strategies.
- Do not rush to answer questions for children.
- Help children learn to problem solve and find resources to address their challenges.
- Define position on at-risk behaviors (e.g., zero tolerance for drug or alcohol use).
- Avoid double standards (e.g., "Do as I say, not as I do"), as modeling is a powerful learning mechanism.
- Don't make excuses for children/teens (if they think there is a problem, there usually is).
- Frequently communicate expectations to children regarding behaviors and school performance.
- Encourage parents to become acquainted with their children's friends and the parents of their children's friends (hold meetings to determine group rules).
- Provide parents with excellent resources for parenting (see the section Internet Resources).
- Caution parents to prevent their children/teens from watching R-rated movies, especially children under 13 years of age.
- Help parents to assist their children in dealing with the current stressful events in their lives and in our society.
- Encourage parents to take time for themselves to rest or relax, and to seek counseling if highly stressed, anxious, or depressed; emphasize to them that their mood state will affect their children.
- Emphasize the importance of daily physical activity and exercise in releasing stress and anxiety for all family members.
- Encourage family activities and outings.

IMPORTANT INFORMATION ABOUT LIMIT SETTING FOR PARENTS

- All feelings are okay; all behaviors are not.
- Work on only one or two limits at a time.
- Make sure that consequences are age appropriate.
- Follow through on limits set.
- Teach parents structured choices.
- Give children at least two choices about something that needs to happen. This increases decision-making ability, cooperation, independence, and self-esteem. For example: "Do you want to do your homework before or after dinner today? You decide—it's up to you."

TEACH PARENTS HOW TO HELP THEIR SCHOOL-AGE CHILDREN AND TEENS

- Problem-solving steps:
  - Identify the problem.
  - Identify the cause of the problem.
  - Generate solutions.
  - Discuss the consequence of each solution.
  - Choose a solution and put it into action.
- Develop positive patterns of thinking:
  - Teach the thinking, behaving, and emotion triangle (i.e., how you think affects how you behave and how you feel. If you think you are stupid, you will feel depressed and not attempt to do better in school). It is necessary to stop the negative thought and turn it into a positive one (e.g., "Okay, I may not have done as well on my math test as I should have, but I'm good at English." The consequence is feeling emotionally better).
  - When a child or teen feels stressed, anxious, depressed, or angry, ask them "What was just going through your mind? Is this type of thinking helpful? Is it true?" Chances are it is not. This exercise helps the child/teen to begin to connect thoughts to feelings.
- Control anger:
  - Help the child identify anger triggers and cues as well as implement cool down strategies, such as:
    - Counting to 10 or saying the alphabet
    - Diaphragmatic breathing using the 4-7-8 method. Breathe in slowly while counting to 4; hold for 7; and breathe out slowly for a count of 8
    - Walking away
    - Positive self-talk (e.g., "I am calming down")
    - Writing it down
    - Talking it out
    - Listening to music
    - Communicating the anger to the person in appropriate ways
    - Telling the other person they are angry, using "I" instead of "You" statements
    - Channeling the anger in appropriate ways (e.g., use physical activity)
    - Learning to accept no for an answer or unchangeable situations (e.g., you cannot change other people, only how to respond to them)

PARENTS AND CHILDREN/TEENS NEED TO KNOW HOW TO ACCESS RESOURCES

- Children/teens and parents need to learn where to turn for help and information.
- It is critical to know your community resources.
- Reinforce to children/teens and parents that you deal with their mental and emotional health just as you deal with their physical health.
- Encourage families to use multiple resources (e.g., the internet, books, school staff, healthcare professionals, extended family, and mental health professionals).

OTHER PREVENTIVE STRATEGIES

- Screen for mental health/psychosocial morbidities at every healthcare encounter.
- Assess parenting competence, style, stressors, and presence of mental health problems.
- Raise awareness of these problems (e.g., use posters in practice settings, distribute handouts, teach parenting classes).
- Build developmental assets in children/teens and parents as well communities (e.g., teach effective communication strategies, problem-solving skills, refusal skills, and coping strategies; provide children and teens with opportunities for involvement in community education).
- Implement preventive strategies for children and teens at highest risk for psychopathology and for those who have experienced traumatic events, including motor vehicle accidents, hospitalization, and rape, as well as family and neighborhood violence.
- Encourage parents to be actively involved in their children's lives, and to monitor their activities (e.g., who, what, when, and where) as well as the things that they are reading, watching, and listening.
- Emphasize to parents the importance of mentoring and modeling healthy behaviors.
- Advise parents to require 48-hours advance notice for sleeping over at a friend's house as most drug and alcohol parties come together at the last minute.
- Encourage parents to spend special time with their children/teens and to listen to them.
- Facilitate mentors for children/teens, as those who have mentors are less likely to use illegal drugs and alcohol and are less likely to skip school.
- Encourage service to others, such as belonging to sport/club/hobby/religious groups.
- Provide opportunities for children to be successful; encourage mastery of skill development; teach coping and problem-solving strategies as well as refusal skills; build relationships with youth.
- Teach children coping and problem-solving skills (e.g., encourage journaling and creative expression with school-age children and teens).
- Detect abuse and neglect early, address poverty, build strong families with supports/resources.
- Use quality resources to promote mental health in your state.

INTERNET RESOURCES

ACT for Youth (Assets Coming Together)

www.actforyouth.net/

The ACT for Youth Center of Excellence is an excellent resource that links research to practice in areas of positive youth development and adolescent sexual health. The Center provides publications and presentations as well as technical assistance and training and education.

Bright Futures Handouts for Families

www.brightfutures.org/

Encounter forms for each well-child visit throughout childhood and adolescence can be accessed at this site:

www.brightfutures.org/mentalhealth/pdf/tools.html#families

Creating Opportunities for Personal Empowerment (COPE)

www.cope2thrive.com

This website provides a variety of evidence-based cognitive behavioral skill-building intervention materials that can be easily delivered to children, teens, and young adults in clinical practice, community settings, and schools and universities after a 4-hour online training seminar. A digitalized interactive version of COPE also is available for adolescents.

NAPNAP

www.dbmhresource.org/topics.html

Resources on Mental Health topics by the Developmental/Behavioral/Mental Health SIG

National Association of Pediatric Nurse Practitioners: www.dbmhresource.org/

The REACH Institute

www.thereachinstitute.org/

The REACH Institute is dedicated to improving the mental health of American children and adolescents with emotional and behavioral challenges. It provides workshops for healthcare providers that teach the best evidence-based therapies, from psychotherapy to pharmacology, to improve the mental health of children and teens. Excellent resources at the website are available for healthcare providers, agencies, and families.

REFERENCES

American Psychiatric Association. (2013). *Diagnostic and statistical manual of mental disorders: DSM-V*. American Psychiatric Association.

Erlich, K. J., Li, J., Dillon, E., Li, M., & Becker, D. F. (2018). Outcomes of a brief cognitive skills-based intervention (COPE) for adolescents in the primary care setting. *Journal of Pediatric Health Care, 33*(4), 415–424. https://doi.org/10.1016/j.pedhc.2018.12.001.

Foy, J. M., Green, C. M., & Earls, M. F. (2019). American Academy of Pediatrics, AAP Committee on Psychosocial Aspects of Child and Family Health, Mental Health Leadership Work Group. Mental Health Competencies for Pediatric Practice. *Pediatrics, 144*(5), e20192757.

Hart Abney, B. G., Lusk, P., Hovermale, R., & Melnyk, B. M. (2019). Decreasing depression and anxiety in college youth using the creating opportunities for personal empowerment program (COPE). *Journal of the American Psychiatric Nurses Association, 25*(2), 89–98. https://doi.org/10.1177/1078390318779205

Hoying, J., & Melnyk, B. M. (2016). COPE: A pilot study with urban-dwelling minority sixth grade youth to improve physical activity and mental health outcomes. *Journal of School Nursing, 32*(5), 347–356. https://doi.org/10.1177/1059840516635713

Hoying, J., Melnyk, B. M., & Arcoleo, K. (2016). Effects of the COPE cognitive behavioral skills building TEEN program on the healthy lifestyle behaviors and mental health of Appalachian early adolescents. *Journal of Pediatric Health Care, 30*(1), 65–72.

ICD–10 (2021). ICD-10-CM/PCS Medical Coding. https://www.icd10data.com

Jellinek, M., Patel, B. P., & Froehle, M. (2002). *Bright futures in practice: Mental health- Vol I. Practice guide*. Arlington, VA: National Center for Education in Maternal and Child Health.

Jellinek, M., Patel, B. P., & Froehle, M. (2002). *Bright Futures in practice: Mental health- Vol II. Tool kit*. Arlington, VA: National Center for Education in Maternal and Child Health.

Kozlowski, J., Lusk, P., & Melnyk, B. M. (2015). Pediatric nurse practitioner management of child anxiety in the rural primary care clinic with the evidence-based COPE. *Journal of Pediatric Health Care, 29*(3), 274–282.

KySS Online Child and Adolescent Mental Health Program. https://nursing.osu.edu/offices-and-initiatives/office-continuing-education/kyss-mental-health-fellowship-child-and

Lusk, P., & Melnyk, B. M. (2011). The brief cognitive-behavioral COPE intervention for depressed adolescents: Outcomes and feasibility of delivery in 30-minute outpatient visits. *Journal of the American Psychiatric Nurses Association*, *17*(3), 226–236.

Melnyk, B. M. (2020). Reducing healthcare costs for mental health hospitalizations with the evidence-based COPE program for child and adolescent depression and anxiety: A cost analysis. *Journal of Pediatric Health Care*, *34*(2), 117–121. https://doi.org/10.1016/j.pedhc.2019.08.002

Melnyk, B. M., & Fineout-Overholt, E. (2019). *Evidence-based practice in nursing & healthcare. A guide to best practice* (4th ed.). Wolters Kluwer/Lippincott Williams & Wilkins.

Melnyk, B. M., Amaya, M., Szalacha, L. A., Hoying, J., Taylor, T. & Bowersox, K. (2015). Feasibility, acceptability and preliminary effects of the COPE on-line cognitive-behavioral skills building program on mental health outcomes and academic performance in freshmen college students: A randomized controlled pilot study. *Journal of Child and Adolescent Psychiatric Nursing*, *28*(3), 147–154. https://doi.org/10.1111/jcap.12119

Melnyk, B. M., Jacobson, D., Kelly, S., Belyea, M., Shaibi, G., Small, L., O'Haver, J., & Marsiglia, F. F. (2013). Promoting healthy lifestyles in high school adolescents: A randomized controlled trial. *American Journal of Preventive Medicine*, *45*(4), 407–415. [Epub ahead of print]. https://doi.org/10.1016/j.amepre.2013.05.013

Melnyk, B. M., Jacobson, D., Kelly, S. A., Belyea, M. J., Shaibi, G. Q., Small, L., O'Haver, J. A., & Marsiglia, F. F. (2015). Twelve-month effects of the COPE healthy lifestyles TEEN program on overweight and depression in high school adolescents. *Journal of School Health*, *85*(12), 861–870.

Melnyk, B. M., Jacobson, D., Kelly, S., O'Haver, J., Small, L., & Mays, M. Z. (2009). Improving the mental health, healthy lifestyle choices and physical health of Hispanic adolescents: A randomized controlled pilot study. *Journal of School Health*, *79*(12), 575–584.

Melnyk, B. M., Kelly, S., & Lusk, P. (2014). Outcomes and feasibility of a manualized cognitive-behavioral skills building intervention: Group COPE for depressed and anxious adolescents in school settings. *Journal of Child and Adolescent Psychiatric Nursing*, *27*(1), 3–13. [Epub ahead of print]. https://doi.org/10.1111/jcap.12058

CHAPTER 3

Holly Brown, Amy Schwab Jerum, Bernadette Mazurek Melnyk, and Jacqueline Hoying

Evidence-Based Assessment and Management of Anxiety Disorders and Obsessive-Compulsive Disorder

FAST FACTS

- Anxiety disorders are the most common mental health problems in children and teens.
- Worries and fears are a normal part of a child's development, but should not be excessive, interfere with functioning, or persist beyond developmentally appropriate periods.
- Fear is the emotional response to a real or perceived impending threat whereas anxiety is anticipation of a future threat.
- Routine mental health screening is recommended at all well-child visits and for presentation of symptoms or concerns.
- Youth with anxiety disorders experience severe and persistent distress that interferes with their daily functioning in school and in social interactions, affecting the child's cognition, emotional regulation, and behavior.
- Anxiety disorders are significantly under-reported, undetected, and under-diagnosed.
- A mechanism for a proactive, preventive approach to care is assessment and brief intervention in the pediatric primary care setting.
- Anxiety disorders are often comorbid with depression, bipolar, obsessive-compulsive, learning/language, eating, attention deficit hyperactivity disorder (ADHD), and substance related disorders.
- Somatic complaints, such as stomach pain, headaches, chest pain, and fatigue are common (see Table 3.1 for common signs of anxiety).

ANXIETY DISORDERS

Like other mental health disorders, anxiety disorders are diagnosed according to the *Diagnostic and Statistical Manual of Mental Disorders*, Fifth Edition (*DSM-5*) (American Psychiatric Association [APA], 2013)™.

Disorders that have features of excessive fear and anxiety along with associated behavioral disorders are categorized as anxiety disorders in the *DSM-5* (APA, 2013).

SEPARATION ANXIETY DISORDER

Children and teens with separation anxiety disorder have excessive fear that is not developmentally appropriate related to separating from people to whom the individual is attached. They must have at least three of the following criteria to meet this diagnosis:

Table 3.1. Common Signs of Anxiety in Children and Teens

Commonly seen symptoms (by age/ developmental level)	Physical	Behavioral	Cognitive
Preschool	Restlessness, irritability, fidgeting	Crying, excessive clinging, temper tantrums, regression (e.g., bedwetting)	Fearful thinking, perseverative thought patterns
School age	Stomachaches, vomiting, headaches, hyperventilating, chest pain, increased heart rate	Refuses sleepovers/camp, school refusal, social withdrawal, insomnia	Fearful/catastrophic thinking, worry about things before they happen
Adolescent	Headaches, fainting, palpitations, pain intolerance	Anger, aggression, insomnia, isolating	Pessimistic/negative thinking, cognitive distortions, poor concentration

- The child/teen becomes excessively distressed when separated (or fearing/anticipating separation) from a person or persons to whom they have a strong attachment. They may even experience distress when separated from places or items associated with that attachment figure (e.g., home, items). The young person's fear of being separated is so elevated, they may refuse to go away from home, even to school, work, or usual activities.
- The child/teen worries excessively and persistently about loss of their attachment figure/person. The worry is persistent and they will often worry that their attachment figure (parent, etc.) will experience harm when they are not there. Often children cite this worry that something will happen to their parent as a reason they can't tolerate going to school.
- The child/teen may have excessive (and persistent) fear about being alone or without major attachment figures at home or in other settings. They may worry about being hurt, getting kidnapped, or becoming ill.
- These children often express reluctance to sleep away from home or to go to sleep without being near a major attachment figure. They might have nightmares about being apart.
- The child/teen may have numerous complaints of physical symptoms (e.g., headaches, or GI symptoms such as stomachaches, nausea, or vomiting) when a separation from major attachment figures is anticipated (or has happened).

These fears/anxiety have to be present for at least 4 weeks in children and teens; cause clinically significant upset or deficits in social, academic, or other key areas of functioning; and cannot be explained by another mental health disorder (APA, 2013).

SELECTIVE MUTISM

Children and teens with selective mutism fail to speak in social situations, such as school, but are able to speak in other social situations.

SPECIFIC PHOBIA

Children and teens affected by specific phobias have excessive fear or anxiety about a specific object or situation (e.g., heights, animals, flying) and often express it by crying, tantrums, freezing, or clinging.

SOCIAL ANXIETY DISORDER (SOCIAL PHOBIA)

Social anxiety disorder or social phobia is categorized by an intense fear of social and performance situations and activities, such as being called on in class or starting a conversation with a peer. The anxiety must occur with peers and not just with adults.

Other criteria include:

- Intense anxiety and fear of being embarrassed, humiliated, rejected, or not accepted in social situations. There is elevated anxiety when in social situations and subsequent avoidance of these social situations. Social situations almost always involve fear or anxiety.
- Intensity of the fear and anxiety are out of proportion to what usually happens in these situations; that is, the actual threat of being embarrassed or rejected.
- The deficits result in functional limitations in effective communication, social participation, social relationships, and academic achievement.
- The onset of the symptoms is in the early development period, but may not fully manifest until social communication demands exceed limited capabilities.
- The symptoms are not caused by another medical or neurological condition or to low abilities in the domains of word structure and grammar, and are not better explained by autism spectrum disorder, intellectual disability, or developmental delay (APA, 2013).

If the fear/anxiety only occurs with speaking or performing in public, it is specified as performance anxiety.

PANIC DISORDER

Children and teens with panic disorder experience recurrent, unexpected, and abrupt feelings of intense fear or panic that quickly escalates. During panic episodes, one of the following symptoms occurs:

- Feeling like their heart is racing, experiencing fast/pounding heart rate.
- Trembling or feeling shaky. Can feel light-headed or dizzy/faint; sweating; trembling, or shaking.
- Shallow, fast breathing. Feeling short of breath and/or experiencing chest discomfort. Shortness of breath; feelings of choking; chest pain, or discomfort.
- Gastrointestinal distress, nausea, and stomachache.
- Feeling detached from one's self or from reality (APA, 2013).

Children and teens who experience panic attacks are followed by at least 1 month of persistent concern about having another attack or a significant change in behavior or routine related to the attacks. Panic attacks can be so severe that fears are present about having a heart attack.

AGORAPHOBIA

Children and teens with agoraphobia have fear or anxiety of being in a situation where escape may be difficult or where help is not available. It often occurs in two or more situations, such as using public transportation or being in a crowded elevator, and being in these situations will be avoided.

GENERALIZED ANXIETY DISORDER

Children and teens with generalized anxiety disorder have excessive worry that is difficult or impossible to control, more often than not, for at least 6 months and occurring in a variety of settings.

One of the following symptoms is required to diagnose generalized anxiety disorder in children (at least three symptoms are required in diagnosis of an adult):

- restlessness;
- irritability;
- trouble concentrating or staying on task;
- often tired; easily fatigued;
- sleep disturbance (falling asleep or staying asleep); and
- muscle tension (APA, 2013).

These symptoms are not caused by a medical condition or the physiological effects of a substance and are not explained by another mental health disorder.

SUBSTANCE/MEDICATION-INDUCED ANXIETY DISORDER

Criteria for the diagnosis of a substance/medication-induced anxiety disorder include the following:

- Anxiety or panic attacks predominate the clinical picture.
- Evidence, including physical exam, labs, and symptom development, correlate with substance use or withdrawal.
- The substance is known to produce symptoms consistent with the presentation.
- Symptoms are not better explained by a medical or mental health condition not related to use of a substance; symptoms do not occur exclusively during a delirium.
- Symptoms cause clinically significant distress or impaired functioning.

OBSESSIVE-COMPULSIVE AND OTHER RELATED DISORDERS

Children and teens with obsessive-compulsive disorder (OCD) have obsessions, compulsions, or both, which are time-consuming (e.g., take more than an hour a day) and cause clinically significant distress or impairment in social, occupational, or other areas of functioning. For this diagnosis, the symptoms are not associated with effects of a substance or another medical condition and are not explained by another mental health disorder.

Obsessions are characterized by: (a) intrusive thoughts, the thoughts are unwanted and recurrent; these thoughts, urges, or images are associated with elevated levels of anxiety or distress; and (b) the child/teen attempts to suppress the thoughts, urges, or images by self-talk or replacing the thought with another thought or action (e.g., performing a compulsion, such as checking a door multiple times to make sure it is locked) (APA, 2013).

Compulsions are characterized by: (a) repetitive behaviors, such as hand washing, ordering, or checking, or mental acts, such as praying or counting, and (b) prevention or decreasing anxiety or distress.

Other related disorders to OCD in children/teens include trichotillomania (hair pulling disorder), excoriation (skin picking disorder).

See Table 3.2 for critical history-taking questions.

Table 3.2. Critical History-Taking Question Domains

Biological	Psychological	Social	Behavioral	Protective
Is there a family history of anxiety disorders in biological relatives?	Is the anxiety developmentally appropriate for the age of the child or teen?	Does the youth have an ACE score? Has this child/teen experienced or witnessed a traumatic event (e.g., has the child been a witness to domestic violence, experienced physical/sexual abuse)?	Does the child have symptoms in response to a specific stimulus (e.g., social situations); is it spontaneous (free-floating or present all the time for no particular reason); or is it anticipatory?	What are the areas of strength for this youth?
Does the child have a chronic medical condition or has the child suffered an injury that may contribute to their symptom experience?	What is the child's temperament and how has that influenced their experience with worries and fears?	What are the social determinant needs for this youth and family? What is the impact of structural racism for this youth and family?	What are the situations or factors that bring the anxiety symptoms on?	What are the strengths of the family?
What impact do the anxiety symptoms have on the child's sleep, energy, appetite, and concentration?	What is the history of attachment for the child and caregiver?	Is there a history of recent stressful life events, marital transition, or family members with mental health disorders?	What are the reinforcements for anxiety symptoms (e.g., school refusal and parent staying home from work)?	What are the strengths of the community where the child resides?
	What is the child's ability to connect thoughts, behaviors and feelings?	Does the anxiety interfere with or impair the child's daily functioning, such as school attendance and grades, social relationships or activities, or family relationships, routines, and family accommodation for anxiety symptoms?	What situations or factors influence the improvement of anxiety symptoms?	
	What is the child's history with self/affect regulation?	What is the parenting style and does it promote anxiety (e.g., overprotective/overcontrolling; rejecting/critical) or aim for competency development?		

ACE, adverse childhood event.

MEDICAL CONDITIONS TO BE RULED OUT

- asthma,
- brain tumor,
- cardiac arrhythmia/valvular disease,
- chronic pain/illness,
- diabetes,
- dysmenorrhea,
- hyperthyroidism,
- hypoglycemia,
- hypoxia,
- lead intoxication,
- migraine headaches,
- pheochromocytoma, and
- seizure disorder.

MEDICATIONS/DRUGS THAT MAY CAUSE ANXIETY

- alcohol (including withdrawal from),
- antidepressants (e.g., Celexa, Prozac, Luvox, Paxil, Zoloft),
- antihistamines,
- antipsychotics (e.g., side effects, such as akathisia),
- bronchodilators,
- caffeine (assess initiation, discontinuation, or changes in use of: carbonated beverages, energy drinks, coffee),
- diet pills,
- marijuana,
- nicotine (including withdrawal from),
- steroids (including anabolic),
- stimulants (e.g., cocaine, ADHD medications), and
- sympathomimetics (e.g., nasal decongestants such as pseudoephedrine).

MENTAL HEALTH CONDITIONS THAT MAY MIMIC ANXIETY

- ADHD (trouble with focus/concentration, restlessness);
- depression (trouble with focus/concentration, insomnia, somatic complaints);
- bipolar disorder (trouble with focus/concentration, irritability, restlessness, insomnia);
- OCD (intrusive thoughts, avoidance, reassurance seeking);
- psychotic disorder (trouble with focus/concentration, restlessness, agitation, social withdrawal);
- autism spectrum disorder (ASD) (social skill deficits, trouble with focus/concentration); and
- learning disorder (worries about school performance).

MANAGEMENT

- Conduct regular screening, careful assessment, and evaluation with the goal of early diagnosis of clinically significant anxiety and its severity of impact on the child's functioning.
- Provide information about common signs and symptoms of anxiety and its management in a manner that accounts for the cognitive, linguistic, and cultural needs of the family and youth.
- Consider environmental changes: promote optimal sleep, exercise, and nutrition habits.
- Understand and address social determinants of health needs.
- Decrease and/or eliminate stressors.
- Establish and/or reinforce predictable schedules and/or routines.
- Encourage parents and their children to get enough snuggle time—physical connection can sometimes be the very thing the child needs.
- Deliver cognitive behavioral therapy (CBT) or cognitive behavioral skills building with the Creating Opportunities for Personal Empowerment (COPE) program (Hart Abney et al., 2019; Hoying & Melnyk, 2016; Kozlowski et al., 2015; Melnyk, 2003; Melnyk, 2020) in youth ages 6+ years (see depressive disorders chapter as first line evidence-based management for children and adolescents with mild to moderate anxiety). COPE can be delivered individually, in small groups, or in classroom format and is reimbursed in primary care settings with the 99214 CPT code.
- Consider combining CBT/skills building with psychopharmacological intervention when symptoms are severe. The combination is safe and more effective than CBT alone and medication alone to reduce severe anxiety in children and teens diagnosed with these disorders (Walter et al., 2020).
- Teach, practice, and reinforce coping skills, such as breathing exercises, mindfulness meditation, visualization, positive self-talk, distraction with music or stories, and exercise, both as a preventive intervention and management.
- Provide behavioral intervention: contingency management (e.g., positive reinforcement, shaping of behaviors, extinction).
- Deliver family interventions:
  - Assist parents in managing their own anxiety.
  - Teach parents to function as co-therapists in the home environment (i.e., the CBT therapist transfers skills to the parents, who then transfer skills to the anxious child in the home environment; parents can learn the cognitive behavioral skills taught in the COPE program with their child so they can be reinforced at home).
- Conduct brief anxiety interventions:

  Engage child and parent in motivational interviewing, as evidenced by:
  - Genuine expression of empathy, developmental appropriate illustration of discrepancy between the patient's current behavior and the treatment goal, rolling with the client's resistance, and support of the patient's self-efficacy.
  - Use of open questions; reflective listening; affirmation such as through compliments or statements of understanding; provision of summary statements to unify and reinforce discussed material; and eliciting change talk.

- Younger children have a limited ability to understand health-related issues in relation to internal rather than external sources—interventions with younger children need to be concrete and focused on behavioral recommendations for the child.
- Brief cognitive behavioral interventions, such as breathing exercises, imagery, modeling, reinforcement, and behavioral rehearsal are well-established treatments for symptoms of anxiety and can be particularly useful in procedural situations, such as immunizations and actual or perceived painful procedures (Stein & Craske, 2019; Stein & Sareen; 2019).

- Pharmacological intervention:
  - First-line: antidepressants (selective serotonin reuptake inhibitors [SSRIs])/anti-anxiety agents and buspirone (Buspar). Although SSRIs are called antidepressants, they are effective for treating anxiety in children and teens.
  - Second-line: venlafaxine (Effexor) and benzodiazepines.
  - Alternatives: duloxetine (Cymbalta; a serotonin and norepinephrine reuptake inhibitor [SNRI] has an FDA indication for generalized anxiety disorder in children 7 years of age and older), alpha-adrenergic agents, beta blockers, or antihistamines.
  - **When starting SSRIs in children and teens, start low and go slow!** Dosing can be increased every 1 to 2 weeks by an amount approximately equal to the starting dose while observing for side effects. A dose change effect may not be observable for 2 to 4 weeks (Riddle, 2019).
  - The most common side effects from SSRIs are upset stomach and/or nausea, which tends to subside in a few days. Another common side effect is agitation or behavioral activation when dosage is increased.
  - Taper SSRIs when discontinuing them except for fluoxetine (Prozac) because of the long half-life; **do not abruptly stop them**. Withdrawal symptoms may include dysphoric mood, irritability, insomnia, agitation, anxiety, headache, emotional lability, and flulike symptoms (Riddle, 2019).

See Table 3.3 for medications used to treat pediatric anxiety disorders. The FDA has only approved SSRIs for obsessive compulsive disorder in children and teens. However, rigorous studies by the National Institutes of Health have supported the safety and efficacy of fluoxetine (Prozac), sertraline (Zoloft), and fluvoxamine (Lexepro) for generalized anxiety disorder, social anxiety disorder, and/ separation anxiety in youth (Riddle, 2019).

Although clinicians should be mindful of cases, particularly in young people, where SSRIs may have a paradoxical effect on suicidality, this should not detract from the evidence that not using antidepressants for moderate to severe depression is likely to promote a greater risk. For health-care professionals, frequent monitoring of suicidality, especially early in a new treatment course, is key.

Table 3.3. Medication Guide for Pediatric Anxiety Disorders

Class/Medication	Indications	Side Effects	Dosing		
			Initial (mg)	**Range (mg/day)**	**Schedule**
Selective Serotonin Reuptake Inhibitors (SSRIs):*	First-line treatment Non addictive Well tolerated	Aggression** Disinhibited behavior** Impulsivity** GI side effects Weight gain or loss Dry mouth Insomnia** Somnolence Headaches Irritability Restlessness** Sexual side effects Sweating Tremor		Use the lowest dose to treat symptoms	
Citalopram (Celexa)			5–20	10–60	QD; QAM
Escitalopram (Lexapro)			5–10	10–20	QD; QAM
Fluoxetine (Prozac)			5–20	10–80	QD; QAM
Fluvoxamine (Luvox)			12.5–50	50–300	BID to TID
Paroxetine (Paxil)			5–10	0–60	QD; QAM or PM
Sertraline (Zoloft) *Carefully consider Black Box warning.*			12.5–25	50–200	QD-BID; QAM
Serotonin-Norepinephrine Reuptake Inhibitors (SNRIs): Duloxetine (Cymbalta) *Has more warnings and precautions than SSRIs.*	FDA approved for treatment of generalized anxiety disorder in children and teens aged 7–17 years.	In addition to side effects seen with SSRIs, additional warnings include hepatotoxicity, orthostatic hypotension, severe skin reactions, alterations in glucose control in diabetes.	30 mg	120	Daily
Non-Benzodiazepine: Buspirone	First-line treatment for generalized anxiety Nonaddictive Well tolerated	Headache Nausea Dizziness Lightheadedness Somnolence	5 mg BID	5–60	BID-TID

(*continued*)

Table 3.3. Medication Guide for Pediatric Anxiety Disorders (*continued*)

Class/Medication	Indications	Side Effects	Dosing		
			Initial (mg)	Range (mg/day)	Schedule
Benzodiazepines: Diazepam (Valium) Clonazepam (Klonopin) Lorazepam (Ativan)	Second-line treatment Addiction potential and cognitive blunting Time-limited circumstances	Sedation Cognitive blunting Dizziness Ataxia Memory disturbance Constipation Diplopia Hypotension	1–2 mg HS 0.125–0.5 mg 0.125–0.5 mg BID	0.25–4 mg 0.125–3 mg 0.125–4 mg	HS-BID HS-BID HS-TID

Adapted from: Ghalib, K. D., Vidair, H. B., Woodcome, H. A., Walkup, J. T. & Rynn, M. A. (2011). Assessment and treatment of child and adolescent anxiety disorders. In A. Martin, L. Scahill, & C. J. Kratochvil (Eds.), *Pediatric psychopharmacology principles and practice* (2nd ed., pp. 480-495). Oxford University Press and Riddle, M. A. (2019). *Pediatric psychopharmacology for primary care*. American Academy of Pediatrics.

Note: *Caution must be exercised when prescribing SSRIs to children and adolescents with psychiatric disorders as studies have shown an increased risk for suicidal thinking (suicidality) in the first few months after starting treatment. Patients started on SSRIs should be monitored weekly for the first four weeks of treatment for increased anxiety symptoms, presence of or increase in suicidality, or unusual changes in behavior. Families should be advised to monitor for these signs/symptoms and alert their provider if present.

**Behavior activation is more common in younger children compared to teens diagnosed with anxiety.

REFERENCES

American Psychiatric Association. (2013). *Diagnostic and statistical manual of mental disorders, fifth edition (DSM-5™)*. American Psychiatric Association.

Birmaher, B., Khetarpal, S., Brent, D., Cully, M., Balach, L., Kaufman, J., & Neer, S. M. (1997). The screen for child anxiety related emotional disorders (SCARED): Scale construction and psychometric characteristics. *Journal of the American Academy of Child and Adolescent Psychiatry, 36*(4), 545–553

Ghalib, K. D., Vidair, H. B., Woodcome, H. A., Walkup, J. T. & Rynn, M. A. (2011). Assessment and treatment of child and adolescent anxiety disorders. In A. Martin, L. Scahill, & C. J. Kratochvil (Eds.), *Pediatric psychopharmacology principles and practice* (2nd ed., pp. 480–495). Oxford University Press.

Hart Abney, B. G., Lusk, P., Hovermale, R., & Melnyk, B. M. (2019). Decreasing depression and anxiety in college youth using the Creating Opportunities for Personal Empowerment Program (COPE). *Journal of the American Psychiatric Nurses Association, 25*(2), 89–98. [Epub ahead of print June 4, 2018].

Hoying, J., & Melnyk, B. M. (2016). COPE: A pilot study with urban-dwelling minority sixth grade youth to improve physical activity and mental health outcomes. *Journal of School Nursing, 32*(5), 347–356. https://doi.org/10.1177/1059840516635713.

Kozlowski, J., Lusk, P., & Melnyk, B. M. (2015). Pediatric nurse practitioner management of child anxiety in the rural primary care clinic with the evidence-based COPE. *Journal of Pediatric Health Care, 29*(3), 274–282

Kroenke, K., Spitzer, R. L., Williams, J. B., et al. (2007). Anxiety disorders in primary care: Prevalence, impairment, comorbidity, and detection. *Annals of Internal Medicine, 146*, 317–325.

Kroenke, K., Spitzer, R. L., Williams, J. B., & Lowe, B. (2010). The patient health questionnaire somatic, anxiety and depressive symptom scales: A systematic review. *General Hospital Psychiatry, 32*(4), 345–359.

Lowe, B., Decker, O., Muller, S., Brahler, E., Schellberg, D., Herzog, W., & Herzberg, P. Y. (2008). Validation and standardization of the Generalized Anxiety Disorder Screener (GAD-7) in the general population. *Medical Care, 46*(3), 266–274.

Melnyk, B. M. (2003). The creating opportunities for personal empowerment programs for children, adolescents and college youth/young adults. COPE2Thrive, LLC.

Melnyk, B. M. (2020). Reducing healthcare costs for mental health hospitalizations with the evidence-based COPE program for child and adolescent depression and anxiety: A cost analysis. *Journal of Pediatric Health Care, 34*(2), 117–121. https://doi.org/10.1016/j.pedhc.2019.08.002

Monga, S., Birmaher, B., Chiappetta, L., Brent, D., Kaufman, J., Bridge, J., & Cully, M. (2000). Screen for child anxiety-related emotional disorders (SCARED): Convergent and divergent validity. *Depression & Anxiety, 12*(2), 85–91.

Riddle, M. A. (2019). *Pediatric psychopharmacology for primary care*. American Academy of Pediatrics.

Runyon, K., Chesnut, S. R., & Burley, H. (2018). Screening for childhood anxiety: A meta-analysis of the screen for child anxiety related emotional disorders. *Journal of Affective Disorders, 240*, 220–229.

Spitzer, R. L., Kroenke, K., Williams, J. B., & Lowe, B. (2006). A brief measure for assessing generalized anxiety disorder: The GAD-7. *Archives of Internal Medicine, 166*(10), 1092–1097.

Stein, M. B., & Craske, M. G. (2017). Treating anxiety in 2017: Optimizing care to improve outcomes. *Journal of the American Medical Association, 318*(3), 235–236.

Stein, M. B., & Sareen, J. (2019). Anxiety disorders. In L. W. Roberts (Ed.), *Textbook of psychiatry* (7th ed., pp. 341–370). American Psychological Association.

Tiirikainen, K., Haravuori, H., Ranta, K., Kaltiala-Heino, R., & Marttunen, M. (2019). Psychometric properties of the 7-item Generalized Anxiety Disorder Scale (GAD-7) in a large representative sample of Finnish adolescents. *Psychiatry Research, 272*, 30–35.

Walter, H. J., Bukstein, O. G., Abright, A. R., Keable, H., Ramtekkar, U., Ripperger-Suhler, J., & Rockhill, C. (2020). Clinical practice guideline for the assessment and treatment of children and adolescents with anxiety disorders. *Journal of the American Academy of Child & Adolescent Psychiatry, 59*(10), 1107–1124. doi: 10.1016/j.jaac.2020.05.005.

INTERNET RESOURCES

About Our Kids

www.kidsmentalhealthinfo.com/link/about-our-kids/

This website contains a wealth of resources for families about child and adolescent mental health and parenting. Resources include science-based articles, newsletters, and manuals; a guide to common mental health problems; lists of recommended books, websites, and organizations; a glossary of medical terms explained in an easy-to-understand format; and an ask-the-expert service. About Our Kids is presented by the New York University School of Medicine Child Study Center.

American Academy of Child and Adolescent Psychiatry

www.aacap.org

This website is an excellent source of information on the assessment and treatment of child and adolescent mental health disorders. Handouts for use with families (i.e., *Facts for Families*) are available on a multitude of social and emotional problems, including anxiety disorders (#47 The Anxious Child). They also are available in a variety of languages.

CARES: UCLA Center for Child Anxiety Resilience Education and Support

www.carescenter.ucla.edu

This website is an excellent resource for providers, teachers, parents, and kids that provides up-to-date evidence-based information regarding diagnosis, self-management, and treatment for childhood anxiety disorders. The content not only identifies treatment but strategies for building resilience in youth across all domains of their life.

Kids Health

www.kidshealth.org

This is an outstanding website that contains health information for healthcare providers, parents, teens, and children. Many of the topics relate to emotions and behaviors (e.g., anxiety, fears, depression) and are developmentally sensitive to specific age groups. Physicians and other healthcare providers review all material before it is posted on this website.

National Institute of Mental Health

www.nimh.gov

This outstanding website offers multiple educational handouts on a variety of mental health disorders, including anxiety disorders, and links to other informative websites.

The REACH Institute

www.thereachinstitute.org/about-REACH.html

The REACH Institute is dedicated to improving the mental health of American children and adolescents with emotional and behavioral challenges. Excellent resources and continuing education at the website are available for healthcare providers, agencies, and families.

Screening Tools for Anxiety in Children and Adolescents Generalized Anxiety Disorder-7 (GAD-7) and Generalized Anxiety Disorder-2 Scales

DESCRIPTION

The Generalized Anxiety Disorder-7 (**GAD-7**) is a self-reported screening questionnaire for anxiety, which has seven items that measure severity of various signs of generalized anxiety disorder according to reported response categories of "not at all," "several days," "more than half the days," and "nearly every day." Assessment is indicated by the total score, which is determined by adding together the scores for the scale all seven items. Although originally developed to diagnose generalized anxiety disorder, the GAD-7 also has good sensitivity and specificity as a screening tool for panic, social anxiety, and post-traumatic stress disorder. It is available in many languages (see www.phqscreeners.com/).

The Generalized Anxiety Disorder-2 (GAD-2) scale consists of the first two questions from the GAD-7. Assessment is indicated by the total score on the two items.

AGE RANGE

Although the majority of psychometric testing has been conducted with adults (Kroenke, 2010), the GAD-7 is being widely used with adolescents.

PSYCHOMETRIC PROPERTIES

Studies have supported the validity and reliability of the GAD-7 as a measure of anxiety in the general population (Kroenke et al., 2010; Lowe et al., 2008; Spitzer et al., 2006). The GAD-7 and GAD-2 (the shorter 2-item questionnaire) has high sensitivity and specificity for generalized anxiety disorder and high specificity for panic disorder, social anxiety disorder, and post-traumatic stress disorder (Kroenke et al., 2007). Tiirikainen et al. (2019) demonstrated that the instrument is a valid and reliable measure for generalized anxiety in adolescents. The psychometric properties for the GAD-7 in adolescents is similar to those reported for adults.

SCORING

Cut points of 5, 10, and 15 represent mild, moderate, and severe levels of anxiety. When screening for anxiety disorders, a recommended cut point for further evaluation is a score of 10 or greater. A total score on the GAD-2 of greater than 3 suggests anxiety disorder or panic disorder (Spitzer et al., 2006).

USE

The GAD-7 and GAD-2 are in the public domain and no permission is required to reproduce, translate, display or distribute the tool. It is available in many different languages.

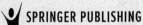

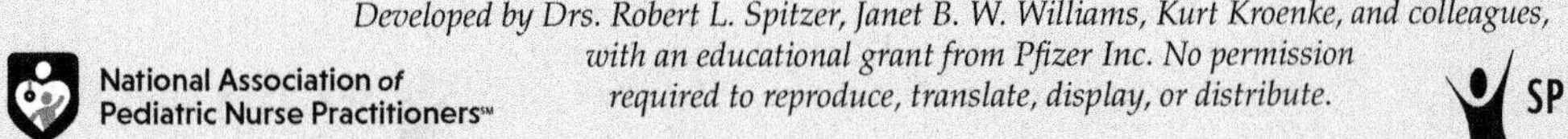
National Association of Pediatric Nurse Practitioners™
Developed by Drs. Robert L. Spitzer, Janet B. W. Williams, Kurt Kroenke, and colleagues, with an educational grant from Pfizer Inc. No permission required to reproduce, translate, display, or distribute.
SPRINGER PUBLISHING

GENERALIZED ANXIETY DISORDER 7-ITEM (GAD-7) SCALE

Over the last 2 weeks, how often have you been bothered by the following problems?	Not at all sure	Several days	Over half the days	Nearly every day
1. Feeling nervous, anxious, or on edge	0	1	2	3
2. Not being able to stop or control worrying	0	1	2	3
3. Worrying too much about different things	0	1	2	3
4. Trouble relaxing	0	1	2	3
5. Being so restless that it's hard to sit still	0	1	2	3
6. Becoming easily annoyed or irritable	0	1	2	3
7. Feeling afraid as if something awful might happen	0	1	2	3
Add the score for each column	+	+	+	
Total score (*add your column scores*) =				

If you checked off any problems, how difficult have these made it for you to do your work, take care of things at home, or get along with other people?

Not difficult at all ____________________

Somewhat difficult ____________________

Very difficult ____________________

Extremely difficult ____________________

Source: Spitzer, R. L., Kroenke, K., Williams, J. B. W., & Lowe B. (2006). A brief measure for assessing generalized anxiety disorder. *Archives of Internal Medicine, 166,* 1092–1097.

Developed by Drs. Robert L. Spitzer, Janet B. W. Williams, Kurt Kroenke, and colleagues, with an educational grant from Pfizer Inc. No permission required to reproduce, translate, display, or distribute.

National Association *of* Pediatric Nurse Practitioners℠

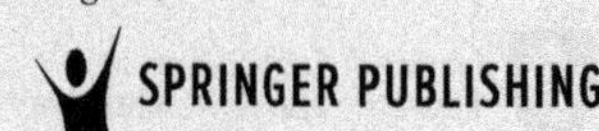

Screen for Child Anxiety Related Disorders (SCARED): Child and Parent Versions

DESCRIPTION

The screen for child anxiety related disorders (SCARED) is a 41-item self-report questionnaire that taps anxiety related disorders. Children answer each of the 41 items (e.g., "When I feel frightened, it's hard to breathe; I get headaches when I am at school") on a 0 to 3 scale from "Not True or Hardly Ever True" or "Somewhat True or Sometimes True" or "Very True or Often True" to describe themselves for the last 3 months.

AGE

The scale is appropriate for use in 8- to 17-year-old children and teens, and their parents.

PSYCHOMETRIC PROPERTIES

The SCARED has established validity and excellent internal consistency reliability (Birmaher et al., 1997; Monga et al., 2000; Runyon et al., 2018). Runyon et al. (2018) found that parent and child versions of the SCARED instrument also demonstrated moderate to large test–retest reliability and parent–child correlations.

SCORING

A total score of ≥25 may indicate the presence of an anxiety disorder. Scores higher than 30 are more specific. Cut off scores on specific items may indicate panic disorder, generalized anxiety disorder, separation anxiety, social anxiety disorder and significant school avoidance (see the SCARED tool on the following pages for the items that are totaled for cut off scores to determine the specific anxiety disorders that may exist).

AVAILABILITY

Free for download on website: www.psychiatry.pitt.edu/research/tools-research/assessment-instruments. At the end of the instrument, there is information regarding scoring the instrument.

From Birmaher, B., Brent, D. A., Chiappetta, L., Bridge, J., Monga, S., & Baugher, M. (1999). Psychometric properties of the Screen for Child Anxiety Related Emotional Disorders (SCARED): A replication study. *Journal of the American Academy of Child and Adolescent Psychiatry, 38*(10), 1230–1236.
The SCARED is available at no cost at www.pediatricbipolar.pitt.edu under resources/instruments.

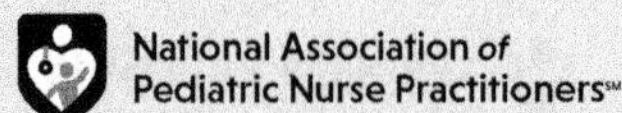

SPRINGER PUBLISHING

SCREEN FOR CHILD ANXIETY RELATED DISORDERS (SCARED)—CHILD VERSION

Screen for Child Anxiety Related Disorders (SCARED) CHILD Version—Page 1 of 2 (To Be Filled Out by the CHILD)

Name: ______________________ Date: ____________

Directions:
Below is a list of sentences that describe how people feel. Read each phrase and decide if it is "Not True or Hardly Ever True" or "Somewhat True or Sometimes True" or "Very True or Often True" for you. Then, for each sentence, check ✓ the box that corresponds to the response that seems to describe you *for the last 3 months.*

	0 **Not True or Hardly Ever True**	1 **Somewhat True or Sometimes True**	2 **Very True or Often True**	
1. When I feel frightened, it is hard to breathe.				**PA/SO**
2. I get headaches when I am at school.				**SCH**
3. I don't like to be with people I don't know well.				**SOC**
4. I get scared if I sleep away from home.				**SEP**
5. I worry about other people liking me.				**GA**
6. When I get frightened, I feel like passing out.				**PA/SO**
7. I am nervous.				**GA**
8. I follow my mother or father wherever they go.				**SEP**
9. People tell me that I look nervous.				**PA/SO**
10. I feel nervous with people I don't know well.				**SOC**
11. I get stomachaches at school.				**SCH**
12. When I get frightened, I feel like I am going crazy.				**PA/SO**
13. I worry about sleeping alone.				**SEP**
14. I worry about being as good as other kids.				**GA**

From Birmaher, B., Brent, D. A., Chiappetta, L., Bridge, J., Monga, S., & Baugher, M. (1999). Psychometric properties of the Screen for Child Anxiety Related Emotional Disorders (SCARED): A replication study. *Journal of the American Academy of Child and Adolescent Psychiatry, 38*(10), 1230–1236.

The SCARED is available at no cost at www.pediatricbipolar.pitt.edu under resources/instruments.

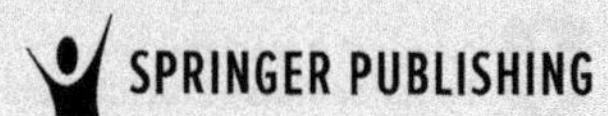

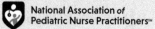

	0 **Not True or Hardly Ever True**	1 **Somewhat True or Sometimes True**	2 **Very True or Often True**	
15. When I get frightened, I feel like things are not real.				**PA/SO**
16. I have nightmares about something bad happening to my parents.				**SEP**
17. I worry about going to school.				**SCH**
18. When I get frightened, my heart beats fast.				**PA/SO**
19. I get shaky.				**PA/SO**
20. I have nightmares about something bad happening to me.				**SEP**
21. I worry about things working out for me.				**GA**
22. When I get frightened, I sweat a lot.				**PA/SO**
23. I am a worrier.				**GA**
24. I get really frightened for no reason at all.				**PA/SO**
25. I am afraid to be alone in the house.				**SEP**
26. It is hard for me to talk with people I don't know well.				**SOC**
27. When I get frightened, I feel like I am choking.				**PA/SO**
28. People tell me that I worry too much.				**GA**
29. I don't like to be away from my family.				**SEP**
30. I am afraid of having anxiety (or panic) attacks.				**PA/SO**
31. I worry that something bad might happen to my parents.				**SEP**
32. I feel shy with people I don't know well.				**SOC**
33. I worry about what is going to happen in the future.				**GA**
34. When I get frightened, I feel like throwing up.				**PA/SO**
35. I worry about how well I do things.				**GA**
36. I am scared to go to school.				**SCH**

From Birmaher, B., Brent, D. A., Chiappetta, L., Bridge, J., Monga, S., & Baugher, M. (1999). Psychometric properties of the Screen for Child Anxiety Related Emotional Disorders (SCARED): A replication study. *Journal of the American Academy of Child and Adolescent Psychiatry, 38*(10), 1230–1236.

The SCARED is available at no cost at www.pediatricbipolar.pitt.edu under resources/instruments.

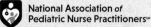

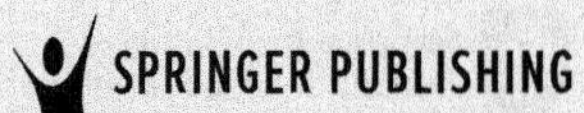

	0 **Not True or Hardly Ever True**	1 **Somewhat True or Sometimes True**	2 **Very True or Often True**	
37. I worry about things that have already happened.				**GA**
38. When I get frightened, I feel dizzy.				**PA/SO**
39. I feel nervous when I am with other children or adults and I have to do something while they watch me (for example: read aloud, speak, play a game, play a sport).				**SOC**
40. I feel nervous when I am going to parties, dances, or any place where there will be people that I don't know well.				**SOC**
41. I am shy.				**SOC**

For children ages 8 to 11, it is recommended that the clinician explain all questions, or have the child answer the questionnaire sitting with an adult in case they have any questions.

From Birmaher, B., Brent, D. A., Chiappetta, L., Bridge, J., Monga, S., & Baugher, M. (1999). Psychometric properties of the Screen for Child Anxiety Related Emotional Disorders (SCARED): A replication study. *Journal of the American Academy of Child and Adolescent Psychiatry, 38*(10), 1230–1236.

The SCARED is available at no cost at www.pediatricbipolar.pitt.edu under resources/instruments.

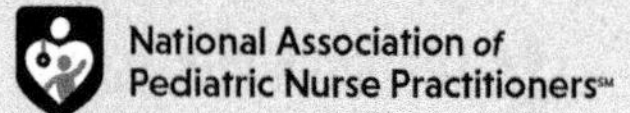

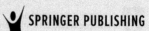

SPRINGER PUBLISHING

Screen for Child Anxiety Related Disorders (SCARED) CHILD Version (To Be Completed by the Clinician)

Name: ________________________________ Date: __________________

Scoring:

A total score of ≥**25** may indicate the presence of an **Anxiety Disorder**. Scores higher than 30 are more specific. **TOTAL =**

A score of **7** for items 1, 6, 9, 12, 15, 18, 19, 22, 24, 27, 30, 34, 38 **may** indicate **Panic Disorder** or **Significant Somatic Symptoms. PA/SO =**

A score of **9** for items 5, 7, 14, 21, 23, 28, 33, 35, 37 **may** indicate **Generalized Anxiety Disorder. GA =**

A score of **5** for items 4, 8, 13, 16, 20, 25, 29, 31 may indicate **Separation Anxiety Disorder. SEP =**

A score of **8** for items 3, 10, 26, 32, 39, 40, 41 may indicate **Social Phobic Disorder. SOC =**

A score of **3** for items 2, 11, 17, 36 may indicate **Significant School Avoidance Symptoms. SCH =**

Developed by Boris Birmaher, MD, Suneeta Khetarpal, MD, Marlane Cully, MEd, David Brent, MD, and Sandra McKenzie, PhD.

From Birmaher, B., Brent, D. A., Chiappetta, L., Bridge, J., Monga, S., & Baugher, M. (1999). Psychometric properties of the Screen for Child Anxiety Related Emotional Disorders (SCARED): A replication study. *Journal of the American Academy of Child and Adolescent Psychiatry, 38*(10), 1230–1236.

The SCARED is available at no cost at www.pediatricbipolar.pitt.edu under resources/instruments.

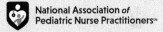

SPRINGER PUBLISHING

SCREEN FOR CHILD ANXIETY RELATED DISORDERS (SCARED)—PARENT VERSION

Screen for Adult Anxiety Related Disorders (SCAARED)
(To Be Completed by the Patient)

Name: ______________________________ Date: ________________

Directions:
Below is a list of sentences that describe how people feel. Read each phrase and decide if it is "Not True or Hardly Ever True" or "Somewhat True or Sometimes True" or "Very True or Often True" for you. Then, for each sentence, check ✓ the box that corresponds to the response that seems to describe you now *or within the past 3 months.*

	0 **Not True or Hardly Ever True**	1 **Somewhat True or Sometimes True**	2 **Very True or Often True**	
1. When I feel nervous, it is hard for me to breathe.				**PA/SO**
2. I get headaches when I am at school, at work or in public places.				**PA/SO**
3. I don't like to be with people I don't know well.				**SOC**
4. I get nervous if I sleep away from home.				**SEP**
5. I worry about people liking me.				**GA**
6. When I get anxious, I feel like passing out.				**PA/SO**
7. I am nervous.				**GA**
8. It is hard for me to stop worrying.				**GA**
9. People tell me that I look nervous.				**PA/SO**
10. I feel nervous with people I don't know well.				**SOC**
11. I get stomachaches at school, at work, or in public places.				**PA/SO**
12. When I get anxious, I feel like I'm going crazy.				**PA/SO**
13. I worry about sleeping alone.				**SEP**
14. I worry about being as good as other people.				**GA**

From Birmaher, B., Brent, D. A., Chiappetta, L., Bridge, J., Monga, S., & Baugher, M. (1999). Psychometric properties of the Screen for Child Anxiety Related Emotional Disorders (SCARED): A replication study. *Journal of the American Academy of Child and Adolescent Psychiatry, 38*(10), 1230–1236.
The SCARED is available at no cost at www.pediatricbipolar.pitt.edu under resources/instruments.

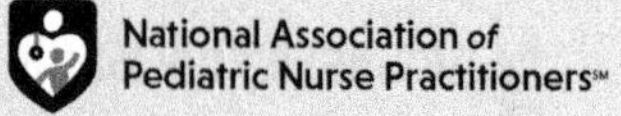

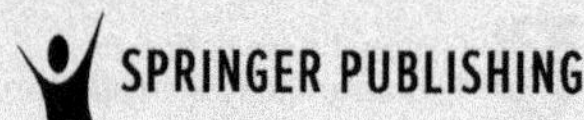

	0 Not True or Hardly Ever True	1 Somewhat True or Sometimes True	2 Very True or Often True	
15. When I get anxious, I feel like things are not real.				**PA/SO**
16. I have nightmares about something bad happening to my family.				**SEP**
17. I worry about going to work or school, or to public places.				**PA/SO**
18. When I get anxious, my heart beats fast.				**PA/SO**
19. I get shaky.				**PA/SO**
20. I have nightmares about something bad happening to me.				**SEP**
21. I worry about things working out for me.				**GA**
22. When I get anxious, I sweat a lot.				**PA/SO**
23. I am a worrier.				**GA**
24. When I worry a lot, I have trouble sleeping.				**GA**
25. I get really frightened for no reason at all.				**PA/SO**
26. I am afraid to be alone in the house.				**SEP**
27. It is hard for me to talk with people I don't know well.				**SOC**
28. When I get anxious, I feel like I'm choking.				**PA/SO**
29. People tell me that I worry too much.				**GA**
30. I don't like to be away from my family.				**SEP**
31. When I worry a lot, I feel restless.				**GA**
32. I am afraid of having anxiety (or panic) attacks.				**PA/SO**
33. I worry that something bad might happen to my family.				**SEP**
34. I feel shy with people I don't know well.				**SOC**
35. I worry about what is going to happen in the future.				**GA**
36. When I get anxious, I feel like throwing up.				**PA/SO**

From Birmaher, B., Brent, D. A., Chiappetta, L., Bridge, J., Monga, S., & Baugher, M. (1999). Psychometric properties of the Screen for Child Anxiety Related Emotional Disorders (SCARED): A replication study. *Journal of the American Academy of Child and Adolescent Psychiatry, 38*(10), 1230–1236.

The SCARED is available at no cost at www.pediatricbipolar.pitt.edu under resources/instruments.

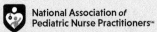

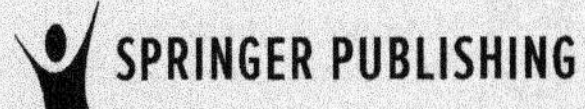

	0 Not True or Hardly Ever True	1 Somewhat True or Sometimes True	2 Very True or Often True	
37. I worry about how well I do things.				**GA**
38. I am afraid to go outside or to crowded places by myself.				**PA/SO**
39. I worry about things that have already happened.				**GA**
40. When I get anxious, I feel dizzy.				
41. I feel nervous when I am with other people and I have to do something while they watch me (for example: speak, play a sport.)				

From Birmaher, B., Brent, D. A., Chiappetta, L., Bridge, J., Monga, S., & Baugher, M. (1999). Psychometric properties of the Screen for Child Anxiety Related Emotional Disorders (SCARED): A replication study. *Journal of the American Academy of Child and Adolescent Psychiatry, 38*(10), 1230–1236.

The SCARED is available at no cost at www.pediatricbipolar.pitt.edu under resources/instruments.

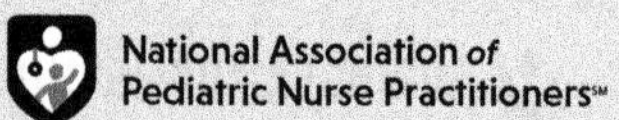

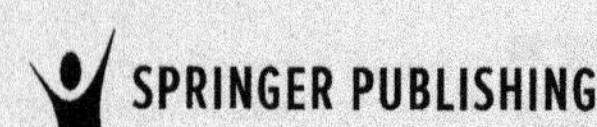

Screen for Adult Anxiety Related Disorders (SCAARED)
(To Be Completed by the Clinician)

Name: ______________________________ Date: ________________

Scoring:

A total score of ≥**23** may indicate the presence of an **Anxiety Disorder. TOTAL** =

A score of **5** for items 1, 2, 6, 9, 11, 12, 15, 17, 18, 19, 22, 25, 28, 32, 36, 38, 40 may indicate **Panic Disorder** or **Significant Somatic Symptoms. PA/SO** =

A score of **12** for items 5, 7, 8, 14, 21, 23, 24, 29, 31, 35, 37, 39, 44 may indicate **Generalized Anxiety Disorder. GA** =

A score of **3** for items 4, 13, 16, 20, 26, 30, 33 may indicate **Separation Anxiety Disorder. SEP** =

A score of **7** for items 3, 10, 27, 34, 41, 42, 43 **may** indicate **Social Phobia Disorder. SOC** =

From Angulo, M., Rooks, B., Sakolsky, D., Goldstein, T., Goldstein, B., Monk, K., Hickey, M., Gill, M., Diler, R., Hafeman, D., Merranko, J., Axelson, D., & Birmaher, B. (In Press). *Psychometrics of the screen for adult anxiety related disorders (SCAARED)-A new scale for the assessment of DSM-5 anxiety disorders*. Psychiatry Research.

The SCAARED is available at no cost at www.pediatricbipolar.pitt.edu under resources/instruments.

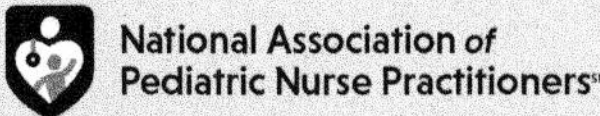

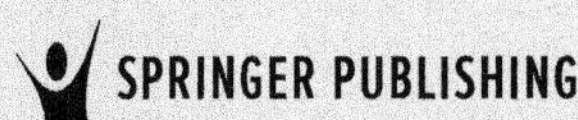

The State-Trait Anxiety Inventory for Children (STAIC)
(C. D. Spielberger, et al.)

DESCRIPTION OF THE STAIC

The STAIC differentiates between anxiety proneness to anxious behavior rooted in personality (trait anxiety) and anxiety as a fleeting emotional state (state anxiety). The instrument is targeted to measure anxiety in upper elementary or junior high school students. It consists of two 20-item Likert scales. The STAIC S-Anxiety scale consists of 20 statements that ask children how they feel at a *particular moment in time*. The STAIC T-Anxiety scale also consists of 20 item statements, but children respond to these items by indicating how they *generally* feel. Examples from the state anxiety questionnaire include:

1. I feel	very relaxed	relaxed	not relaxed
2. I feel	very upset	upset	not upset

AGE RANGE

While especially constructed to measure anxiety in 9- to 12-year-old children, the STAIC also may be used for younger children with average or above reading ability and for older children who are below average in ability.

PSYCHOMETRIC PROPERTIES OF THE STAIC

Studies have supported the validity and internal consistency of the STAIC. Normed scores are available for fourth-, fifth-, and sixth-grade elementary school children.

ORDERING INFORMATION

The STAIC can be obtained from Mind Garden online at www.mindgarden.com/ or by calling 650-261-3550.

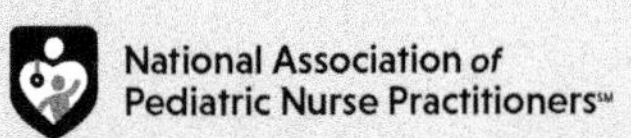

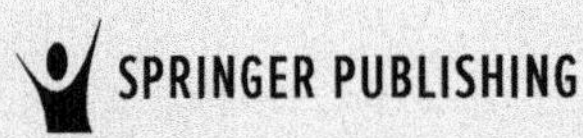

The State-Trait Anxiety Inventory (STAI) for Adults
(C. D. Spielberger, et al.)

DESCRIPTION OF THE STAI

The STAI also differentiates between proneness to anxious behavior rooted in personality (trait anxiety) and anxiety as a fleeting emotional state (state anxiety). The instrument is targeted to measure anxiety in adults as well as in high school and college-age students. It consists of two 20-item Likert scales and can be administered in 10 minutes. The STAI S-Anxiety scale consists of 20 statements that ask individuals how they feel at a *particular moment in time*. The STAI T-Anxiety scale also consists of 20 item statements, but individuals respond to these items by indicating how they *generally* feel.

Examples from the state anxiety questionnaire include:

1	2	3	4
Almost Never	Sometimes	Often	Almost Always

A. I feel at ease	1	2	3	4
B. I feel upset	1	2	3	4

Examples from the T-anxiety scale include:

1	2	3	4
Almost Never	Sometimes	Often	Almost Always

A. I am a steady person	1	2	3	4
B. I lack self-confidence	1	2	3	4

AGE RANGE

Adults as well as high school and college-age students.

PSYCHOMETRIC PROPERTIES

The STAI is a valid and highly reliable tool for measuring anxiety. Normed scores are available for adults as well as for high school and college students.

ORDERING INFORMATION

Both of these scales can be obtained from Mind Garden online at www.mindgarden.com/ or by calling 650-261-3550.

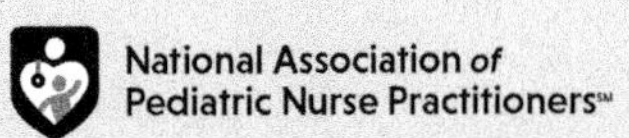

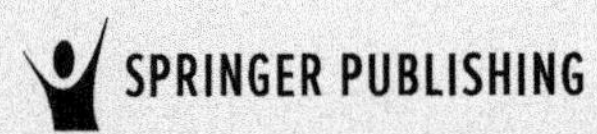

KySS Worries Questionnaire (Ages 10–21 Years)

(© Bernadette Mazurek Melnyk and Zendi Moldenhauer)

DESCRIPTION OF THE KySS WORRIES QUESTIONNAIRE

The KySS Worries Questionnaire is a 15-item Likert-scale questionnaire that taps common worries in older school-age children and youth. A parent version of the scale also is available. The original scale consisted of 13 items. Since the original scale was created, two additional items (#14-weight and #15-level of activity/exercise) were added to the scale.

AGE RANGE

The worries questionnaire is targeted for use with older school-age children and teens, between the ages of 10 and 21 years of age. A separate scale targets the worries of parents of school-age children and teens.

PSYCHOMETRIC PROPERTIES

Content validity was established by pediatric and mental health experts. Face validity was established by 15 parents as well as 15 children and teens, between 10 and 20 years of age. Cronbach's alpha with a sample of 621 school-age children and teens was .87 for the first 13 items on the scale. Cronbach's alpha with a sample of 603 parents was .90 for the first 13 items on the scale.

USE

These instruments are in the public domain and may be reproduced and used without permission from the authors.

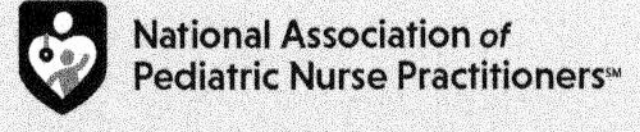

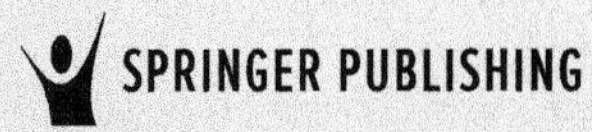

KySS Worries Questionnaire (Ages 10–21 Years)

(© Bernadette Mazurek Melnyk and Zendi Moldenhauer)

Please answer each of the following questions by circling your answers.

Do you worry about any of the following for yourself?

	Not at All	Sometimes	Often	Nearly Always	Always
1. Depression	1	2	3	4	5
2. Anxiety	1	2	3	4	5
3. Parents separating or divorcing	1	2	3	4	5
4. Violence/being hurt	1	2	3	4	5
5. Physical abuse/neglect	1	2	3	4	5
6. Sexual abuse/rape	1	2	3	4	5
7. Sexual activity	1	2	3	4	5
8. Substance abuse	1	2	3	4	5
9. Eating disorders	1	2	3	4	5
10. Problems with your self-esteem	1	2	3	4	5
11. Your relationship with your parents	1	2	3	4	5
12. Knowing how to cope with things that stress you	1	2	3	4	5
13. Being made fun of by your friends	1	2	3	4	5
14. Your weight	1	2	3	4	5
15. Your level of activity/exercise	1	2	3	4	5

16) Do you have any other worries? If yes, please describe them.

____

____

17) Do your worries interfere with your ability to do school work? ___ Yes ___ No

18) Do your worries affect your relationship with your friends? ___ Yes ___ No

This handout may be distributed to families.

From Melnyk, B. M., & Lusk, P. (2022). *A Practical Guide to Child and Adolescent Mental Health Screening, Evidence-Based Assessment, Intervention, and Health Promotion* (3rd ed.).

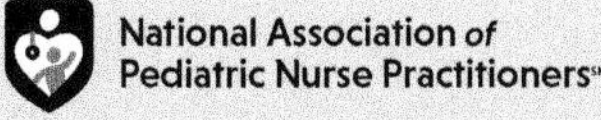

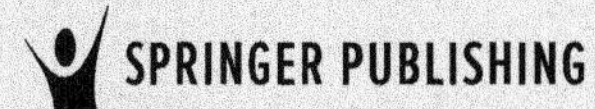

KySS Worries Questionnaire for Parents

(© Bernadette Mazurek Melnyk and Zendi Moldenhauer)

Please answer each of the following questions by circling your answers.

Do you worry about any of the following for your child?

	Not at All	Sometimes	Often	Nearly Always	Always
1. Depression	1	2	3	4	5
2. Anxiety	1	2	3	4	5
3. Parents separating or divorcing	1	2	3	4	5
4. Violence/being hurt	1	2	3	4	5
5. Physical abuse/neglect	1	2	3	4	5
6. Sexual abuse/rape	1	2	3	4	5
7. Sexual activity	1	2	3	4	5
8. Substance abuse	1	2	3	4	5
9. Eating disorders	1	2	3	4	5
10. Self-esteem	1	2	3	4	5
11. Your relationship with your child	1	2	3	4	5
12. How your child copes with stressful things	1	2	3	4	5
13. Being "bullied" by classmates	1	2	3	4	5
14. Your child's weight	1	2	3	4	5
15. Your child's level of activity/exercise	1	2	3	4	5

16) Do you have any other worries about your child? If yes, please describe them.

____

____

17) Do your child's worries interfere with their ability to do school work? ___ Yes ___ No

18) Do your child's worries interfere with their friendships? ___ Yes ___ No

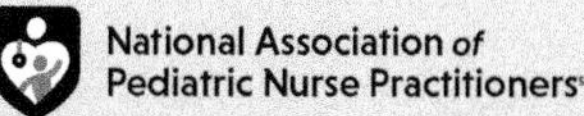

SPRINGER PUBLISHING

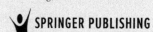

Information for Parents About Anxiety in Children and Teens

FAST FACTS

- Fear and anxiety are a normal part of growing up, but they should not interfere with your child's daily activities.
- Anxiety disorders are among the most common mental health problems in children and teens.
- Children and teens with anxiety experience severe and persistent distress that interferes with their daily functioning; often these disorders are under-diagnosed.
- You might describe your child as a "worrier."
- Children and teens will often report physical complaints or describe "feeling sick" (e.g., stomach pain, headaches, chest pain, fatigue).
- Many times, children with anxiety also have problems with paying attention/staying focused at school; they may have problems being "moody."
- Many times, healthcare providers will mistake anxiety symptoms for attention deficit symptoms.

See Table 3.4 for common signs of anxiety in children and teens.

Table 3.4. Common Signs of Anxiety in Children and Teens

Physical	**Behavioral**	**Thoughts**
Restlessness and irritability (very common in younger children) Headaches Stomachaches, nausea, vomiting, diarrhea Feeling tired Palpitations, increased heart rate, increased blood pressure Hyperventilation/shortness of breath Muscle tension Difficulty sleeping Dizziness, tingling fingers, weakness Tremors	Escape/avoidant behaviors Crying Clinging to/fear of separating from parents Speaking in a soft voice Variations in speech patterns Nail-biting Thumb-sucking Always "checking out" surroundings Freezing Regression (bedwetting, temper tantrums) Anger/irritability	Worry about "what ifs . . ." Always thinking something terrible will happen Unreasonable, rigid thinking

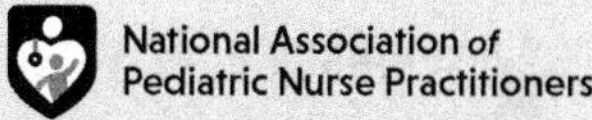

SPRINGER PUBLISHING

MEDICAL PROBLEMS THAT MIMIC ANXIETY SYMPTOMS

- low blood sugar,
- thyroid problems,
- seizures,
- irregular heartbeat,
- migraine headaches, and
- breathing problems.

MEDICATIONS/DRUGS THAT MAY CAUSE ANXIETY SYMPTOMS

- caffeine,
- nicotine,
- antihistamine (Benadryl),
- medications for asthma,
- marijuana,
- nasal decongestants, such as pseudoephedrine,
- stimulant medication (e.g., Ritalin),
- street drugs (e.g., cocaine), and
- steroids.

Prescribed medications to treat anxiety, when started, can cause effects that mimic anxiety symptoms, but these symptoms often subside after a few days.

MANAGEMENT

- Talk to your primary care provider if you have concerns; describe what you are noticing about your child.
- Ask your primary care provider for things to read or websites to visit to learn more about your child's symptoms.
- Therapy might be recommended to help treat your child's symptoms. It could involve individual, group, or family work (cognitive behavioral therapy or skills building is the type of therapy that is supported by research to be effective for children and teens experiencing anxiety and/or depression).
- Help your child to practice mindfulness (staying in the present moment).
- Consider what could be changed at home or in school to help your child deal with their worries (e.g., set a regular bedtime routine or think about which activities are stressful for your child and think about ways to handle them differently).
- Medication is often recommended as an alternative treatment if symptoms are interfering with your child's day-to-day activities. Your provider may recommend a class of medicines called SSRIs, short for selective serotonin reuptake inhibitors.

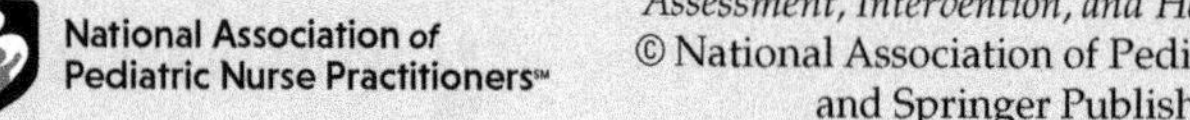

- Be sure to ask:
  - What symptoms will the medication treat?
  - How long will my child have to take this medication?
  - How much medication will my child have to take, and how many times a day will they have to take it?
  - How often will we see and/or talk to you about how my child is doing on the medication?
  - What happens if my child misses a dose of medication?
  - How do we stop the medication?
- SSRIs sometime take weeks to see the positive benefit; it is important for your child to take the medication as prescribed. The most common side effects when starting an SSRI is stomach upset/nausea, which tends to subside in a few days.
- Watch your child for any suicidal behaviors when being started on an SSRI.
- Never have your child abruptly stop the medication if placed on an SSRI.

- Your level of anxiety and stress will affect your child so seek help if you also are experiencing anxiety to the point where it is interfering with your concentration, judgment, or functioning.
- Teach, practice, and reinforce coping skills, such as breathing exercises, mindfulness meditation, visualization, positive self-talk, distraction with music or stories, and exercise.

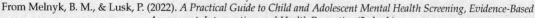

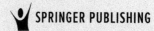

Information for Parents on How to Help Your Child/Teen Cope With Stressful Events or Uncertainty

The most important thing that you can do to help your child/teen cope with stressful events is to remain as calm as possible when you are with them. Children pick up on their parents' anxiety very quickly. If they sense you are anxious, they will be anxious as well. Therefore, if you are having difficulty coping with a stressful situation, it is a good idea to reach out to resources to help you, such as friends, family members, support groups, clergy, or healthcare professionals. Taking care of your own stress so that you are less anxious will help your child to stay calm.

RECOGNIZE SIGNS OF ANXIETY/STRESS IN YOUR CHILD

- Children and teens typically regress when stressed. That is, they go back to doing things they did when they were younger to help themselves feel more comfortable and secure. For instance, a preschool child may go back to sucking their thumb and a school-age child or teen may act more dependent upon the parents or have difficulty separating from them.
- Other common signs of anxiety in *young children* include: restlessness/hyperactivity, temper tantrums, nightmares, clinging behaviors, difficulty separating, and distress around new people.
- Common signs of anxiety in *older school age-children and teens* include: difficulty concentrating and sleeping, anger/irritability, restlessness/hyperactivity, worry, and physical complaints, such as stomachaches or headaches.
- At age 9 years, children realize that death is permanent. Fears of death or physical violence and harm are often common after this age.
- Signs and symptoms of anxiety such as these are usually healthy, temporary coping strategies that help your child to deal with stress. However, if these symptoms persist for several weeks or interfere with your child's functioning, talk to your child's primary healthcare provider about them. Your child's doctor or nurse practitioner will know what to do to help.
- Be honest and give age-appropriate and developmentally appropriate explanations about stressful events when they occur.
- For young children (under 8 years of age), only provide answers to questions they are asking and do not overwhelm them with too much detail. Use language that young children can understand. Do not expose young children to visual images in the newspapers or on television that may be terrifying.
- It may be easier for young children to express how they are feeling by asking them to talk about how their stuffed animals or dolls are feeling or thinking.
- Help children and teens to express how they are feeling about what they have seen or heard. If children have difficulty verbally expressing their feelings, ask them to make a drawing about how they are feeling. Older school-age children and teens can benefit from writing about how they feel.

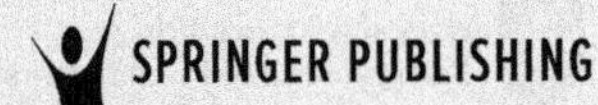

- Ask your child/teen, "What is the scariest or worst thing about this event for you?" or "What is worrying you the most right now?" and take time to really listen to what they have to say.
- Reassure children that they did nothing wrong to cause what happened. Toddlers and preschool children especially feel guilty when stressful events happen.
- Tell children and teens that what they are feeling (e.g., anger, anxiety, helplessness) is normal and that others feel the same way.
- Decrease anxiety in your child by reassuring them that you will get through this together. Emphasize that adults are doing everything possible to take care of the stressful situation and that they are not alone.
- Help your child/teen to release tension by encouraging daily physical exercise and activities.
- Continue to provide as much structure to your child's schedules and days as possible.
- Recognize that added stress/anxiety usually increases psychological or physical symptoms (e.g., headaches or abdominal pain) in children/teens that are already anxious or depressed.
- Young children who are depressed typically have different symptoms (e.g., restlessness and excessive motor activity) from those experienced by older school-age children or teens who are depressed (e.g., sad or withdrawn affect; anger/irritability, difficulty sleeping, or eating; talking about feeling hopeless).
- Use this opportunity as a time to work with your child on their coping skills (e.g., relaxation techniques, positive reappraisal, prayer). Children watch how their parents cope and often take on the same coping strategies. Therefore, showing your child that you use positive coping strategies to deal with stress will help them to develop healthy ways of coping.
- Be sure to have your child or teen seen by a healthcare provider or mental health professional for signs or symptoms of persistent anxiety, depression, recurrent pain, persistent behavioral changes, or if they have difficulty maintaining routine schedules or the symptoms are interfering with functioning.
- Remember that stressful times can be an opportunity to build future coping and life skills as well as to bring your family closer together.

Information for Helping Children, Teens, and Their Families Cope With War and/or Terrorism

1. Be honest and give age-appropriate and developmentally appropriate explanations about the traumatic event.
    - For young children in particular only provide answers to questions they are asking and do not overwhelm them with too much detail.
    - Use language that young children can understand.
    - It may be easier for young children to express how they are feeling by asking them to talk about what their stuffed animals or dolls are feeling or thinking.
    - Help children and teens to express how they are feeling about what they have seen or heard. If children have difficulty verbally expressing their feelings, ask them to make a drawing about how they are feeling. Older school-age children and teens can benefit from writing about how they feel.
    - Ask children and teens, "What is the scariest or worst thing about this for you?" or "What is worrying you the most?"
2. Do not expose young children to visual images in the newspapers or on television that are potentially terrifying.
3. Reassure children that they did nothing wrong to cause what happened.
    - Toddlers and preschool children especially feel guilty when something tragic happens.
4. Tell children and teens that what they are feeling (e.g., anger, anxiety, helplessness) is normal and that others feel the same way.
5. Alleviate some of their anxiety by reassuring children that you will get through this *together* and will be stronger as a result of what you have been through. Emphasize that adults will be there to help them through this and that they are not alone.
6. Spend some special time with your child every day, even if only 15 minutes.
7. Help children and teens to release their tension by encouraging daily physical exercise and activities.
8. Continue to provide structure to children's schedules and days.
9. Recognize that war or a tragic event could elevate psychological or physical symptoms (e.g., headaches, abdominal pain or chest pain, nightmares), especially in children and teens who are already depressed or anxious.
    - Remember that young children who are depressed typically have different symptoms (e.g., restlessness, excessive motor activity) from those experienced by older school-age children or teens who are depressed (e.g., sad or withdrawn affect, difficulty sleeping or eating, talking about feeling hopeless).
    - Anger/irritability can be a sign of anxiety in children and teens.

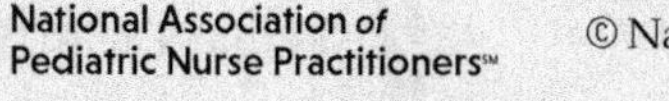

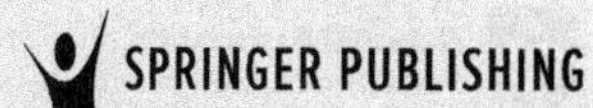

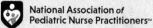

- Children, even teens, who are stressed typically regress (e.g., revert to doing things that they did when they were younger, such as sucking their thumbs, bedwetting, or acting dependent upon their parents). This is a healthy temporary coping strategy. However, if these symptoms persist for several weeks, talk to your healthcare provider about them.

10. Use this opportunity as a time to work with children on their coping skills.
    - Use coping strategies that you know are typically helpful for your child, since each child copes in a way that is best for them (e.g., prayer, doing things to help other people, listening to music).
11. As a parent, remember that emotions are contagious. If you are highly upset or anxious, there is a good chance that your child also will feel the same way. If you are having difficulty coping with stress or with what is going on in the world around you, it is important to talk with someone who can help you to cope. You being calm will help your child to stay calm.
12. Be sure to have your child or teen seen by a healthcare provider or mental health professional for signs or symptoms of depression, persistent anxiety, recurrent pain, persistent behavioral changes, or if they have difficulty maintaining routine schedules, or if symptoms are interfering with functioning.
13. Remember that this can be an opportunity to build future coping and life skills as well as to bring your family unit closer together.

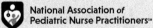

SPRINGER PUBLISHING

Information for School-Age Children and Teens About Stress and Anxiety

FAST FACTS

- It is common for older children and teens to struggle with feelings of anxiety or stress and to worry about things (real or made up).
- These feelings can make it hard to go to school, talk with teachers, or hang out with friends.
- Your parents, teachers, and friends might describe you as a "worrier."
- Your body feels worry too. You might not feel good and may have headaches, stomachaches, or feel tired, especially when you have to do something that stresses you.
- Worry can make it hard to pay attention at school. It can even make you feel sad, angry/grumpy, or frustrated!
- Most people, at some time in their lives, need help to deal with stress. There is nothing to be ashamed of in asking for help with how you feel.
- There are many things you can do to help feel less stressed and worried.
- It is important to see a doctor or practitioner to talk about your worries and to undergo a check-up, as it is important to make sure that there is not a medical reason for why you are feeling the way that you do.

WHAT YOU CAN DO ABOUT WORRY AND STRESS

- Talk to someone you trust about how you are feeling.
- If you have trouble talking, write down how you feel in a journal and then share it with someone.
- Try to do relaxing exercises (imagine being at your favorite place; take slow deep breaths and, when you breathe out, imagine all of your stress leaving you; listen to calming music).
- Do positive self-talk every morning and night, before you go to bed (e.g., "I am feeling calmer; I am going to handle this well").
- Stay focused in the present moment (try not to feel guilty about something that has happened in the past or worry about the future, because most things we worry about don't ever happen). When you start to worry, turn your head slowly from left to right and notice what you are seeing, hearing, and feeling.
- Exercise for at least 30 minutes, 5 days a week (this is a great way to release stress!).
- Don't take certain medications or drugs that can cause you to feel anxiety. These include caffeine, which is found in drinks such as Pepsi, Mountain Dew, energy drinks, coffee, and tea; nicotine in cigarettes; marijuana; nasal decongestants (e.g., Sudafed); stimulant medication (e.g., Ritalin), or street drugs (e.g., cocaine).

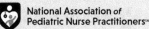

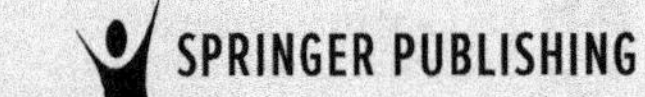

WHEN WHAT YOU ARE DOING ISN'T HELPING

- Talk to your parent(s), your doctor, or nurse practitioner if you think you worry too much about things. Describe how you think and feel.
- Ask your primary care provider for things to read or websites to visit so you and your parents can learn more about how you are feeling.
- Your doctor or practitioner might want you to meet with a counselor to help you with your worries. You might meet with the counselor alone, with your family, or in a group with other kids who have the same problems.
- Medication may help to stop your worry. Ask your doctor or practitioner how this could help.

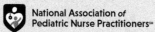

SPRINGER PUBLISHING

CHAPTER 4

Bernadette Mazurek Melnyk, Holly Brown, and Pamela Lusk

Evidence-Based Assessment and Management of Depressive Disorders

FAST FACTS

- Depressive disorders include major depressive disorder, persistent depressive disorder (dysthymia), disruptive mood dysregulation disorder, premenstrual dysphoric disorder, substance/medication-induced depressive disorder, and depressive disorder due to another medical condition (American Psychiatric Association, 2013).
- The common feature of depressive disorders is the presence of sad, empty, or irritable mood, which is associated with somatic and cognitive changes that **interfere with functioning** at home, in school, and/or with peers.
- An estimated 5% of children (males and females equally) and 10% to 20% of teens (females are three times as often affected as males in adolescence).
- The mean age of onset for a major depressive disorder is 14 years, and 8 years for dysthymia.
- Recurrence is as high as 60% to 70%; often recurs in adulthood if first major episode of major depressive disorder is not effectively treated.
- The risk in children/teens is increased if one or more parents are depressed.
- An estimated 40% to 70% of affected children/teens have mental health comorbidities (e.g., anxiety disorders, substance use, conduct disorders, attention deficit hyperactivity disorder [ADHD]).
- Detection is low, <20% of cases.
- Approximately only 50% of affected children and adolescents receive treatment.
- The average length of an untreated episode of major depressive disorder is 7 to 9 months.
- Depression is a risk factor for other high-risk behaviors and often precedes substance abuse by about 4 years.
- Depression is often misdiagnosed as ADHD in young children as they may present with inattention, impulsivity, and hyperactivity.
- The causes of depressive disorders can be multifactorial, including:
  - biological changes in chemistry of the brain, such as imbalances in serotonin, dopamine, and/or norepinephrine or excess cortisol;
  - genetic;
  - environmental (e.g., stressful situations);
  - depressogenic cognition (i.e., a negative pattern of thinking);
  - physical; or
  - drug related.

RISK FACTORS FOR DEPRESSIVE DISORDERS

- parental depression or other family mental health problems;
- family dysfunction, including domestic violence and marital conflict;
- societal or family violence or abuse, physical or sexual abuse;
- acute or chronic illness;
- life stressors and changes, trauma, and/or losses;
- low self-esteem;
- poor coping skills;
- attachment issues;
- adverse childhood events (ACES);
- lack of social or peer support/social isolation;
- substance abuse or other psychopathology; or
- overweight/obesity.

DEPRESSIVE DISORDERS ARE A MAJOR RISK FACTOR FOR SUICIDE

- Suicide is the second leading cause of death in 10- to 34-year-olds (5%–10% of high school students make attempts every year).
- According to the Centers for Disease Control and Prevention (CDC), the suicide rate for children ages 10 to 14 nearly tripled from 2007 to 2017.
- Suicidality increases with age.
- The age group with the highest incidence of suicide is older male teens.
- Girls make more attempts at suicide, but males are more successful.

PREDICTORS/MAJOR RISK FACTORS FOR SUICIDE

- degree of hopelessness (the #1 predictor of suicide);
- family history of suicide or recent suicide in school;
- method available (e.g., gun, medications);
- prior history of self-harming behaviors or impulsivity;
- depression and/or a sudden change in mood;
- drug and alcohol abuse;
- inability to establish a safety plan;
- serious medical illness;
- family violence;
- giving away treasured items; or
- thoughts that one is a burden to others.

COMMON PRESENTATION MODES OF DEPRESSIVE DISORDERS BY AGE GROUP

- **Infants:** Feeding difficulties, sleep disturbances, irritability, poor eye contact, irritable or apathetic
- **Toddlers and preschoolers:** Behavior problems, excessive tantrums, aggression, irritability, regression.

- **School-age children:** Sadness, irritability, impulsivity, crying spells, loss of pleasure or interest in activities, sleep problems, frequent complaints that *no one likes me,* somatic complaints (i.e., stomachaches or headaches), externalizing (i.e., acting out) behaviors.
- **Adolescents:** Sadness, hopelessness, self-hatred, anger, withdrawn, loss of pleasure/interest in activities, neurovegetative symptoms (e.g., decrease or increase in sleep and appetite, lack of concentration), drug and alcohol use common, comorbidity with anxiety common.

SCREENING FOR DEPRESSION

As with all mental health disorders, depression should not be diagnosed solely by a screening tool. Screening tools raise "red flags" that should be investigated further by sensitive clinical interviews.

The U.S. Preventive Services Task Force (USPSTF) recommends screening all adolescents (12–18 years of age) for major depressive disorder (MDD). Systems should be in place to ensure accurate diagnosis, psychotherapy (cognitive behavioral or interpersonal), and follow-up (see www.uspreventiveservicestaskforce.org/uspstf/document/RecommendationStatementFinal/depression-in-children-and-adolescents-screening (Siu, 2016).

Two questions recommended by the USPSTF for adults that are appropriate for older adolescents, especially if time is limited, include:

1. Over the past 2 weeks, have you ever felt down, depressed, or hopeless?
2. Over the past 2 weeks, have you felt little interest or pleasure in doing things?

Tools for depression screening that are free and in the public domain include:

- ***The Patient Health Questionnaire-9 (PHQ-9) Modified for Teens:*** A nine-item depression scale for screening and monitoring depression, which has been found to be effective for screening adolescents as young as 13 years of age. The PHQ-9 is based directly on the diagnostic criteria for major depressive disorder in the *DSM-5*. Download at:

  www.aacap.org/App_Themes/AACAP/docs/member_resources/toolbox_for_clinical_practice_and_outcomes/symptoms/GLAD-PC_PHQ-9.pdf

  If youth answer the ninth item positively on the PHQ-9 for suicidal thoughts, an in-depth suicidal screen and assessment must be conducted.

  The Patient Health Questionnaire-9 can be used for 18- to 24-year-olds.
- ***The Center for Epidemiological Studies Depression Scale* (*CES-DC*) for Children**: A valid and reliable instrument for depression screening in older school-age children and teens; 20 items on a 4-point Likert scale from 0 *(Not at all)* to 3 *(A lot)* (e.g., During the past week, I felt down and unhappy); scores over 15 indicate significant levels of depression. This scale is free and in the public domain; can be downloaded at www.brightfutures.org/mentalhealth/pdf/professionals/bridges/ces_dc.pdf
- ***The Patient Health Questionnaire-2 (PHQ-2):*** Uses the first two questions from the PHQ-9, including:
  1. Over the past 2 weeks, how often have you been bothered by any of the following:

     (1) little interest or pleasure doing things.

     (2) feeling down, depressed, or hopeless.

  Download at: PatientHealthQuestionnaire-2_v1.0_2014Jul2.pdf

SCREENING FOR SUICIDE

All youth who screen positive for depression also should be screened for suicide.

Assess for Suicidal Ideation/Intent, Plan, and Means

If depression is suspected or patients make self-harming comments, **ALWAYS** ask about:

- suicidal ideation;
- plan and means; and
- intent.

Suicide warning signs: no hope for the future, change in behavior (giving away treasured items), mood (sudden upswing in mood), thinking (preoccupation with death), major life changes (major illness or death of a loved one).

The Ask Suicide Questions (ASQ) tool is in the public domain and can be downloaded from: and contains the following questions:

www.nimh.nih.gov/research/research-conducted-at-nimh/asq-toolkit-materials/index.shtml Choose the Youth toolkit (for outpatient clinics)

www.nimh.nih.gov/research/research-conducted-at-nimh/asq-toolkit-materials/youth-asq-toolkit.shtml#outpatient

It contains the following questions:

1. In the past few weeks, have you wished you were dead? ❍ Yes ❍ No
2. In the past few weeks, have you felt that you or your family would be better off if you were dead? ❍ Yes ❍ No
3. In the past week, have you been having thoughts about killing yourself? ❍ Yes ❍ No
4. Have you ever tried to kill yourself? ❍ Yes ❍ No

   If yes, how?

   If the patient answers yes to any of the above, ask the following question:
5. **Are you having thoughts of killing yourself right now?** ❍ Yes ❍ No

   If yes, please describe: [ ]

Next steps:

- If patient answers "No" to all questions 1 through 4, screening is complete (not necessary to ask question #5). No intervention is necessary. (*Note: Clinical judgment can always override a negative screen.*)
- **If patient answers "Yes" to any of questions 1 through 4, or refuses to answer, they are considered a positive screen. Ask question #5 to assess acuity:**
  - **"Yes"** to question #5 = **acute positive screen** (imminent risk identified)
    - **Patient requires a STAT safety/full mental health evaluation. Patient cannot leave until evaluated for safety.**
    - Keep patient in sight. Remove all dangerous objects from room. Alert physician or clinician responsible for patient's care.
  - **"No"** to question #5 = **non-acute positive screen** (potential risk identified)
    - **Patient requires a brief suicide safety assessment to determine if a full mental health evaluation is needed. Patient cannot leave until evaluated for safety.**
    - Alert healthcare provider responsible for the patient's care.

Management of Suicidal Ideation

- Option if low risk for suicide: Mobilize social supports.
- Options if high-risk for suicide: Call 911; transport to the emergency department.
- Access in-home crisis intervention programs.
- Depending on severity, consider outpatient counseling, inpatient hospitalization, or residential programs.
- **Provide resources to all patients:**
  - 24/7 National Suicide Prevention Lifeline 1-800-273-TALK (8255) En Español: 1-888-628-9454
  - 24/7 Crisis Text Line: Text "HOME" to 741-741
  - The ASQ Suicide Screening Tool Kit–Youth is in the public domain and downloadable from the National Institute for Mental Health at:

    www.nimh.nih.gov/research/research-conducted-at-nimh/asq-toolkit-materials/youth-asq-toolkit.shtml#outpatient

    www.nimh.nih.gov/research/research-conducted-at-nimh/asq-toolkit-materials/index.shtml

Assessment of Depression

Consider:

- onset and development of symptoms; context in which symptoms occur/are sustained;
- biological/psychosocial stressors;
- comorbid psychopathology;
- impact of symptoms on activities of daily living and family;
- parent–child interactions;
- developmental history; and
- coping behaviors and styles, sleep, and rhythmicity.

Medical History

- medical visits/hospitalizations (e.g., recurrent pain syndromes); and
- medical disorders (e.g., hypothyroidism, anemia, chronic illness) and medications.

School History

- academic, athletic, social, and behavioral functioning;
- potential versus actual achievements; and
- pattern of attendance and school nurse visits.

Social History

- environmental stressors, separations, and losses; and
- involvement with peers/withdrawal, giving away prized possessions.

Family History

- family mental health history (e.g., anxiety/mood disorders);
- family medical history (e.g., headaches, chronic illness, recurrent pain); and
- parental responses to medications (e.g., selective serotonin reuptake inhibitors [SSRIs]).

Interviewing the Child/Adolescent

Consider:

- the child's/adolescent's report of symptoms and sense of functional impairment;
- objective signs of depression (e.g., loss/gain of weight, hypo/hyperactivity); and
- depending on development, engaging the child in play, drawing, or other artistic expression; also, obtain history from collateral contacts.

Specific Assessment Questions for Children and Adolescents

- **Mood:** Have you been feeling sad, down, blue, or grouchy most of the day, more days than not? Do you find yourself crying a lot? Have you been getting into arguments more than usual?
- **Anhedonia:** Are you able to enjoy things you used to enjoy? Do you feel bored or tired a lot of the time?
- **Negative self-concept:** How do you feel about yourself on a scale of 0 (meaning you do not feel good about yourself at all) to 10 (meaning you feel really good about yourself)?
- **Guilt:** Do you feel badly or guilty about things you have done? Do you feel you are a burden to others?
- **Relationships with friends:** Do you have friends? Are you liked by other kids?
- **Neurovegetative signs:** Do you have trouble falling asleep or staying asleep? Do you have trouble concentrating in school? How is your appetite? Are you eating more or less than usual?
- **Somatic symptoms:** Do you have a lot of headaches or stomachaches?
- **Suicidal ideations:** Do you ever wish you were dead? Do you think about death or make plans to hurt yourself? Have you ever hurt yourself?
- **Current health and medications:** Certain illnesses and medications can cause or present like mood disorders.
- **Alcohol and drug use:** How much alcohol do you drink? What drugs are you taking? How often?

Specific Assessment Questions for Parents

- **Mood/affect:** How is your child's mood and emotions? Is this a change from how they usually are?
- **Neurovegetative signs:** Is your child having trouble falling or staying asleep? Has their appetite changed and how if yes?
- **Suicidal ideation:** Has your child ever talked about wanting to hurt him- or herself or die? Is there a history of self-harm?
- **Impaired functioning at school or with peers:** Is there a change with how your child has been functioning at school, home or with peers?

Special Assessment Findings With Bipolar Disorder

All youth who screen positive for depression should be assessed for bipolar disorder, which can occur at any age in childhood or adolescence. Bipolar disorder can cause mood swings from the highs of hyperactivity, extreme irritability, or euphoria (mania) to the lows of serious depression.

For a diagnosis of bipolar I disorder, **there must be at least one manic episode**. Findings include:

- Expansive mood. Mood may be very elevated, euphoric or mood may be predominantly irritable in mania (not always euphoric mood). In mania, the person is abnormally active. Has increased energy and feels driven to be involved in goal-directed activity. These symptoms of mania last at least a week and are present most of the day (APA, 2013).
- Grandiose sense of self, one's self- esteem, thoughts of self- importance/influence are inflated.
- Decreased need for sleep. Can report going without sleep for days, without feeling tired.
- Speech rate and rhythm are fast. Talkative, so much more than usual that others notice. Pressured speech, can barely finish one thought before on to another. Does not pause; others have difficulty interjecting questions or comments.
- Racing thoughts. Feeling like their thoughts are so fast, they can't keep up with them.
- Easily distracted, quickly switches to new/different thought/focus/or topic of interest.
- Increase in projects and goal-directed, purposeful activities (socially, at work, at school). These activities might be re-decorating, rearranging office or home, and so forth.
- Inability to be still, overactive/in constant motion, may exhibit hypersexual behaviors.
- Risky behaviors, involvement in activities that have great potential for painful consequences (e.g., buying sprees, gambling, promiscuity, substance use).

A hypomanic episode is a period of persistently elevated or irritable mood with persistently increased activity or energy and activity lasting at least 4 consecutive days (APA, 2013).

For a diagnosis of bipolar II disorder, there must be at least one hypomanic episode and at least one major depressive episode, but no history of a manic episode.

Physical Diagnoses That Should Be Ruled Out With Depression if Suspected From History

- hypothyroidism (obtain TSH, FT4);
- anemia (obtain CBC with differential);
- mononucleosis or chronic fatigue syndrome (obtain monospot);
- eating disorders;
- substance use or withdrawal; for example, alcohol, cocaine, amphetamines, opiates (obtain toxicology screen);
- premenstrual syndrome;
- diabetes (obtain fasting serum glucose);
- head trauma or CNS lesions;
- cushing syndrome;
- HIV/AIDS;
- mitral valve prolapse;
- systemic lupus erythematosus;
- developmental delay;
- failure to thrive;
- seizures;

- lead intoxication (obtain lead level); and
- medication side effects; for example, benzodiazepines, beta-blockers, clonidine, corticosteroids, Accutane, and oral contraceptives.

Conditions That Should Be Ruled Out With a Bipolar Manic Episode if Suspected From History

- hyperthyroidism;
- asthma medication; and
- steroid use.

Diagnostic Criteria for Major Depressive Disorder

To meet *DSM-5* criteria for MDD the depressive symptoms need to be a change from previous functioning, and interfere with functioning now at home/school, or in social situations and have been present for 2 weeks. There has been either: (a) depressed mood or (b) loss of interest or pleasure in activities that one used to enjoy (APA, 2013)

Additional symptoms include:

- sad, depressed mood most of the day or nearly every day; in children and teens, irritability is a symptom of depression and is often present;
- weight changes, either weight loss or weight gain;
- sleeping too little or sleeping too much most days; and
- more active or less active than usual; may feel fatigue and loss of energy most every day.
- feelings of worthlessness, thoughts of being a burden to others or excessive guilt;
- Difficulty concentrating or making decisions;

Recurrent thoughts of death (not just fear of dying), and/or recurrent suicidal ideation (with or without plan or previous suicide attempt).

In order to make the diagnosis of MDD, the above symptoms are not due to substance use or another medical condition. And for the diagnosis of MDD (vs. another mood disorder) there has never been a manic episode (or hypomanic episode).

Diagnostic Criteria for Persistent Depressive Disorder (Dysthymia)

- Depressed or irritable mood for most of the day, for more days than not (either by subjective report or observation) for at least 1-year.
- Presence, while depressed, of at least two of the following:
  - poor appetite or overeating;
  - insomnia or hypersomnia;
  - low energy or fatigue;
  - low self-esteem;
  - poor concentration or difficulty making decisions; and
  - feelings of hopelessness.
- During the 1-year period, the youth has never been without the symptoms for more than 2 months at a time.
- There has never been a manic episode or a hypomanic episode.

- The disturbance is not better explained by a persistent schizoaffective disorder, schizophrenia, delusional disorder, or other specified or unspecified schizophrenia spectrum and other psychotic disorder.
- The symptoms are not due to the physiological effects of a substance or other medical condition.
- The symptoms cause clinically significant distress or impairment in social, school, or other important areas of functioning (*DSM-5*).

Evidence-Based Management of Depression

- Assess for suicidal ideation (conduct a risk assessment). Teach about suicide warning signs. Caution families to remove drugs, alcohol, and weapons from the home (i.e., means restriction).
- Educate the family about the depressive condition and support the child and family.
- Because of the gaps in guidelines that existed for primary care providers to manage adolescent depression, researchers from the United States and Canada established the Guidelines for Adolescent Depression-Primary Care (GLAD-PC) with clinical management flow charts (Cheung et al., 2007). These were updated in 2018 (Cheung, Zuckerbrot, Jensen, et al., 2018) to assist primary care providers to put the recommendations into practice. Each of the following recommendations was graded on the level of supporting evidence based on the Oxford Centre for Evidence-Based Medicine grades of evidence (A–D) system (see www.cebm.net/levels_of_evidence.asp). See the GLAD-PC tool kit for support materials at www.thereachinstitute.org/images/pdfs/glad-pc-toolkit-2018.pdf.

Initial Management of Depression

- ***Recommendation I:*** Clinicians should educate and counsel families and patients about depression and options for the management of the disorder (grade of evidence: 5; strength of recommendation: very strong). Clinicians should also discuss the limits of confidentiality with the adolescent and family (grade of evidence: 5; strength of recommendation: very strong).
- ***Recommendation II:*** After appropriate training, clinicians should develop a treatment plan with patients and families (grade of evidence: 5; strength of recommendation: very strong) and set specific treatment goals in key areas of functioning, including home, peer, and school settings (grade of evidence: 5; strength of recommendation: very strong).
- ***Recommendation III:*** Management should include the establishment of a safety plan, which includes restricting lethal means; engaging a concerned third party; and developing an emergency communication mechanism should the patient deteriorate, become actively suicidal or dangerous to others, or experience an acute crisis associated with psychosocial stressors, especially during the period of initial treatment when safety concerns are the highest (grade of evidence: 3; strength of recommendation: very strong) (Cheung, Zuckerbrot, Jensen, Laraque et al., 2018; Stanley & Brown, 2012).

Treatment Recommendations for Depression

- ***Recommendation I:*** Clinicians should work with administration to organize their clinical settings to reflect best practices in integrated and/or collaborative care models (e.g., facilitating contact with psychiatrists, case managers, embedded therapists) (grade of evidence: 4; strength of recommendation: very strong).
- ***Recommendation II:*** After initial diagnosis, in cases of mild depression, clinicians should consider a period of active support and monitoring before starting evidence-based treatment (grade of evidence: 3; strength of recommendation: very strong).

- ***Recommendation III:*** If a clinician identifies an adolescent with moderate or severe depression or complicating factors and/or conditions such as coexisting substance abuse or psychosis, consultation with a mental health specialist should be considered (grade of evidence: 5; strength of recommendation: strong). Appropriate roles and responsibilities for ongoing co management by the clinician and mental health clinician(s) should be communicated and agreed on (grade of evidence: 5; strength of recommendation: strong). The patient and family should be active team members and approve the roles of the primary care and mental health clinicians (grade of evidence: 5; strength of recommendation: strong).
- ***Recommendation IV:*** Clinicians should recommend scientifically tested and proven treatments (i.e., psychotherapies, such as cognitive behavior therapy or interpersonal therapy and/or antidepressant treatment, such as SSRIs) whenever possible and appropriate to achieve the goals of the treatment plan (grade of evidence: 1; strength of recommendation: very strong).
- ***Recommendation V:*** Clinicians should monitor for the emergence of adverse events during antidepressant treatment (SSRIs) (grade of evidence: 3; strength of recommendation: very strong) (Cheung et al., 2018).

School and after-care personnel should be involved; interdisciplinary collaboration is important.

Careful and regular follow-up with the family is crucial.

Cognitive Behavioral Therapy–Based Programs for Children and Teens

- **The American Academy of Child and Adolescent Psychiatry recommends psychotherapy as the first treatment approach for depressed youth with mild to moderate depression.**

  Cognitive behavior therapy (CBT), which teaches that how a person thinks affects how they feel and how they behave, and interpersonal therapy have been supported by research as effective treatments for depression, anxiety, and other mental health disorders (family therapy also may be indicated). Two manualized reproducible evidence-based intervention programs that are based on CBT include:

  1. The Adolescent Coping with Depression Course by G. N. Clarke and P. M. Lewinsohn; see www.kpchr.org/public/acwd/acwd.html) or;
  2. COPE (Creating Opportunities for Personal Empowerment) for Children, Adolescents and Young Adults by Bernadette Mazurek Melnyk (Melnyk, 2004) is an evidence-based manualized seven-session cognitive behavioral skills building program that has been shown to decrease stress, anxiety, depression, and suicidal ideation as well as improve self-esteem, healthy lifestyle behaviors, and academic competence (Erlich et al., 2018; Hart Abney et al., 2019; Hoying & Melnyk, 2016; Hoying, Melnyk, & Arcoleo, et al., 2016; Kozlowski et al., 2015; Lusk & Melnyk, 2011, 2013; Melnyk et al., 2007, 2009, 2013, 2014, 2015). The program can be delivered by non-mental health clinicians, including primary care providers who are receiving reimbursement with the 99214 CPT code (Melnyk, 2020), teachers and social workers, after completing an on-line training workshop. A digitalized on-line interactive version of the program also is available for adolescents. More information about the COPE program is provided in Chapter 17, Brief Evidence-Based Interventions for Child and Adolescent Mental Health, and at www.COPE2Thrive.com.

- Medications should be reserved for severe depression or moderate depression not responding to cognitive behavioral therapy/skills building and should be prescribed in conjunction with counseling therapy.

- Children and teens with depression respond to antidepressants at a rate of approximately 50% to 60% (Riddle, 2019).
- SSRIs (e.g., Prozac, Celexa, Paxil, Zoloft, Effexor, Lexapro) are the recommended first-line treatment (see Table 4.1), but only fluoxetine and escitalopram have U.S. Food and Drug Administration (FDA) approval for depression in children (fluoxetine) and adolescents (fluoxetine and escitalopram) (Riddle, 2019).
- Medication guides and patient information is available at Dwyer & Bloch, 2019 www.ncbi.nlm.nih.gov/pmc/articles/PMC6738970/
- There is an FDA Black Box Warning for antidepressant use in children, adolescents, and young adults.

  www.medpagetoday.org/psychiatry/depression/210?vpass=1. This link discusses the warning, provides guidelines for prescribing antidepressants, and gives key safety points to address Black Box warning.
- Generic medications are available for SSRIs and are typically less expensive than brand medications.
- It is extremely important to start antidepressant medication at LOW doses in children and adolescents and increase dosage SLOWLY. A trial of 8 weeks is recommended; it usually takes 2 to 4 weeks to see an effect, sometimes longer. Families should be educated to observe for serotonin syndrome with the start of SSRIs, including insomnia and agitation. As a general rule of thumb, antidepressants should be used for 6 to 9 months after target symptoms are relieved, weaned slowly, and never stopped abruptly. Avoid tricyclic antidepressants (e.g., amitriptyline, nortriptyline) whenever possible, especially in patients with suicidal ideation due to the potential for cardiac toxicity with overdose. In a classic landmark study (the Treatment for Adolescents with Depression Study), the group that received combined therapy of fluoxetine and individual cognitive behavioral therapy showed a 71% response rate versus a 35% response in adolescents who were taking placebo and receiving weekly clinical monitoring (March et al., 2004).

WARNING: SSRIs MAY INCREASE SUICIDAL IDEATION IN CHILDREN AND ADOLESCENTS/ YOUNG ADULTS.

FDA Black Box Warning www.medpagetoday.org/psychiatry/depression/210?vpass=1

Refer when there is:

1. Poor or incomplete response to two interventions or no improvement with psychosocial interventions in 2 months.
2. Increase in symptoms despite treatment.
3. A recurrent episode within 1 year of previous episode.
4. The patient or families request referral.

Special Notes on the Management of Bipolar Disorder

- Manic episodes in children and adolescents are treated as they are in adults.
- Lithium is the only medication that is FDA approved for manic episodes in teens, 12 years of age and older.
- Divalproex (Depakote) is commonly used as a mood stabilizer to treat bipolar disorder in children and adolescents.

Table 4.1. Prescribing Information for the Selective Serotonin Reuptake Inhibitors (SSRIs) Used for the Treatment of Major Depressive Disorder

SSRI (Recommended Order of Preference)	Usual Starting Dose (SD) and Target Dosage (TD) per Day		Side Effects	Important Considerations for Use of SSRIs
- Fluoxetine (Prozac)	(SD): (TD):	5–10 mg 20–60 mg	**Common:** Nausea, diarrhea, constipation, dry mouth, decreased or increased appetite, restlessness, diaphoresis, headaches, sleep changes (usually see symptoms quickly but they diminish over time) **Rare/Serious Side Effects:** Prolonged QT interval, hyponatremia, seizures, serotonin syndrome, induction of mania, suicidality	Prozac is the FDA-approved antidepressant for major depressive disorder in children as young as 8 years of age; onset of therapeutic action typically takes 2–4 weeks (true for other SSRIs); consider increasing the dose if it is not improving symptoms in 6–8 weeks or switching to another SSRI. SSRIs can be stimulating in children and adolescents. **Use cautiously and observe for activation of known or unknown bipolar disorder and/or suicidal ideation.** If activating, have the medication taken in the morning to decrease insomnia. Prozac is contraindicated with the use of MAOIs or within 2 weeks of MAOI use (true for all SSRIs). Prozac has a long half-life (13–15 days), which may potentiate interactions with another drug if introduced too early after discontinuation. Because of the long half-life, it has an advantage in children/teens with adherence problems.

(*continued*)

Table 4.1. Prescribing Information for the Selective Serotonin Reuptake Inhibitors (SSRIs) Used for the Treatment of Major Depressive Disorder (*continued*)

SSRI (Recommended Order of Preference)	Usual Starting Dose (SD) and Target Dosage (TD) per Day		Side Effects	Important Considerations for Use of SSRIs
- Citalopram (*Celexa*)	(SD): (TD):	5–10 mg 20–40 mg	**Common:** Same as Prozac, also may have flu-like rhinitis, abdominal pain, back pain, fatigue; less activating than Prozac **Rare/Serious Side Effects:** Same as Prozac	**Monitor children/teens and their symptoms in person regularly on a weekly basis during the first 4 weeks of treatment.** Assess therapeutic levels when initiating and increasing dosage. Use with caution in patients with a history of seizures (true for all SSRIs). Taper is usually not necessary due to the drug's long half-life.
- Sertraline (*Zoloft*)	(SD): (TD):	12.5–25 mg 50–100 mg	**Common and Rare/ Serious Side Effects:** Same as Prozac	Same as Prozac. Taper is usually not necessary, yet tapering is a prudent approach to avoid withdrawal symptoms. As with Prozac, taper to avoid withdrawal symptoms, such dizziness, nausea, stomach cramps, and sweating. A good approach to tapering is a 50% reduction for 3 days, then another 50% reduction for 3 days, followed by discontinuation.
- Paroxetine (*Paxil*)	(SD): (TD):	5–10 mg 20–40 mg	**Common and Rare/ Serious Side Effects:** Same as Prozac; sedation is common; may be less activating than other SSRIs	Not specifically approved for depression, however, preliminary evidence suggests efficacy for depressed children and adolescents. Often preferred for patients with depression and comorbid anxiety. Taper to avoid withdrawal effects. If sedating, advise to take at bedtime.

(*continued*)

Table 4.1. Prescribing Information for the Selective Serotonin Reuptake Inhibitors (SSRIs) Used for the Treatment of Major Depressive Disorder (*continued*)

SSRI (Recommended Order of Preference)	Usual Starting Dose (SD) and Target Dosage (TD) per Day		Side Effects	Important Considerations for Use of SSRIs
- Fluvoxamine (*Luvox*)	(SD): (TD):	25 mg 50–200 mg	**Common and Rare/ Serious Side Effects:** Same as Prozac; sedation is common	Useful for patients with comorbid depression and anxiety. Divide doses above 50 mg/ day into two doses and give the larger dose at bedtime. Taper to avoid withdrawal effects.
- Escitalopram (*Lexapro*)	(SD): (TD):	5–10 mg 10–20 mg	**Common and Rare/Serious Side Effects:** Same as those associated with Prozac; sedation is unusual	Well tolerated. FDA approved for MDD in youth, starting at age 12 years. Useful for depression and comorbid anxiety disorder. Tapering is not usually necessary, but it is helpful for many patients to avoid withdrawal symptoms.

Important Note: Caution must be exercised when prescribing SSRIs to children and adolescents (up to age 25 years) with psychiatric disorders as studies have shown an increased risk of suicidal thinking and behavior (suicidality) in the first few months of starting treatment. Patients started on SSRIs should be observed closely for worsening of symptoms, suicidality, or unusual changes in behavior. Families should be advised to monitor for these signs/ symptoms and alert the provider if they are present (Stahl, 2019).

- Atypical antipsychotic medications (e.g., olanzapine [Zyprexa]; risperidone [Risperdal], aripiprazole [Abilify]) are also used in combination with divalproex. Olanzapine is approved for use in manic/mixed episodes in teens, 13 years and older. Risperidone is approved for acute mania/mixed mania in children 10 years of age and older. Aripiprazole is approved for bipolar maintenance.
- Many atypical antipsychotic medications (e.g., olanzapine, risperidone) contribute to substantial weight gain in children and adolescents and, therefore, are often discontinued by individuals. Sedation also is common and may help if taken at bedtime. These medications also may increase risk for diabetes and dyslipidemia. Weight gain is less frequent and severe with aripiprazole.
- Due to multiple challenges in the management of children and adolescents with bipolar disorder, involvement of a psychiatric mental health provider is essential.

Special Notes on Post-Partum Depression

- The USPSTF recommends screening for depression in adults, including pregnant and post-partum women.
- Post-partum depression (PPD) occurs in approximately 10% to 15% of women within 4 weeks after delivery of a child (specify postpartum onset).

- Of every 1,000 women who give birth, between 1 and 2 experience postpartum psychosis.
- When delusions are present, it often involves the infant (e.g., being possessed by the devil).
- PPD is often accompanied by severe anxiety and panic attacks.
- Many mothers go untreated.
- Routine screening in the first 4 weeks after delivery is important.

Post-Partum Blues

- PPD must be differentiated from post-partum blues that typically occur 3 to 7 days after birth.
- Affects 70% to 80% of women.
- Peaks at 3 to 5 days.
- Predominantly positive mood with labile and intense episodes of irritability.
- Lasts from hours to several days.
- Resolves without significant consequences.
- May be related to hormonal shifts after delivery.

Screening Tools for Post-Partum Depression

- Edinburgh Post-Natal Depression Scale (EPDS): Quick screen with 10 items; in the public domain and free.
- Center for Epidemiologic Study Depression (CES-D) scale: In the public domain and free.

Parental Depression

- Has multiple negative adverse outcomes on children.
- Ask parents if they are having difficulty in caring for their child/children.
- Ask about support systems.
- Ask about current stressors.
- Ask about past depression and outcomes.
- Ask permission to speak to other family members.
- Assess risk for suicidal behavior.
- Help parents plan for how to talk to their children and family members about their depression.
- Assess how the child is dealing with the parent's depression.
- Refer parent to a mental health provider.

Resources for Families

- Depression and Bipolar Support Alliance: www.dbsalliance.org/site/PageServer?pagename=home
- National Alliance for the Mentally Ill: www.nami.org
- National Mental Health Association: 703-684-7722; www.nmha.org

REFERENCES

American Psychiatric Association. (2013). *Diagnostic and statistical manual of mental disorders* (5th ed.). (DSM-IV). Author.

Cheung, A., Zuckerbrot, R. A., & Jensen, P. S. (2018). *Guidelines for adolescent depression in primary care (GLAD-PC Toolkit)*. Reach Institute. See https://www.thereachinstitute.org/images/pdfs/glad-pc-toolkit-2018.pdf

Cheung, A. H., Zuckerbrot, R. A., Jensen, P. S., Ghalib, K., Laraque D., Stein, R. E. K., & GLAD-PC Steering Group. (2007). Guidelines for adolescent depression in primary care (GLAD-PC): II. Treatment and ongoing management. *Pediatrics, 230*, e1313–e1326. https://doi.org/10.1542/peds.2006-1395

Cheung, A. H., Zuckerbrot, R. A., Jensen, P. S., Laraque, D., & Stein, R. E. K. (2018). Guidelines for adolescent depression in primary care (GLAD-PC): II. Treatment and ongoing management. *Pediatrics, 141*(3), e20174082. https://doi.org/10.1542/peds.2017-4082

Dwyer, J. B., & Bloch, M. H. (2019). Antidepressants for pediatric patients. *Current Psychiatry, 18*(9), 26F–42F.

Erlich, K. J., Li, J., Dillon, E., Li, M., & Becker, D. F. (2018). Outcomes of a brief cognitive skills-based intervention (COPE) for adolescents in the primary care setting. *Journal of Pediatric Health Care, 33*(4), 415–424. https://doi.org/10.1016/j.pedhc.2018.12.001

Hart Abney, B. G., Lusk, P., Hovermale, R., & Melnyk, B. M. (2019). Decreasing depression and anxiety in college youth using the creating opportunities for personal empowerment program (COPE). *Journal of the American Psychiatric Nurses Association, 25*(2), 89–98. https://doi.org/10.1177/1078390318779205

Hoying, J., & Melnyk, B. M. (2016). COPE: A pilot study with urban-dwelling minority sixth grade youth to improve physical activity and mental health outcomes. *Journal of School Nursing, 32*(5), 347–356. https://doi.org/10.1177/1059840516635713

Hoying, J., Melnyk, B. M., & Arcoleo, K. (2016). Effects of the COPE cognitive behavioral skills building TEEN program on the healthy lifestyle behaviors and mental health of Appalachian early adolescents. *Journal of Pediatric Health Care, 30*(1), 65–72. https://doi.org/10.1016/j.pedhc.2015.02.005

Kozlowski, J., Lusk, P., & Melnyk, B. M. (2015). Pediatric nurse practitioner management of child anxiety in the rural primary care clinic with the evidence-based COPE. *Journal of Pediatric Health Care, 29*(3), 274–282. https://doi.org/10.1016/j.pedhc.2015.01.009

Lusk, P., & Melnyk, B. M. (2011). The brief cognitive-behavioral COPE intervention for depressed adolescents: Outcomes and feasibility of delivery in 30-minute outpatient visits. *Journal of the American Psychiatric Nurses Association, 17*(3), 226–236. https://doi.org/10.1177/1078390311404067

Lusk, P., & Melnyk, B. M. (2013). COPE for depressed and anxious teens: A brief cognitive-behavioral skills building intervention to increase access to timely, evidence-based treatment. *Journal of Child and Adolescent Psychiatric Nursing, 26*(1), 23–31. https://doi.org/10.1111/jcap.12017

March, J., Silva, S., Petrycki, S., Curry, J., Wells, K., Fairbank, J., Burns, B., Domino, M., McNulty, S., Vitiello, B., Severe, J., Treatment for Adolescents With Depression Study (TADS) Team. (2004). Fluoxetine, cognitive-behavioral therapy, and their combination for adolescents with depression: Treatment for adolescents with depression study (TADS) randomized controlled trial. *Journal of the American Medical Association, 292*(7), 807–820. https://doi.org/10.1001/jama.292.7.807

Melnyk, B. M. (2004). *COPE (Creating opportunities for personal empowerment) for children, Teens and young adults: A 7-session cognitive behavioral skills building program*. COPE2thrive.

Melnyk, B. M. (2020). Reducing healthcare costs for mental health hospitalizations with the evidence-based COPE program for child and adolescent depression and anxiety: A cost analysis. *Journal of Pediatric Health Care, 34*(2), 117–121. +* https://doi.org/10.1016/j.pedhc.2019.08.002

Melnyk, B. M., Jacobson, D., Kelly, S. A., Belyea, M. J., Shaibi, G. Q., Small, L., O'Haver, J. A., & Marsiglia, F. F. (2013). Promoting healthy lifestyles in high school adolescents: A randomized controlled trial. *American Journal of Preventive Medicine, 45*(4), 407–415. September 10, 2013. [Epub ahead of print]. https://doi.org/10.1016/j.amepre.2013.05.013

Melnyk, B. M., Jacobson, D., Kelly, S. A., Belyea, M. J., Shaibi, G. Q., Small, L., O'Haver, J. A., & Marsiglia, F. F. (2015). Twelve-month effects of the COPE healthy lifestyles TEEN program on overweight and depression in high school adolescents. *Journal of School Health, 85*(12), 861–870. https://doi.org/10.1111/josh.12342

Melnyk, B. M., Jacobson, D., Kelly, S. A., O'Haver, J., Small, L., & Mays, M. Z. (2009). Improving the mental health, healthy lifestyle choices and physical health of Hispanic adolescents: A randomized controlled pilot study. *Journal of School Health, 79*(12), 575–584.

Melnyk, B. M., Kelly, S., & Lusk, P. (2014). Outcomes and feasibility of a Manualized cognitive-behavioral skills building intervention: Group COPE for depressed and anxious adolescents. *Journal of Child and Adolescent Psychiatric Nursing, 27*(1), 3–13. https://doi.org/10.1111/jcap.12058

Melnyk, B. M., Small, L., Morrison-Beedy, D., Strasser, A., Spath, L., Kreipe, R., Crean, H., Jacobson, D., Kelly, S., & O'Haver, J. (2007). The COPE healthy lifestyles TEEN program: Feasibility, preliminary, efficacy, and lessons learned from an after-school group intervention with overweight adolescents. *Journal of Pediatric Health Care, 21*(5), 315. https://doi.org/10.1016/j.pedhc.2007.02.009

Richardson, L. P., McCauley, E., Grossman, D. C., McCarty, C. A., Richards, J., Russo, J. E., Rockhill, C., & Katon, W. (2010). Evaluation of the patient health questionnaire-9 item for detecting major depression among adolescents. *Pediatrics, 126*(6), 1117–1123. https://doi.org/10.1542/peds.2010-0852

Riddle, M. A. (2019). *Pediatric psychopharmacology for primary care* (2nd ed.). American Academy of Pediatrics.

Siu, A. L. (2016). On behalf of the U.S. Preventive Services Task Force Screening for depression in children and adolescents: U.S. Preventive Services Task Force recommendation statement. *Pediatrics, 137*(3), e20154467. https://doi.org/10.1542/peds.2015-4467

Stahl, S. (2019). *Essential psychopharmacology prescriber's guide; Children and adolescents*. Cambridge University Press.

Stanley, B., & Brown, G. K. (2012). Safety planning intervention: A brief intervention to mitigate suicide risk. *Cognitive and Behavioral Practice, 19*, 256–264. https://doi.org/10.1016/j.cbpra.2011.01.001

Screening Tools for Child and Adolescent Depression

As with other disorders, depression should not be diagnosed solely by a screening tool. Further evaluation in the form of a clinical interview is necessary for children and adolescents identified as depressed through a screening process. Further evaluation also is warranted for children or adolescents who exhibit depressive symptoms but who do not screen positive.

There are a few valid and reliable depression screening tools for children and adolescents. The U.S. Preventive Services Task Force (USPSTF) recommends screening all adolescents (12–18 years of age) for major depressive disorder (MDD) when systems are in place to ensure accurate diagnosis, psychotherapy (cognitive behavioral or interpersonal) and follow-up, and concludes that the evidence is insufficient to assess the balance of benefits and harms of screening of children (7–11 years)

www.uspreventiveservicestaskforce.org/uspstf/recommendation/depression-in-children-and-adolescents-screening

In adults, the USPSTF recommends asking the following two questions, which may be as effective as using longer screening instruments. These questions may be indicated when interviewing teens, especially if time is limited for the use of longer screening instruments.

1. Over the past 2 weeks, have you ever felt down, depressed, or hopeless?
2. Over the past 2 weeks, have you felt little interest or pleasure in doing things?

National Association of Pediatric Nurse Practitioners™

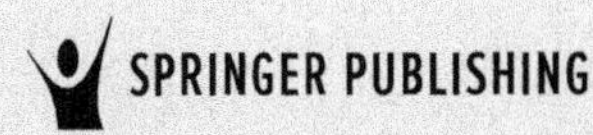

Center for Epidemiological Studies Depression Scale for Children (CES-DC)
(L.S. Radloff)

DESCRIPTION

The Center for Epidemiological Studies Depression Scale for Children (CES-DC) (see the instrument on the following page) is a 20-item self-report depression inventory with possible scores ranging from 0 to 60. Each response to an item is scored as follows:

0 = Not at all

1 = A little

2 = Some

3 = A lot

However, items 4, 8, 12, and 16 are phrased positively, and thus are scored in the opposite order:

3 = Not at all

2 = A little

1 = Some

0 = A lot

Higher CES-DC scores indicate increasing levels of depression. Weissman et al. (1980), the developers of the CES-DC, have used the cut-off score of 15 as being suggestive of depressive symptoms in children and adolescents. That is, scores over 15 can be indicative of significant levels of depressive symptoms.

PSYCHOMETRIC PROPERTIES

The CES-DC has been found to be a valid and reliable tool for depression screening in older school-age children and adolescents (Faulstich et al., 1986).

REFERENCES

Faulstich, M. E., Carey, M. P., Ruggiero, L., Enyart, P., & Gresham, F. (1986). Assessment of depression in childhood and adolescence: An evaluation of the center for epidemiological studies depression scale for children (CES-DC). *American Journal of Psychiatry*, *143*(8), 1024–1027. https://doi.org/10.1176/ajp.143.8.1024

Weissman, M. M., Orvaschel, H., & Padian, N. (1980). Children's symptom and social functioning self-report scales: Comparison of mothers' and children's reports. *Journal of Nervous Mental Disorders*, *168*(12), 736–740. https://doi.org/10.1097/00005053-198012000-00005

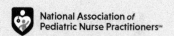

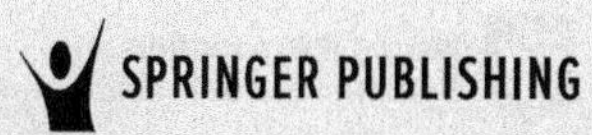

BRIGHT FUTURES TOOL FOR PROFESSIONALS

Center for Epidemiological Studies

Depression Scale for Children (CES-DC)

Number ____________________

Score ______________________

INSTRUCTIONS

Below is a list of the ways you might have felt or acted. Please check how *much* you have felt this way during the *past week*.

DURING THE PAST WEEK	Not at all	A little	Some	A lot
1. I was bothered by things that usually don't bother me.				
2. I did not feel like eating, I wasn't very hungry.				
3. I wasn't able to feel happy, even when my family or friends tried to help me feel better.				
4. I felt like I was just as good as other kids.				
5. I felt like I couldn't pay attention to what I was doing.				
DURING THE PAST WEEK	**Not at all**	**A little**	**Some**	**A lot**
6. I felt down and unhappy.				
7. I felt like I was too tired to do things.				
8. I felt like something good was going to happen.				
9. I felt like things I did before didn't work out right.				
10. I felt scared.				
DURING THE PAST WEEK	**Not at all**	**A little**	**Some**	**A lot**
11. I didn't sleep as well as I usually sleep.				
12. I was happy.				
13. I was more quiet than usual.				
14. I felt lonely, like I didn't have any friends.				
15. I felt like kids I know were not friendly or that they didn't want to be with me.				
DURING THE PAST WEEK	**Not at all**	**A little**	**Some**	**A lot**
16. I had a good time.				
17. I felt like crying.				
18. I felt sad.				
19. I felt people didn't like me.				
20. It was hard to get started doing things.				

From: Bright Futures at Georgetown University, available at www.brightfutures.org

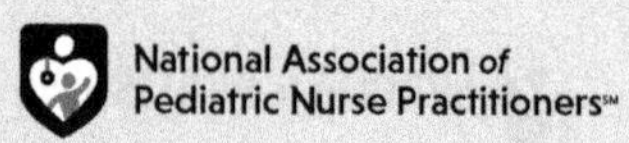

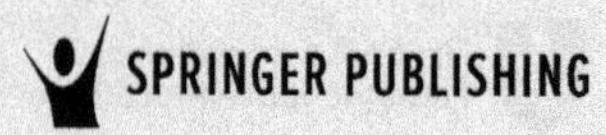

Patient Health Questionnaire-9 (PHQ-9) and PHQ-9 Modified for Teens

The Patient Health Questionnaire-9 (PHQ-9) assists clinicians in identifying individuals who may be affected by depression. It is available in the public domain and free for use in multiple languages at www.phqscreeners.com/overview.aspx. The instrument has been modified for use with adolescents 12 to 18 years of age (i.e., PHQ-9 Modified for Teens).

DESCRIPTION

These nine-item self-report instruments can be administered in less than 5 minutes. The tools are used as a brief screen for depression; they identify adults and adolescents at risk for depression so that healthcare providers can conduct a clinical interview for definitive diagnosis and treatment.

PSYCHOMETRIC PROPERTIES

The PHQ-9 has been established as valid and reliable across culturally diverse populations and a variety of medical conditions. In a recent study with 442 adolescents 13 to 17 years of age, a PHQ-9 score of 11 or more had a sensitivity of 89.5% and a specificity of 77.5% for detecting youth who met the *Diagnostic and Statistical Manual of Mental Disorders* criteria for major depression. Increasing PHQ-9 scores were significantly correlated with increasing levels of functional impairment as well as reports of psychosocial problems by the teens' parents (Richardson et al., 2010).

SCORING

Item scores are summed. Total scores equal to or more than 11 indicates a positive screen. Regardless of the total score on the nine items, endorsement of serious suicidal ideation or past suicide attempt (questions 12 and 13) should be interpreted as a positive screen.

1 to 4: Minimal depression

5 to 9: Mild depression

10 to 14: Moderate depression (≥11 positive score)

15 to 19: Moderately severe depression

20 to 27: Severe depression

CODING FOR REIMBURSEMENT

The following codes can be used for mental health screening:

96110- Mental health screening

99420- Health risk assessment

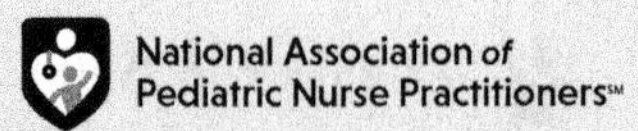

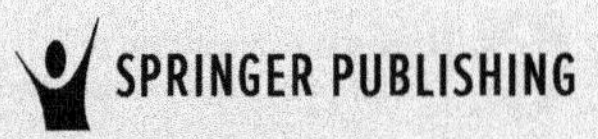

PATIENT HEALTH QUESTIONNAIRE-9 (PHQ-9)

Over the last 2 weeks, how often have you been bothered by any of the following problems? (*Use "✓" to indicate your answer*)	Not at all	Several days	More than half the days	Nearly every day
1. Little interest or pleasure in doing things	0	1	2	3
2. Feeling down, depressed, or hopeless	0	1	2	3
3. Trouble falling or staying asleep, or sleeping too much	0	1	2	3
4. Feeling tired or having little energy	0	1	2	3
5. Poor appetite or overeating	0	1	2	3
6. Feeling bad about yourself — or that you are a failure or have let yourself or your family down	0	1	2	3
7. Trouble concentrating on things, such as reading the newspaper or watching television	0	1	2	3
8. Moving or speaking so slowly that other people could have noticed? Or the opposite — being so fidgety or restless that you have been moving around a lot more than usual	0	1	2	3
9. Thoughts that you would be better off dead or of hurting yourself in some way	0	1	2	3

FOR OFFICE CODING ___*0*___ + ________ + ________ + ________

= Total Score: ________

If you checked off any problems, how difficult have these problems made it for you to do your work, take care of things at home, or get along with other people?			
Not difficult at all	**Somewhat difficult**	**Very difficult**	**Extremely difficult**

Developed by Drs. Robert L. Spitzer, Janet B. W. Williams, Kurt Kroenke, and colleagues, with an educational grant from Pfizer Inc. No permission required to reproduce, translate, display or distribute.

PHQ-9: MODIFIED FOR TEENS

Name:________________________ Clinician:______________________ Date:________________

Instructions: How often have you been bothered by each of the following symptoms during the past **2 weeks?** For each symptom put an "X" in the box beneath the answer that best describes how you have been feeling.

	0 **Not at all**	1 **Several days**	2 **More than half the days**	3 **Nearly every day**
1. Feeling down, depressed, irritable, or hopeless?				
2. Little interest or pleasure in doing things?				

National Association of Pediatric Nurse Practitioners℠

SPRINGER PUBLISHING

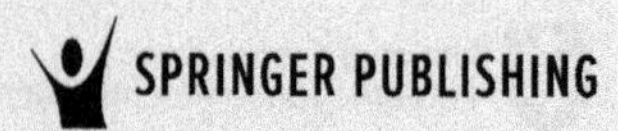

	0 **Not at all**	1 **Several days**	2 **More than half the days**	3 **Nearly every day**
3. Trouble falling asleep, staying asleep, or sleeping too much?				
4. Poor appetite, weight loss, or overeating?				
5. Feeling tired, or having little energy?				
6. Feeling bad about yourself – or feeling that you are a failure, or that you have let yourself or your family down?				
7. Trouble concentrating on things like schoolwork, reading, or watching TV?				
8. Moving or speaking so slowly that other people could have noticed? Or the opposite – being so fidgety or restless that you were moving around a lot more than usual?				
9. Thoughts that you would be better off dead, or of hurting yourself in some way?				

In the **past year** have you felt depressed or sad most days, even if you felt okay some days?

[ ] **Yes** [ ] **No**

If you are experiencing any of the problems on this form, how **difficult** have these problems made it for you to do your work, take care of things at home or get along with other people?

[ ] Not difficult at all [ ] Somewhat difficult [ ] Very difficult [ ] Extremely difficult

Has there been a time in the **past month** when you have had serious thoughts about ending your life?

[ ] Yes [ ] No

Have you **EVER**, in your WHOLE LIFE, tried to kill yourself or made a suicide attempt?

[ ] Yes [ ] No

***If you have had thoughts that you would be better off dead or of hurting yourself* in some way, please discuss this with your health care clinician, go to a hospital emergency room or call 911.

Office use only **Severity score:**

Modified with permission by the GLAD-PC team from the PHQ-9 (Spitzer et al., 1999) and Revised PHQ-A (Johnson, 2002).

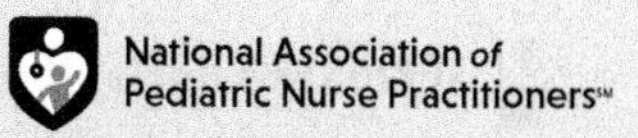

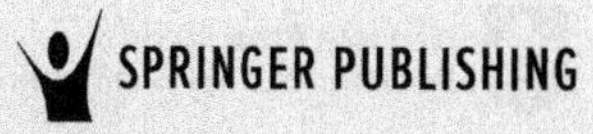

REFERENCES

Johnson J. G., Harris, E. S., Spitzer, R. L., & Williams, J. B. (2002). The patient health questionnaire for adolescents: validation of an instrument for the assessment of mental disorders among adolescent primary care patients. *Journal of Adolescent Health, 30*(3), 196–204. doi: 10.1016/s1054-139x(01)00333-0

Spitzer, R. L., Kroenke, K., & Williams, J. B. (1999). Validation and utility of a self-report version of PRIME-MD: The PHQ primary care study. Primary care evaluation of mental disorders. Patient health questionnaire. *JAMA, 282*(18), 1737–1744. doi: 10.1001/jama.282.18.1737

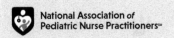

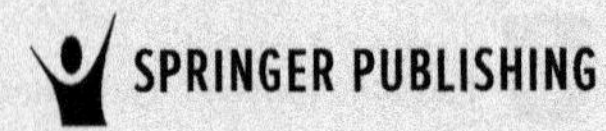

Edinburgh Postnatal Depression Scale

The Edinburgh Postnatal Depression Scale (EPDS) assists clinicians in identifying mothers suffering from postpartum depression early and easily. It is in the public domain and free for use in clinical settings.

DESCRIPTION

This 10-item, widely used self-report instrument can be administered in less than 5 minutes. Used as a brief screening tool, the EPDS identifies women who are at high risk for postpartum depression so that healthcare professionals can then refer them for definitive diagnosis and treatment. Mothers respond using a 4-point Likert scale to the items, which tap various clinical depression symptoms, such as guilt, sleep disturbance, low energy, and suicidal ideation. The EPDS is available in multiple languages and also can be used for depression screening during pregnancy.

PSYCHOMETRIC PROPERTIES

Multiple studies have supported the scale's validity and excellent reliability.

ADMINISTRATION AND SCORING

The EPDS can be used across various specialties, including obstetrics, pediatrics, psychiatry, psychology, and social work.

Response categories are scored 0, 1, 2, and 3 according to increased severity of the symptom. Items 3, 5–10 are reverse scored (i.e., 3, 2, 1, and 0). The total score is calculated by adding together the scores for each of the 10 items. Mothers who score above 13 are likely to be suffering from a depressive illness of varying severity.

EDINBURGH POSTNATAL DEPRESSION SCALE[1] (EPDS)

Name: ______________________ Address: ______________________

Your Date of Birth: ______________ ______________________

Baby's Date of Birth: ______________ Phone: ______________________

____

As you are pregnant or have recently had a baby, we would like to know how you are feeling. Please check the answer that comes closest to how you have fell **IN THE PAST 7 DAYS**, not just how you feel today.

Sources: Cox, J.L., Holden, J.M., and Sagovsky, R. 1987. Detection of postnatal depression: Development of the 10-item Edinburgh Postnatal Depression Scale. *British Journal of Psychiatry* 150:782–786; Postpartum. (2002). Depression. *New England Journal of Medicine* 347(3): 194–199.

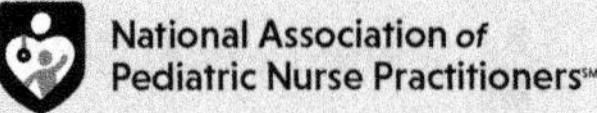

SPRINGER PUBLISHING

Here is an example, already completed.

I have felt happy:

☐ Yes, all the time

☑ Yes, most of the time This would mean: "I have felt happy most of the time" during the past week

☐ No, not very often Please complete the other questions in the same way.

☐ No, not at all

In the past 7 days:

1. I have been able to laugh and see the funny side of things
- ☐ As much as I always could
- ☐ Not quite so much now
- ☐ Definitely not so much now
- ☐ Not at all

2. I have looked forward with enjoyment to things
- ☐ As much as I ever did
- ☐ Rather less than I used to
- ☐ Definitely less than I used to
- ☐ Hardly at all

***3.** I have blamed myself unnecessarily when things went wrong
- ☐ Yes, most of the time
- ☐ Yes, some of the time
- ☐ Not very often
- ☐ No, never

4. I have been anxious or worried for no good reason
- ☐ No, not at all
- ☐ Hardly ever
- ☐ Yes, sometimes
- ☐ Yes, very often

***5.** I have felt scared or panicky for no very good reason
- ☐ Yes, quite a lot
- ☐ Yes, sometimes
- ☐ No, not much
- ☐ No, not at all

Sources: Cox, J.L., Holden, J.M., and Sagovsky, R. 1987. Detection of postnatal depression: Development of the 10-item Edinburgh Postnatal Depression Scale. *British Journal of Psychiatry* 150:782–786; Postpartum. (2002). Depression. *New England Journal of Medicine* 347(3): 194–199.

National Association of Pediatric Nurse Practitioners™

SPRINGER PUBLISHING

***6.** Things have been getting on top of me

- ☐ Yes, most of the time I haven't been able to cope at all
- ☐ Yes, sometimes I haven't been coping as well as usual
- ☐ No, most of the time I have coped quite well
- ☐ No, I have been coping as well as ever

***7.** I have been so unhappy that I have had difficulty sleeping

- ☐ Yes, most of the time
- ☐ Yes, sometimes
- ☐ Not very often
- ☐ No, not at all

***8.** I have felt sad or miserable

- ☐ Yes, most of the time
- ☐ Yes, quite often
- ☐ Not very often
- ☐ No, not at all

***9.** I have been so unhappy that I have been crying

- ☐ Yes, most of the time
- ☐ Yes, quite often
- ☐ Only occasionally
- ☐ No, never

***10.** The thought of harming myself has occurred to me

- ☐ Yes, quite often
- ☐ Sometimes
- ☐ Hardly ever
- ☐ Never

Administered/reviewed by ________________________________ Date ______________

Sources: Cox, J.L., Holden, J.M., and Sagovsky, R. 1987. Detection of postnatal depression: Development of the 10-item Edinburgh Postnatal Depression Scale. *British Journal of Psychiatry* 150:782–786; Postpartum. (2002). Depression. *New England Journal of Medicine* 347(3): 194–199.

National Association of Pediatric Nurse Practitioners℠

SPRINGER PUBLISHING

EDINBURGH POSTNATAL DEPRESSION SCALE[1] (EPDS)

Postpartum depression is the most common complication of childbearing. The 10-question Edinburgh Postnatal Depression Scale (EPDS) is a valuable and efficient way of identifying patients at risk for "perinatal" depression. The EPDS is easy to administer and has proven to be an effective screening tool.

Mothers who score above 13 are likely to be suffering from a depressive illness of varying severity. The EPDS score should not override clinical judgment. A careful clinical assessment should be carried out to confirm the diagnosis. The scale indicates how the mother has felt during the previous week. In doubtful cases it may be useful to repeat the tool after 2 weeks. The scale will not detect mothers with anxiety neuroses, phobias, or personality disorders.

Women with postpartum depression need not feel alone. They may find useful information on the web sites of the National Women's Health Information Center ?(www.4women.gov) and from groups such as Postpartum Support International (www.chss.iup.edu/postpartum) and Depression after Delivery (www.depressionafterdelivery.com).

SCORING

QUESTIONS 1, 2, & 4 (without an *)
Are scored 0, 1, 2, or 3 with top box scored as 0 and the bottom box scored as 3.

QUESTIONS 3, 5–10 (marked with an *)
Are reverse scored, with the top box scored as a 3 and the bottom box scored as 0.

Maximum score: 30
Possible depression: 10 or greater
Always look at item 10 (suicidal thoughts)

Instructions for using the Edinburgh Postnatal Depression Scale:

1. The mother is asked to check the response that comes closest to how she has been feeling in the previous 7 days.
2. All the items must be completed.
3. Care should be taken to avoid the possibility of the mother discussing her answers with others. (Answers come from the mother or pregnant woman.)
4. The mother should complete the scale herself, unless she has limited English or has difficulty with reading.

Source: Cox, J. L., Holden, J. M., & Sagovsky, R. (1987). Detection of postnatal depression: Development of the 10-item. Edinburgh Postnatal Depression Scale. *British Journal of Psychiatry* 150, 782–786.

Source: Wisner, K. L., Parry, B. L., & Piontek, C. M. (2020, July 18). Postpartum depression. *The New England Journal of Medicine, 347*(3), 194–199.

Sources: Cox, J.L., Holden, J.M., and Sagovsky, R. 1987. Detection of postnatal depression: Development of the 10-item Edinburgh Postnatal Depression Scale. *British Journal of Psychiatry 150*:782–786; Postpartum. (2002). Depression. *New England Journal of Medicine* 347(3): 194–199.

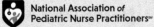

SPRINGER PUBLISHING

Information on Depression for Parents

WHAT IS DEPRESSION?

Depression is an unhappy mood that affects daily functioning, including thoughts, feelings, behavior, and overall health. When depression is too severe or lasts too long, it is considered an illness that can be treated. Left untreated, depression can take the joy out of life and even take away the desire to live. Everyone experiences minor upsets, but this does not mean that everyone is depressed. To have true depression, the symptoms must be present for at least 2 weeks.

HOW COMMON IS DEPRESSION?

Depression in children and teens is far more common than most people realize and affects school-age girls and boys equally. After puberty, girls are twice as likely as boys to be depressed. Ten out of 100 teens get seriously depressed each year, and many more have mild levels of sadness or the blues. About one in 10 children without known problems has suicidal thoughts.

WHAT ARE THE SIGNS OF DEPRESSION?

The most important signs to look for are feelings of sadness and hopelessness. While every child or teen is sad some of the time, no child should feel sad all of the time. If you notice that your child is unhappy and can't seem to have fun, think of this as a sign of depression. To be hopeless or without hope means to feel that nothing can go right, that nothing will change, and that no one can help.

Poor self-esteem is another important sign of depression. This is the teen or child's attitude toward himself or herself. If your child's self-esteem is poor, he or she may feel stupid, ugly, or worthless. Another sign is a change in school performance. If your child was a good student and now wants to stay home, or if his/her grades suddenly fall, he/she may be depressed. Other signs include sleep problems, appetite changes, irritability, anger, crying, and aches and pains, such as headaches or stomachaches.

What would your child say if he or she is depressed? Don't expect your child to say much, because you can't count on him/her telling you how he/she feels. While your child may talk of being unhappy, he or she probably won't say, "I'm depressed" the way an adult will. So, you want to be aware of the signs.

WHAT IF MY CHILD SHOULD MENTION SUICIDE?

Sometimes a child mentions that he or she does not want to live. **If your child mentions suicide: Take it seriously**. Talk to your child. Ask if he or she has made a plan for suicide. If so, it is more serious. If suicide is mentioned or if an attempt is made, seek professional help immediately. Do not assume your child is just looking for attention. Don't ever dare a youngster who mentions suicide to "go ahead." You may think it's a bluff, but he or she may take the dare.

HOW CAN A PARENT HELP?

You can be very helpful to your depressed child. Some suggestions include: Be supportive – listen to what your child has to say. Encourage him or her to keep talking. If your child can't talk well with you, perhaps he or she can talk with a sibling, aunt, friend, teacher, or healthcare provider. Encourage

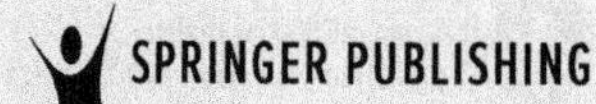

your child to describe or write down how he or she feels. Don't get angry if he/she describes unhappy feelings. **If the problem is severe, worrisome, or lasts more than 2 weeks, get professional help. Talk to your child's healthcare provider if you have any concern that your child may be depressed.**

WHAT ARE THE CAUSES OF DEPRESSION IN CHILDREN?

There is no single answer to the cause of depression. It is probable that several factors combine to create the condition. The child's environment, especially if it is unhappy and stressful, is often a major cause. Depression also may be triggered by difficult situations, such as a death or divorce in the family or abuse. Another possible contributing factor is heredity. Studies show that depression frequently runs in families, so genetics may play a part in the depression of some children. Yet other reasons are a lack of a certain chemical in the brain, called serotonin, and a negative pattern of thinking (e.g., I can't do anything right; everything is bad).

WHAT ARE THE TREATMENTS FOR DEPRESSION?

- Treatment is possible and helpful. The choice of treatment depends on the cause of the problem, the severity of the depression, and whether suicidal thoughts are present. Psychotherapy, such as cognitive behavior therapy, is the primary treatment. By meeting regularly with a therapist, your child can find out the causes of his/her depression, and then learn ways to help deal with it. It is usually good for the family to become involved in the treatment.
- Medication can be an effective part of treatment. Antidepressants have few side effects and are not habit-forming or addictive.
- Finally, you should not feel guilty if your child is depressed. The important point is to realize that there is a problem and to get help for it. If you are concerned, be sure to talk to your child's healthcare provider. Remember, depression in children and teens is treatable.

WHAT CAN I DO TO PREVENT OR HELP MY CHILD WITH DEPRESSION?

- Stay involved in your child's life. Spend time with your child regularly, even if it's only a family dinner. Too often, parents respond to growing teenagers' wishes for independence by withdrawing from their teens' lives. The most important thing for parents to do is to be aware of and involved in their teen's life.
- Support positive relationships by encouraging your teen to get involved in school, clubs, or community events. Help your teen find interests and activities where he or she can connect with other teens. Also, know where your teen is and what he/she is doing when they go out.
- Talk to your teen and listen when he/she talks to you! Parents should talk to their children as often as possible so teens can talk about their problems and worries. Ask your teen about school and friends. Listen to his/her troubles and help find solutions.
- Teach your child coping and problem-solving skills; it also is important for you to role model positive ways of coping and dealing with stress.

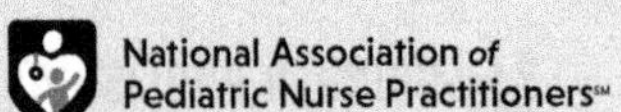

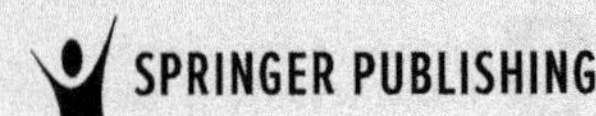

- Know the warning signs of depression and be aware if your child shows any of these signs while talking to you, especially if he or she mentions suicide. Praise your teen's accomplishments rather than finding fault with things he/she does. Teens need to feel that their parents care about them and that what they are doing is recognized.
- It is mainly your job to make sure that your child receives the treatment he or she needs. Make sure that your teen takes his/her medication and goes to counseling. Be supportive.
- For more information about depression, contact the school counselor, psychologist, or social worker at your child's school, or contact your child's doctor or nurse practitioner.

This handout may be distributed to families.
From Melnyk, B. M., & Lusk, P. (2022). *A Practical Guide to Child and Adolescent Mental Health Screening, Evidence-Based Assessment, Intervention, and Health Promotion* (3rd ed.).

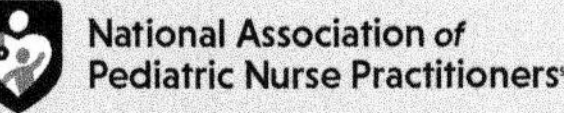

SPRINGER PUBLISHING

Information on Depression for Teens

WHAT IS DEPRESSION?

Depression is a common and serious condition that can affect your thoughts, feelings, behavior, and overall health. Approximately 10 to 20 out of 100 teens get seriously depressed each year, and many more have mild levels of sadness or the blues. There is hope for teens with depression because it can be treated.

WHEN YOU'RE DEPRESSED, YOU MIGHT THINK, FEEL OR ACT IN SOME OF THESE WAYS

- You feel sad or cry a lot and it doesn't go away.
- You feel guilty easily; you feel like you are no good; you've lost your confidence.
- Life seems empty or like nothing good is ever going to happen again.
- You tend to think negatively, like believing that you can't do anything right.
- You have a negative attitude a lot of the time, or it seems like you have no feelings.
- You don't feel like doing a lot of the things you used to enjoy—like playing music, sports, being with friends, going out – and you want to be left alone most of the time.
- It's hard to make up your mind. You forget lots of things, and it's hard to concentrate.
- You get angry often. Little things make you lose your temper; you overreact.
- Your sleep pattern changes; you start sleeping a lot more or you have trouble falling asleep at night. Or you wake up really early most mornings and can't get back to sleep.
- Your eating habits change; you've lost your appetite, or you eat a lot more.
- You feel restless and tired most of the time.
- You think about death, or feel like you're dying, or have thoughts about hurting yourself or committing suicide.

Some teens who are depressed also can get "manic" at times, which may be a sign of bipolar disorder. When you're manic, you may feel or act in some of these ways

- You feel high as a kite... like you're "on top of the world."
- You get unreal ideas about the great things you can do—things that you really can't do.
- Thoughts go racing through your head and you talk a lot.
- You're a nonstop party, constantly running around.
- You do too many wild or risky things, like reckless driving, spending money, and having sex with multiple partners.

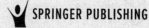

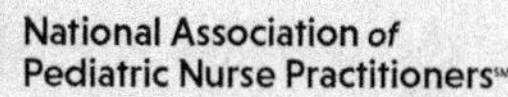

- You're so "up" that you don't need much sleep.
- You're rebellious or irritable and can't get along at home or school, or with your friends.

IF YOU THINK YOU'RE DEPRESSED... TALK TO SOMEONE!

If you have had some of these symptoms and they have lasted a couple of weeks or have caused a big change in your routine, you should talk to someone who can help, like a psychologist, nurse, or doctor, or your school counselor!

TREATMENT FOR DEPRESSION

Having depression doesn't mean that a person is weak, or a failure, or isn't really trying ... it means they need treatment. Most people with depression can be helped with counseling, and some are helped with counseling and medicine. Cognitive behavioral and interpersonal therapies are the best evidence-based type of therapy for depression.

Counseling means talking about feelings with a special healthcare provider who can help you with the relationships, thoughts, or behaviors that are causing the depression. Don't wait; ask your parents or your school counselor for help today. Medicine is used to treat more serious depression. These medications are not "uppers" and are not addictive. When depression is so bad that you can't focus on anything else, when it interferes with your life, medication might be necessary along with counseling. But most often, counseling alone works. With treatment, most depressed people start to feel better in just a few weeks.

WHAT ABOUT SUICIDE?

Most people who are depressed do not kill themselves. But depression increases the risk for suicide or suicide attempts. It is NOT true that people who talk about suicide do not attempt it. Suicidal thoughts, remarks, or attempts are ALWAYS SERIOUS ... if any of these happen to you or a friend, you must tell a responsible adult IMMEDIATELY .... It's better to be safe than sorry.

The National Suicide Prevention hotline has people available to talk to anyone who is suicidal 24 hours a day and can be reached at 1-800-273-8255.

WHY DO PEOPLE GET DEPRESSED?

Sometimes people get seriously depressed after something like a divorce in the family, major money problems, the death of someone they love, a messed-up home life, or breaking up with a boyfriend or girlfriend. Sometimes depression happens because of negative patterns of thinking so learning to turn negative thoughts to positive helps. Other times, depression just happens. Often, teens react to the pain of depression by getting into trouble: trouble with alcohol, drugs, or sex; trouble with school or bad grades; problems with family or friends. This is another reason why it's important to get treatment for depression before it leads to other trouble.

MYTHS ABOUT DEPRESSION

- MYTH: It's normal for teens to be moody; teens don't suffer from "real" depression.

  FACT: Depression is more than just being moody; and it affects people at any age.

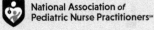

- MYTH: Telling an adult that a friend might be depressed is betraying a trust. If someone wants help, he or she will get it.

  FACT: Depression, which saps energy and self-esteem, interferes with a person's ability or wish to get help. It is an act of true friendship to share your concerns with an adult who can help. No matter what you "promised" to keep secret, your friend's life is more important than a promise.

- MYTH: Talking about depression only makes it worse.

  FACT: Talking about your feelings to someone who can help, like a psychologist or nurse practitioner, is the first step toward beating depression. Talking to a close friend also can provide you with the support and encouragement you need to talk to your parents or school counselor about getting help for depression.

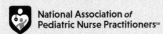

Resources for Child and Adolescent Depressive Disorders

American Academy of Child and Adolescent Psychiatry (AACAP)

www.aacap.org

This website contains information about research, legislative activities, and meetings regarding child and adolescent mental health; policy statements; clinical practice guidelines; and a directory of child and adolescent psychiatrists. It also offers a set of FACT SHEETS for families in English, Spanish, and several other languages on a variety of topics that include ADHD, bullying, depression, and suicide.

Centers for Disease Control and Prevention (CDC)

www.cdc.gov/childrensmentalhealth/data.html

Data and Statistics on Children's Mental Health (Current Prevalence and Treatment Rates)

COPE (Creating Opportunities for Personal Empowerment) for Children, Adolescents and Young Adults

The COPE Program is an evidence-based 7-session manualized cognitive behavioral skills building intervention program, based on the 12 key components of cognitive behavior therapy (CBT), which can be used for mild to moderate depression and anxiety with children, adolescents, and young adults in primary care, specialty clinics, schools, universities, and community health settings. The program can be delivered in individual, small group, classroom, or virtual formats. Healthcare providers delivering the program in primary care receive reimbursement with the 99214 CPT code. A 15-session version also is available, which contains seven CBT skills building sessions along with sessions on nutrition and physical activity for delivery by health professionals in primary care, school-based health centers and community health settings, as well as teachers in classroom settings. An on-line interactive version is available for adolescents. A workshop that can be completed on-line is required prior to delivering the COPE programs. See www.COPE2Thrive.com.

National Institute of Mental Health

www.nimh.nih.gov/health/statistics/major-depression.shtml#part_155721

This outstanding website offers multiple educational handouts on a variety of mental health disorders, including mood disorders, and links to other informative websites. This is the website page for major depression in adolescents.

Youth Depression Treatment and Prevention Group Programs

www.kpchr.org/public/acwd/acwd.html

The following downloadable evidenced-based cognitive behavioral group intervention programs for adolescents, developed by Lewinsohn, Clark, and colleagues are available free of charge. These programs were developed for use by mental health professionals with groups of adolescents who are depressed or at risk for future depression.

- The Adolescent Coping with Depression [CWD-A] Course. This is an evidence-based treatment intervention for actively depressed adolescents. The program also includes a separate intervention for the parents of these depressed adolescents.

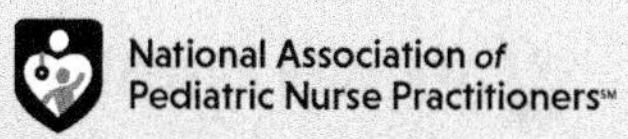

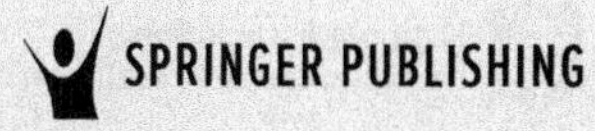

- The Adolescent Coping with Stress [CWS] Course. This is an evidence-based group prevention intervention for youth at risk for future depression.
- A brief, individual treatment program (five to nine sessions) for depressed youth who also are receiving SSRI antidepressant medication is available.

The REACH Institute

www.thereachinstitute.org/

The REACH Institute is dedicated to improving the mental health of American children and adolescents with emotional and behavioral challenges. It provides workshops for healthcare providers that teach the best evidence-based therapies, from psychotherapy to pharmacology, to improve the mental health of children and teens. Excellent resources at the website are available for healthcare providers, agencies, and families.

U.S. Preventive Services Task Force

www.ahrq.gov/clinic/uspstfix.htm

www.uspreventiveservicestaskforce.org/uspstf/recommendation/depression-in-children-and-adolescents-screening

The U.S. Preventive Services Task Force (USPSTF) is an independent group of national experts in prevention and evidence-based practice that works to improve the health of all Americans by making evidence-based recommendations about clinical preventive services such as screenings, counseling services, or preventive medications. The USPSTF is made up of 16 volunteer members from the fields of preventive medicine and primary care, including internal medicine, family medicine, pediatrics, behavioral health, obstetrics/gynecology, and nursing.

Suicide Prevention Resource Center

sprc.org/

(800)-273-TALK

Patient Safety Plan Template: sprc.org/resources-programs/patient-safety-plan-template

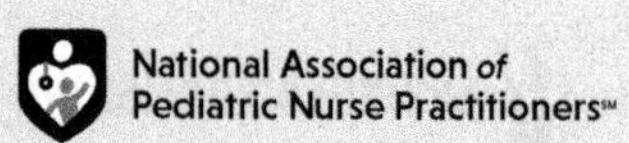

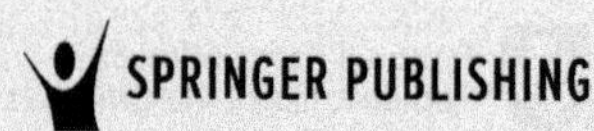

PATIENT SAFETY PLAN TEMPLATE

Step 1: Warning signs (thoughts, images, mood, situation, behavior) that a crisis may be developing:

1. ______________________________

2. ______________________________

3. ______________________________

Step 2: Internal coping strategies: Things I can do to take my mind off my problems without contacting another person (relaxation technique, physical activity):

1. ______________________________

2. ______________________________

3. ______________________________

Step 3: People and social settings that provide distraction:

1. Name ____________________ Phone ____________________

2. Name ____________________ Phone ____________________

3. Place ____________________

4. Place ____________________

Step 4: People whom I can ask for help:

1. Name ____________________ Phone ____________________

2. Name ____________________ Phone ____________________

3. Name ____________________ Phone ____________________

Step 5: Professionals or agencies I can contact during a crisis:

1. Clinician Name ____________________ Phone ____________________

Clinician Pager or Emergency Contact # ____________________

2. Clinician Name ____________________ Phone ____________________

Clinician Pager or Emergency Contact # ____________________

3. Local Urgent Care Services ____________________

Urgent Care Services Address ____________________

Urgent Care Services Phone ____________________

4. Suicide Prevention Lifeline Phone: 1-800-273-TALK (8255)

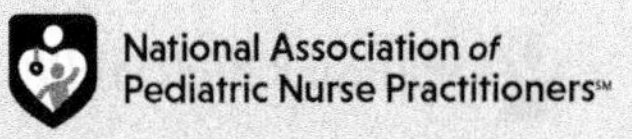

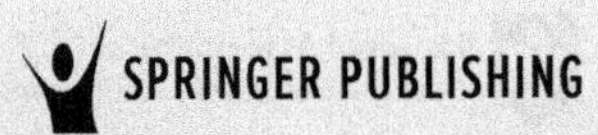

Step 6: Making the environment safe:

1. ______________________________

2. ______________________________

The one thing that is most important to me and worth living for is:

____

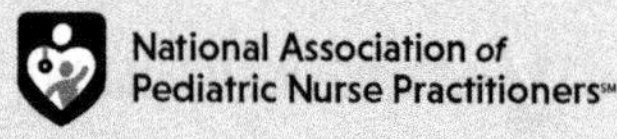

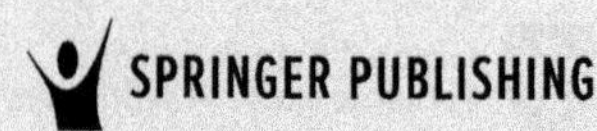

CHAPTER 5

Ann Guthery

Evidence-Based Assessment and Management of Attention Deficit Hyperactivity Disorder (ADHD)

FAST FACTS

- ADHD is the most common chronic behavior disorder in children.
- ADHD is present in 4% to 12% of school-age children.
- Worldwide, it is estimated to affect 5% of children.
- ADHD is more common in males than in females (3–6:1).
- It typically presents during early childhood, before 7 years of age, although changes in the *DSM-5* have noted that most lifetime cases are captured with an onset of age 12 to 14.
- The disorder involves a persistent pattern of inattention, hyperactivity, and impulsiveness, or all three.
- Children with ADHD often have comorbid disorders (e.g., anxiety disorders, depressive disorders, learning disorders, and oppositional defiant disorder) (Posner et al., 2020).

Co-Morbidities Important for Assessment

- specific learning disabilities (10%–40%);
- oppositional defiant disorder (30%–60%);
- depression/anxiety disorders;
- post-traumatic stress disorder (PTSD);
- bipolar disorder;
- fetal alcohol syndrome;
- substance abuse disorders;
- tourette's disorder; and
- psychosocial morbidities.

Mimics of ADHD

- language disorder;
- learning disability;
- anxiety/obsessive compulsive disorder;
- PTSD;
- depressive and bipolar disorders;

- oppositional defiant disorder;
- iron deficiency anemia;
- malnutrition;
- side effects of medication;
- substance abuse;
- sleep disorder;
- child abuse/neglect;
- stressful home environment;
- parenting problem;
- parental psychopathology; and
- inadequate educational setting.

Medical Conditions Associated With ADHD

- seizure disorder,
- thyroid disorder,
- traumatic brain injury,
- fetal alcohol syndrome, and
- lead poisoning.

Testing to Be Considered

- vision;
- hearing;
- CBC with differential (to rule out anemia);
- TSH, FT4 (to rule out thyroid disorders);
- lead screen;
- genetic screen;
- toxicology screen;
- functional MRI suggests impaired function of the prefrontal cortex, striatum, and cerebellum, but are not fully elucidated; and
- EKG to rule out cardiac conditions before starting a stimulant medication.

Rating Scales

Rating scales (e.g., the Vanderbilt, Clinical Attention Profile, SNAP IV) can be a useful adjunct in the diagnosis of ADHD and in the monitoring of response to treatment. The Swan is another tool that can be used to determine strengths, weaknesses, and symptoms of ADHD and normal behaviors. Other helpful tools for ADHD can be downloaded as part of the National Initiative for Children's Healthcare Quality and the American Academy of Pediatrics' toolkit at www.nichq.org/resources/toolkit.

Multiple Sources of Information

Information from parents, the child, teachers, primary care providers, and other caretakers is important for diagnostic consideration.

Referral and Collaboration

It is important to refer a child with ADHD to a mental health provider when the condition has not improved in 3 months or if other comorbid conditions exist (e.g., anxiety disorder, oppositional defiant disorder).

Psycho-Education and Follow-up

Psycho-education with the child, parents, and teachers is important as part of the management strategy. Careful follow-up is imperative, especially in monitoring initial response to medication therapy (Chang et al., 2020).

Psychosocial Therapies

In the latest American Academy of Pediatrics Clinical Practice Guideline for ADHD in Children and Adolescents (Wolraich et al., 2019), behavioral therapy is recommended as the first-line treatment for preschoolers. Behavioral therapy is defined as: "parent training in behavioral management."

For school-age children, stimulant medications methylphenidate and amphetamines in their various forms are the initial treatment (Steele & Roberts, 2020).

DSM-5 Diagnostic Criteria for Attention Deficit Hyperactivity Disorder

The *DSM-5* criteria are divided into two sections. The first section addresses persistent patterns of inattention and the second section focuses on hyperactivity-impulsivity. Both sections assess for interference in functioning or development:

- **Inattention:** The following list of symptoms are associated with inattentive type attention deficit disorder (ADD). For young children usually six symptoms are present and for older adolescents and adults five symptoms are present. The symptoms are persistent and have been experienced for at least 6 months. Children with these difficulties have had disturbances in how they met developmental tasks and function in social/academic and work situations. **Note:** Inattentive ADD symptoms aren't due to the child's oppositional or defiant behaviors, or an inability to understand directions for tasks:
  - Makes careless mistakes or does not pay attention to details.
  - Difficult sustaining attention.
  - Does not seem to listen.
  - Does not follow through on things.
  - Has difficulty organizing tasks and activities.
  - Avoids things that requires sustained mental effort.
  - Lose things.
  - Are distracted.
  - Are forgetful.
- **Hyperactivity and impulsivity:** Six or more of the following symptoms that have persisted for at least 6 months (for older adolescents age 17 years and older, five symptoms) and have negatively impacted developmental level and interfered with social, academic and/or work/occupational functioning. **Note:** The symptoms aren't due to the child's oppositional or defiant behaviors, or an inability to understand directions for tasks:
  - Not able to sit still.
  - Leaves seat in situations when being seated is expected.
  - Runs about or climbs in situations where it is inappropriate.

- Is unable to be quiet.
- Is restless and "on the go."
- Talks excessively.
- Blurts out answers.
- Is impatient and not able to wait turn.
- Interrupts or intrudes.

Specify if the child has an (1) inattentive presentation, (2) hyperactive/impulsive presentation, or (3) combined inattentive and hyperactive/ impulsive presentation.

Pharmacotherapy treatments for children and adolescents with ADHD are detailed in Table 5.1.

Table 5.1. Pharmacotherapy Treatments of Children and Adolescents with ADHD: Initial Dose, Kinetics, and Side Effects

Drug	Dose	Kinetics	Side Effects/Comments
Methylphenidate HCl: short acting (Ritalin/Methylin) 5-, 10-, 20-mg tablets	Start: 0.3 mg/kg/dose or 2.5–5 mg before 8:00 AM and 12:00 noon. May increase by 0.1 mg/kg/dose weekly up to 0.3; until 1.0 mg/kg/dose is reached. Maximum dose is 2 mg/kg/24 hrs or 80 mg/24 hrs. Not recommended for children <5 years	Onset: 30 min Peak: 1.9 hrs Duration: 4–6 hrs	Nervousness, insomnia, anorexia, weight loss, decreased height velocity, tics, stomachaches, headaches. Use with caution with underlying seizure disorder. Contraindicated: Monoamine oxidase inhibitors (MAOIs). Monitor height, weight, blood pressure. Avoid caffeine and decongestants. Avoid doses after 4:00 PM. Consider drug holidays. Also avoid taking stimulants with citrus drinks as it can inactivate them.
Methylphenidate HCl: intermediate acting (Ritalin-SR, Metadate ER, Methylin ER) 10-, 20-mg tablets	Starting dose: 10 mg QD Maximum dose: 80 mg/day	Onset: 30–90 min Peak: 4.7 hrs Duration: 8 hrs	Do not crush or chew tablets. See comments for methylphenidate.

(continued)

Table 5.1. Pharmacotherapy Treatments of Children and Adolescents with ADHD: Initial Dose, Kinetics, and Side Effects (*continued*)

Drug	Dose	Kinetics	Side Effects/Comments
Methylphenidate HCl: long acting (Metadate CD, 20-mg tablets) (Concerta, 18-, 36-, 54-mg tablets) (Daytrana Patch, 10 mg, 15 mg, 20 mg, 30 mg) (Quillivant XR liquid 25 mg/5 mL) (Quilivant chewable tabs 20 mg) (Aptensio - 10 mg capsules) Jornay is a newer medication that is given at night and helps when AM routines are challenging; it continues to work throughout the day.	Starting dose: 20 mg QD or 18 mg for Concerta Maximum dose: 80 mg/day of Metadate or 54 mg/day of Concerta Starting dose for Daytrana is 10 mg max dose 30 mg Quillavant can start at 2 mL = 10 mg to max dose of 12 mL = 60 mg per day Jornay can start at 20 mg with doses not to exceed 100 mg. Recommendation give dose at 8 PM, but could be given between 6:30–9:30 PM	Onset: 30–90 min Peak: 4.7 hrs Duration: 8–12 hrs Leave patch on for 9 hours and it will still work up to 12 hrs Jornay onset 10–12 hrs and then last an additional 10–12 hrs	Do not crush or chew tablets. Exception is the Quillavant chewable tablets. See comments for methylphenidate. Adhesive may cause skin irritation with the patch, use of olive oil to remove adhesive or use of a cortisone cream can help with irritation.
Dextroamphetamine: short acting (Dexedrine, Dextrostat) 5-, 10-, 15-mg tablets, 5 mg/mL elixir	3–5 years: 2.5 mg/24 hrs every morning. Increase by 2.5 mg/24 hrs weekly ≥6 years: 5 mg/24 hrs every morning. Increase by 5 mg/24 hrs at weekly intervals Maximum dose: 40 mg/24 hrs	Onset: 20–60 min Peak: 2 hrs Duration: 4–6 hrs	See comments for methylphenidate. Medication should generally not be used <5 years because ADHD diagnosis should be made only with specialist consultation.
Dextroamphetamine: intermediate acting (Adderall, Dexedrine Spansule) 5-, 10-, 15-, 20-mg tablets	3–5 years: 2.5–5 mg QD or 0.3 mg/kg/dose. Increase by 2.5–5 mg every week ≥6 years: 5 mg/24 hrs. QD or 0.3 mg/kg/dose Maximum dose: 40 mg/24 hrs	Onset: 30–90 min Peak: 6–8 hrs	See comments for methylphenidate.

(*continued*)

Table 5.1. Pharmacotherapy Treatments of Children and Adolescents with ADHD: Initial Dose, Kinetics, and Side Effects (*continued*)

Drug	Dose	Kinetics	Side Effects/Comments
Dextroamphetamine: long acting (Adderall XR) (5, 10, 15, 20, 25, 30 mg) (Vyvanse 20, 30, 40, 50, 60, 70 mg) (Adzenys XR 6.3–12.5 mg) (Mydayis 12.5–24 mg)	≥6 years Starting dose: 5 mg QD for Adderall XR or 0.3 mg/kg/dose Maximum dose: 40 mg/24 hrs For Vyvanse starting dose is 20 mg to max of 70 mg	Onset: 30–90 min Duration: >8 hrs Often Vyvanse can last for 12–13 hrs	See comments for methylphenidate. Adderall XR has long and short acting beads in the capsule. Vyvanse is a pro-drug and is not active until L-lysine interacts with it in the intestinal tract.

Note: Stimulants work best when given regularly. Adjust dose of stimulant medication as the child grows.

There is a risk of abuse with stimulants.

Caution: Use stimulants cautiously in children with marked anxiety, tension, or agitation since these symptoms may be aggravated. Stimulants are contraindicated in children with motor tics or with a family history or diagnosis of Tourette's syndrome, although comorbid diagnosis of ADHD and Tourette's syndrome is rare. Avoid giving nasal decongestants with stimulants.

Adapted from Stahl, S. M. (2021). *Essential psychopharmacology prescribers guide*. Cambridge University Press; Wilens, T. E., & Hammerness, P. G. (2016). *Straight talk about psychiatric medications for kids* (4th ed.). The Guilford Press.

NON-STIMULANTS USED TO TREAT ADHD

Strattera (Atomoxetine HCL)

Doses: 10, 18, 25, 40, 60, 80, and 100 mg. Starting dose is 0.5 mg/kg/day and titrate up 1.5 mg/kg/day

Can take 2 to 4 weeks to see results

Common side effects include upset stomach, decreased appetite, nausea or vomiting, dizziness, tiredness and mood swings.

If a patient has serious heart problems, Strattera should be avoided as it could make increases in heart rate and blood pressure worse.

Strattera can cause liver injury in some patients.

There is a Black Box warning stating: In some children and teens, Strattera increased the risk of suicidal thoughts or actions. Results from Strattera clinical studies with over 2,200 child or teenage ADHD patients suggest that some children and teenagers may have a higher chance of having suicidal thoughts or actions. Although no suicides occurred in these studies, four out of every 1,000 patients developed suicidal thoughts.

Intuniv (Guanfacine)

Doses: 1, 2, 3, 4 mg. Starting dose is 1 mg to a maximum dose of 4 mg.

Intuniv should be swallowed whole with liquid, without crushing, chewing, or breaking the tablet. Intuniv should not be taken with a high-fat meal. Regular checks of the child's blood pressure and heart rate are recommended.

Serious side effects can include low blood pressure and low heart rate. Medicine needs to be tapered as withdrawal symptoms could occur including increased blood pressure, headache, increased heart rate, and lightheadedness.

Common side effects include sleepiness, tiredness, trouble sleeping, low blood pressure, nausea, stomach pain, and dizziness.

Intuniv can be used alone or in combination with a stimulant. One 9-week study included 455 children who were on a stable stimulant dose for at least 4 weeks and had some improvement, but still had ADHD symptoms. These children then took either Intuniv or a placebo with their stimulant. Researchers saw a 30% improvement in the ADHD symptoms when Intuniv was added as compared to placebo.

Immediate release guanfacine can also be used, but it is not FDA approved for ADHD.

Doses: 1 to 4 mg; can be started as low as 0.25 mg when cutting the pills. Side effects from immediate release guanfacine are the same as listed for Intuniv, but at times can be more sedating. Can be helpful for poor impulse and frustration control.

Kapvay (Clonidine HCL)

Doses: 0.1, 0.2 mg. Starting dose is 0.1 mg QHS, titrate to 0.1 mg BID to a max dose of 0.1 mg QAM and 0.2 mg QHS.

Kapvay should be swallowed whole with liquid, without crushing, chewing, or breaking the tablet. Regular checks of the child's blood pressure and heart rate are recommended. It can be taken with and without food.

Serious side effects include low blood pressure and low heart rate.

Common side effects include sleepiness, tiredness, cough, sneezing, runny nose, sore throat, stuffy nose, irritability, trouble sleeping, nightmares, change in mood, constipation, increased body temperature, dry mouth, ear pain.

Suddenly stopping Kapvay may cause withdrawal symptoms, including increased blood pressure, headache, increased heart rate, lightheadedness, tightness in the chest, and nervousness.

Immediate release clonidine also can be used, but it is not approved for ADHD.

Doses: 0.003 to 0.005 mg/kg/day PO in divided doses from BID-QID.

Side effects for Clonidine are the same as listed for Kapvay, but at times, it can be more sedating; it can be helpful for poor impulse and frustration control.

Other nonstimulant medications that can be used second and third line include Wellbutrin, Imipramine and Provigil. These are not FDA approved for children and, if needed, should be prescribed by a psychiatric provider but are listed here for additional information.

Adapted from Eli Lilly and Company, Shire Inc. and Shionogi, Inc; Stahl, S. M. (2020). *Essential psychophamacology prescribers guide*. Cambridge University Press; Wilens, T. E., & Hammerness, P.G. (2016). *straight talk about Psychiatric medications for kids* (4th ed.). The Guilford Press.

Additional Management

It is important for families to know that ADHD is a psychiatric disorder with biological underpinnings that are not the child's fault. When caregivers understand that the child's difficulty in completing schoolwork, paying attending sitting still, or behaving in other ways as desired is not just the child being lazy or oppositional.

Putting the child's energy to productive use pays off. Physical activity can help with ADHD symptoms and should become a part of the family routine when possible.

Children with ADHD are likely to have more difficulty getting and staying organized than their same-aged peers and will need more help as a result. Organizational aids, structure, and accountability can be helpful.

Capitalize on existing pro-social and supportive relationships to support self-esteem. Encourage families to catch the youth doing good things as often these children receive frequent criticism and redirections.

Individual, family therapy, pharmacotherapy or some combination may be warranted. Often because of worries or stress due to side effects, stigma, or cultural experiences families may not want these services. It is important to listen to the family's concerns and provide information that is open, accurate, and clear.

Educating families and caregivers on topics such as giving concise, clear, and concrete directions to the child and having eye contact is helpful. Telling children that are hyper to stop may not be as effective as finding ways to redirect the energy into a preferable behavior.

Encourage a comprehensive assessment that can include psychological testing to rule out learning disorders or other comorbid disorders.

Make sure parents are aware of their rights for 504 plans and Individualized Education Plans (IEPs) and having good communication with the school for accommodations and to help with academic progression.

Caring for a child with ADHD can be stressful. Encouraging parents and caregivers to manage their own anxiety, depression or ADHD will benefit the child.

Adapted from Vinson, S. Y. (Ed.). (2018). *Pediatric mental health for primary care providers*. Springer International Publishing. Chapter 12.

NAPNAP has created an excellent resource that will help teens and families answer common questions about ADHD. View a variety of patient/provider scenarios that answer questions about ADHD. Check out these valuable resources on YouTube with the links provided:

- ADHD Conversations: Introduction
- ADHD Conversations: Symptoms
- ADHD Conversations: Medications: How They Work
- ADHD Conversations: Medication Dosing
- ADHD Conversations: Medication in School
- ADHD Conversations: School Accommodations for ADHD
- ADHD Conversations: Medication Holidays
- ADHD Conversations: Medication Management in College
- ADHD Conversations: Driving and ADHD
- ADHD Conversations: Bullying and ADHD
- ADHD Conversations: Emergency Scenarios

Adapted from the https://www.napnap.org/behavioral-and-mental-health-resources/

REFERENCES

Chang, J. G., Cimion, F. M., & Gossa, W. (2020). ADHD in children: Common questions and answers. *American Family Physician*, *102*(10), 592–602.

Posner, J., Polanczyk, G. V., & Sonuga-Barke, E. (2020). Attention-deficit hyperactivity disorder review. *Lancet*, *395*(10222), 450–462. https://doi.org/10.1016/S0140-6736(19)33004-1

Stahl, S. M. (2021). *Essential psychopharmacology prescribers guide*. Cambridge University Press.

Steele, R. G., & Roberts, M. C. (Eds.). (2020). *Handbook of evidence-based therapies for children and adolescents*. Springer Publishing Company.

Vinson, S. Y., & Vinson, E. S. (Eds.). (2018). *Pediatric mental health for primary care providers*. Springer Publishing Company.

Wilens T. E., & Hammerness, P. G. (Ed.). (2016). *Straight talk about psychiatric medications for kids*. The Guilford Press.

Wolraich, M. L., Hagan, J. F., Allen, C., Chan, E., Davison, D., Earls, M., Evans, S. W., Flinn, S. K., Froehlich, T., Frost, J., Holbrook, J. R., Lehrman, C. U., Lessin, H. R., Okechukwu, K., Pierce, K. L., Winner, J. D., & Zurhellen, W. (2019). Subcommittee on children and adolescents with attention-deficit /hyperactivity disorder. Clinical practice guidelines for the diagnosis, evaluation and treatment of attention-deficit/hyperactivity disorder in children and adolescents. *Pediatrics*, *144*(4), e20192528. https://doi.org/10.1542/peds.2019-2528

Screening Tools for ADHD
The National Initiative for Children's Healthcare Quality (NICHQ)
Vanderbilt Assessment Scale for ADHD-Teacher as Initial Informant
(M. Wolraich et al.)

DESCRIPTION

The National Initiative for Children's Healthcare Quality (NICHQ) and American Academy of Pediatrics (AAP) have sponsored a set of tools for evaluating children with ADHD developed at Vanderbilt University. The initial evaluation scale monitors 43 symptoms for ADHD and other disorders and school performance as reported by a teacher.

PARAMETERS

(1) Symptoms (35)

(2) Performance (8) - academic (3) and classroom behavioral (5)

SYMPTOMS

(1) Fails to give attention to details or makes careless mistakes in schoolwork.

(2) Has difficulty sustaining attention to tasks or activities.

(3) Does not seem to listen when spoken to directly.

(4) Does not follow through on instructions and fails to finish schoolwork (not due to oppositional behavior or failure to misunderstand).

(5) Has difficulty organizing tasks and activities.

(6) Avoids, dislikes, or is reluctant to engage in tasks that require sustained mental effort.

(7) Loses things necessary for tasks or activities (e.g., school assignments, pencils, books).

(8) Is easily distracted by extraneous stimuli.

(9) Is forgetful in daily activities.

(10) Fidgets with hands or feet or squirms in seat.

(11) Leaves seat in classroom or in other situations in which remaining seated is expected.

(12) Runs about or climbs excessively in situations in which remaining seated is expected.

(13) Has difficulty playing or engaging in leisure activities quietly.

(14) Is "on the go" or often acts as if "driven by a motor."

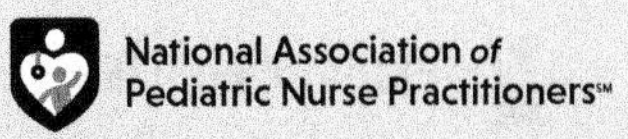

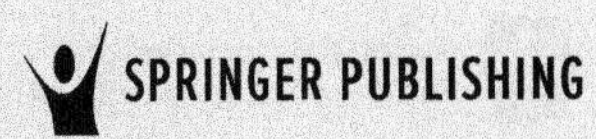

(15) Talks excessively.
(16) Blurts out answers before questions have been completed.
(17) Has difficulty waiting in line.
(18) Interrupts or intrudes on others (butts into conversations or games).
(19) Loses temper.
(20) Actively defies or refuses to comply with adults' requests or rules.
(21) Is angry or resentful.
(22) Is spiteful and vindictive.
(23) Bullies, threatens, or intimidates others.
(24) Initiates physical fights.
(25) Lies to obtain goods for favors or to avoid obligations ("cons" others).
(26) Is physically cruel to people.
(27) Has stolen items of nontrivial value.
(28) Deliberately destroys others' property.
(29) Is fearful, anxious, or worried.
(30) Is self-conscious and easily embarrassed.
(31) Is afraid to try new things for fear of making mistakes.
(32) Feels worthless or inferior.
(33) Blames self for problems; feels guilty.
(34) Feels lonely, unwanted, or unloved; complains that "no one loves him or her."
(35) Is sad, unhappy, or depressed.

Symptoms	Points
Never	0
Occasionally	1
Often	2
Very often	3

ACADEMIC PERFORMANCE

(1) Reading,
(2) Mathematics, and
(3) Written expression.

CLASSROOM BEHAVIORAL PERFORMANCE

(1) Relationship with peers,
(2) Following directions,

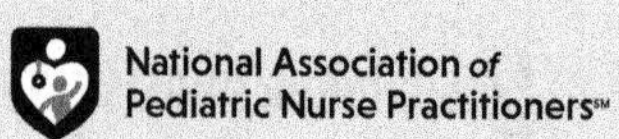

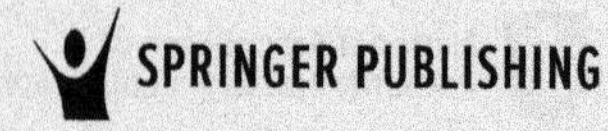

(3) Disrupting classes,
(4) Assignment completion, and
(5) Organizational skills.

Performance Responses	Points
Excellent	1
Above average	2
Average	3
Somewhat of a problem	4
Problematic	5

TALLIES

(1) Total questions answered 2 or 3 in symptom questions 1 to 9.
(2) Total questions answered 2 or 3 in symptom questions 10 to 18.
(3) Total questions answered 2 or 3 in symptom questions 19 to 28.
(4) Total questions answered 2 or 3 in symptom questions 29 to 35.
(5) Total questions answered 4 or 5 in performance questions 1 to 8.

Total symptom score for questions 1 to 18 = SUM (points for symptoms questions 1 to 18); average performance score = SUM (points for all eight performance questions)/8

Diagnosis	Symptom Questions	Performance Questions
Predominantly inattentive subtype ADHD	Score ≥2 in 6 of 9 from questions 1 to 9	Score 4 or 5 on ≥1
Predominantly hyperactive impulsive ADHD	Score ≥2 in 6 of 9 from questions 10 to 18	Score 4 or 5 on ≥1
ADHD-combined inattention hyperactivity	Score ≥2 in 6 of 9 from questions 1 to 9 AND 6 of 9 from questions 10 to 18	Score 4 or 5 on ≥1
Oppositional defiant/conduct disorder screen	Score ≥2 in 3 of 10 from questions 19 to 28	Score 4 or 5 on ≥1
Anxiety/depression screen	Score ≥2 in 3 of 7 from questions 29 to 35	Score 4 or 5 on ≥1

Source: The National Initiative for Children's Healthcare Quality (NICHQ) Vanderbilt Assessment Scales. Available at http://www.uacap.org/clinicians-toolkit.html

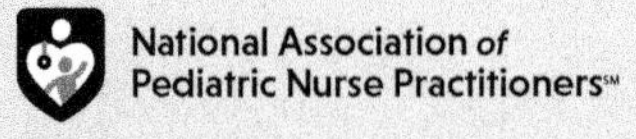

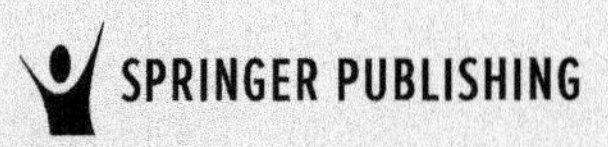

Swanson, Nolan, and Pelham (SNAP-IV-C) (Swanson et al.)

The *Swanson, Nolan, and Pelham Scales-IV Revised (SNAP IV-C)* is an instrument that uses observer ratings and self-report ratings to help assess ADHD and evaluate problem behavior in children and adolescents. The CRS-R instruments are used for routine screenings in schools, mental health clinics, residential treatment centers, pediatric offices, juvenile detention facilities, child protective agencies, and outpatient settings.

INSTRUMENT(S) DESCRIPTION

SNAP IV-Teacher and Parent Rating Scale

The SNAP IV-C contains 90 items. It is typically used with teachers and parents or caregivers when comprehensive information and *DSM-IV* consideration are required.

Scales include:

- Oppositional disorder
- Conduct disorder
- Intermittent explosive disorder
- Stereotypic movement disorder
- Cognitive problems/inattention
- Hyperactivity
- Anxious/shy
- PTSD
- OCD
- Perfectionism
- Narcolepsy
- Personality disorders (histrionic, narcissistic, and borderline)
- Social problems
- Adjustment disorder
- Psychosomatic
- Depression
- Dysthmia
- Mania
- Conners' Global Index
- *DSM-IV* Symptom Subscales
- ADHD Index

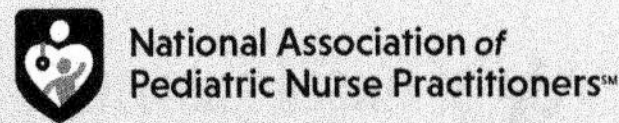

James M. Swanson, PhD., University of California, Irvine, California

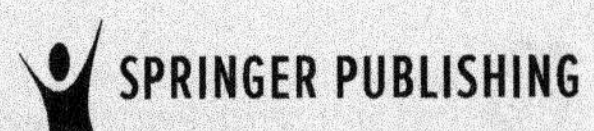

SAMPLE ITEMS

The SNAP-IV-C provides a series of statements that the parent or teacher responds to regarding the child's behavior for the past month. The response is in a Likert type format, using the following categories:

- Not true at all (Never, Seldom).
- Just a little true (Occasionally).
- Pretty much true (Often, Quite a bit).
- Very much true (Very often, Very frequent).

SCORING

The first nine items for the SNAP-IV-C cover inattention symptoms of ADHD. Examples of questions are listed below. A score of 18 or more shows inattention.

1. Makes careless mistakes.
2. Can't pay attention.
3. Doesn't listen.
4. Fails to finish work.
5. Disorganized.
6. Can't concentrate.
7. Loses things.
8. Distractible.
9. Forgetful.

The next nine questions focus on hyperactivity and impulsivity. A score of 18 or more shows hyperactivity.

Questions 19 to 26 focus on ODD and a score of 18 or more shows ODD symptoms.

The remainder of the questions lets you know if there may be comorbid issues along with ADHD that should be explored. For example, if Questions 66 to 73 were scored 2 or higher there may be symptoms of depression. Or if Questions 51 to 56 were scored 2 or higher then there may be anxiety.

VALIDITY/NORMS

The SNAP was originally developed with the *DSM-III* and has done revisions with *DSM-IV* and has been used in numerous ADHD and genetic clinical trials. It has shown excellent internal consistency, but data on norms for age and gender have been sparse. One study (Bussing et al., 2008) looked at over 12,000 kindergarten to fifth grade students in a north central Florida public school district during the 1998 **to** 1999 school year. The SNAP was given to both teachers and parents. Reliability for parent ratings and teacher ratings showed statistical significance ($p < .001$). The findings did not suggest a difference based on age, gender, or race, but did state that this school district was known for high poverty rates and limited diversity.

ADMINISTER TO

For the SNAP-IV-C: Parents and teachers of children and adolescents ages 5 to 17.

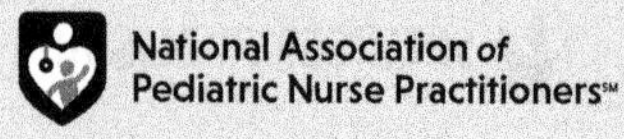

James M. Swanson, PhD., University of California, Irvine, California

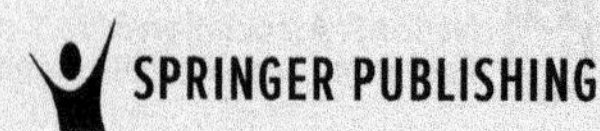

SNAP-IV-C Rating Scale

Child's name: ____________________ Gender______ Age: _____ Grade: ______Date: _________

Ethnicity (check one that best applies) African American Asian Caucasian Hispanic Other ___________________

Completed by: ____________________ Type of class: ________________ Class size: ___________

For each of the 90 items, check the column that best describes this child.

Items		Not at all	Just a little	Quite a bit	Very much
1.	Often fails to give close attention to details or makes careless mistakes in schoolwork, work, or other activities.				
2.	Often has difficulty sustaining attention in tasks or play activities.				
3.	Often does not seem to listen when spoken to directly.				
4.	Often does not follow through on instructions and fails to finish schoolwork, chores, or duties.				
5.	Often has difficulty organizing tasks and activities.				
6.	Often avoids, dislikes, or is reluctant to engage in tasks that require sustained mental effort (e.g., schoolwork or homework).				
7.	Often loses things necessary for tasks or activities (e.g., toys, school assignments, pencils, books, or tools).				
8.	Often is distracted by extraneous stimuli.				
9.	Often is forgetful in daily activities.				
10.	Often has difficulty maintaining alertness, orienting to requests, or executing directions.				
11.	Often fidgets with hands or feet or squirms in seat.				
12.	Often leaves seat in classroom or in other situations in which remaining in seat is expected.				
13.	Often runs about or climbs excessively in situations in which it is inappropriate.				
14.	Often has difficulty playing or engaging in leisure activities quietly.				

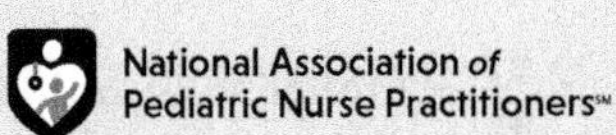

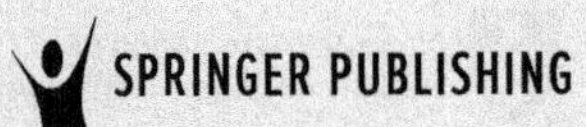

Items		Not at all	Just a little	Quite a bit	Very much
15.	Often is "on the go" or often acts as if "driven by a motor."				
16.	Often talks excessively.				
17.	Often blurts out answers before questions have been completed.				
18.	Often has difficulty awaiting turn.				
19	Often interrupts or intrudes on others (e.g., butts into conversations/games.				
20.	Often has difficulty sitting still, being quiet, or inhibiting impulses in the classroom or at home.				
21.	Often loses temper.				
22.	Often argues with adults.				
23.	Often actively defies or refuses adult requests or rules.				
24.	Often deliberately does things that annoy other people				
25.	Often blames others for his or her mistakes or misbehavior.				
26.	Often touchy or easily annoyed by others.				
27.	Often is angry and resentful.				
28.	Often is spiteful or vindictive.				
29.	Often is quarrelsome.				
30.	Often is negative, defiant, disobedient, or hostile toward authority figures.				
31.	Often makes noises (e.g., humming or odd sounds).				
32.	Often is excitable and impulsive.				
33.	Often cries easily.				
34.	Often is uncooperative.				
35.	Often acts "smart."				
36.	Often is restless or overactive.				
37.	Often disturbs other children.				
38.	Often changes mood quickly and drastically.				
39.	Often easily frustrated if demands are not met immediately.				

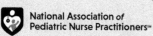

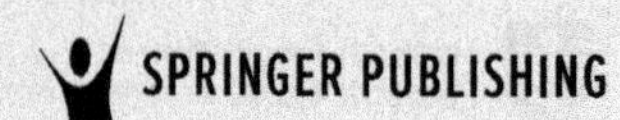

Items		Not at all	Just a little	Quite a bit	Very much
40.	Often teases other children and interferes with their activities.				
41.	Often is aggressive to other children (e.g., picks fights or bullies).				
42.	Often is destructive with property of others (e.g., vandalism).				
43.	Often is deceitful (e.g., steals, lies, forges, copies the work of others, or "cons").				
44.	Often and seriously violates rules (e.g., is truant, runs away, or completely ignores class rules).				
45.	Has persistent pattern of violating the basic rights of others or major societal norms.				
46.	Has episodes of failure to resist aggressive impulses (to assault others or to destroy property).				
47.	Has motor or verbal tics (sudden, rapid, recurrent, non-rhythmic motor, or verbal activity).				
48.	Has repetitive motor behavior (e.g., hand waving, body rocking, or picking at skin).				
49.	Has obsessions (a persistent and intrusive inappropriate ideas, thoughts, or impulses).				
50.	Has compulsions (repetitive behaviors or mental acts to reduce anxiety or distress).				
51.	Often is restless or seems keyed up or on edge.				
52.	Often is easily fatigued.				
53.	Often has difficulty concentrating (mind goes blank).				
54.	Often is irritable.				
55.	Often has muscle tension.				
56.	Often has excessive anxiety and worry (e.g., apprehensive expectations).				
57.	Often has daytime sleepiness (unintended sleeping in inappropriate situations).				
58.	Often has excessive emotionality and attention-seeking behavior.				
59.	Often has need for undue admiration, grandiose behavior, or lack of empathy.				

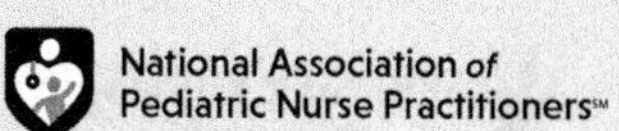

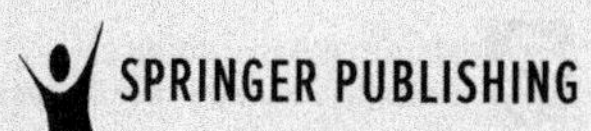

Items		Not at all	Just a little	Quite a bit	Very much
60.	Often has instability in relationships with others, reactive mood, and impulsivity.				
61.	Sometimes, for at least a week, has inflated self-esteem or grandiosity.				
62.	Sometimes, for at least a week, is more talkative than usual or seems pressured to keep talking.				
63.	Sometimes, for at least a week, has flight of ideas or says that thoughts are racing.				
64.	Sometimes, for at least a week, has elevated, expansive or euphoric mood.				
65.	Sometimes, for at least a week, is excessively involved in pleasurable but risky activities.				
66.	Sometimes, for at least 2 weeks, has depressed mood (sad, hopeless, and discouraged).				
67.	Sometimes, for at least 2 weeks, has irritable or cranky mood (not just when frustrated).				
68.	Sometimes, for at least 2 weeks, has markedly diminished interest or pleasure in most activities.				
69.	Sometimes, for at least 2 weeks, has psychomotor agitation (even more active than usual).				
70.	Sometimes, for at least 2 weeks, has psychomotor retardation (slowed down in most activities).				
71.	Sometimes, for at least 2 weeks, is fatigued or has loss of energy.				
72.	Sometimes, for at least 2 weeks, has feelings of worthlessness or excessive, inappropriate guilt.				
73.	Sometimes, for at least 2 weeks, has diminished ability to think or concentrate.				
74.	Chronic low self-esteem most of the time for at least a year.				
75.	Chronic poor concentration or difficulty making decsisions most of the time for at least a year.				
76.	Chronic feelings of hopelessness most of the time for at least a year.				
77.	Currently is hypervigilant (overly watchful or alert) or has exaggerated startle response.				

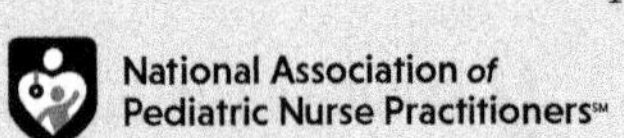

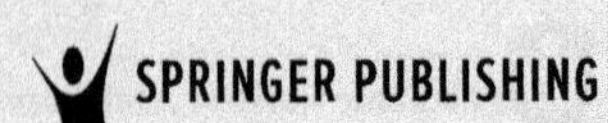

Items		Not at all	Just a little	Quite a bit	Very much
78.	Currently is irritable, has anger outbursts, or has difficulty concentrating.				
79.	Currently has an emotional (e.g., nervous, worried, hopeless, tearful) response to stress.				
80.	Currently has a behavioral (e.g., fighting, vandalism, truancy) response to stress.				
81.	Has difficulty getting started on classroom assignments.				
82.	Has difficulty staying on task for an entire classroom period.				
83.	Has problems in completion of work on classroom assignments.				
84.	Has problems in accuracy or neatness of written work in the classroom.				
85.	Has difficulty attending to a group classroom activity or discussion.				
86.	Has difficulty making transitions to the next topic or classroom period.				
87.	Has problems in interactions with peers in the classroom.				
88.	Has problems in interactions with staff (teacher or aide).				
89.	Has difficulty remaining quiet according to classroom rules.				
90.	Has difficulty staying seated according to classroom rules.				
	Sections below are to be completed by healthcare provider. The following are items that make up various subscales. First four rows provide the cut-offs for ADHD and ODD subscales. See instructions below for further information.	Sum of Items for Each Scale	Average Rating per Item for Each Scale	Teacher 5% Cutoff	Parent 5% Cutoff
	Average score for ADHD-inattention (items 1–9)			2.56	1.78
	Average score for ADHD-hyperactivity-impulsivity (items 11–19).			1.78	1.44
	Average score for ADHD-combined type (items 1–9 and 11–19).			2.00	1.67
	Average score for oppositional items (sum of items 21–28).			1.38	1.88

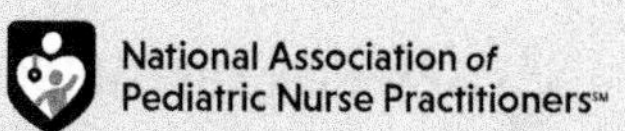

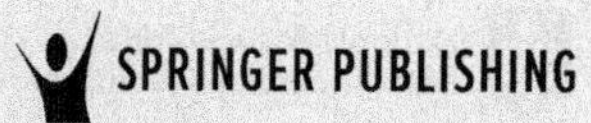

Items		Not at all	Just a little	Quite a bit	Very much
	Average score for inattention/overactivity items (items 4, 8, 11, 31, and 32).				
	Average score for aggression/defiance items (items 21, 23, 29, 34, and 35).				
	Average score for Conners' Index items, which is a general index of childhood problems (items 4, 8, 11, 21, 32, 33, 36, 37, 38, and 39).				
	Conduct disorder (items 41, 42, 43, 44, and 45).				
	Intermittent explosive disorder (item 46).				
	Stereotypic movement disorder (item 48).				
	Obsessive-compulsive disorder (items 49 and 50).				
	Generalized anxiety disorder (items 51, 52, 53, 54, 55, and 56).				
	Narcolepsy (item 57).				
	Histrionic personality disorder (item 58).				
	Narcissistic personality disorder (item 59).				
	Borderline personality disorder (item 60).				
	Manic episode (items 61, 62, 63, 64, and 65).				
	Dysthymic disorder (items 74, 75, and 76).				
	Posttraumatic stress disorder (items 77 and 78).				
	Adjustment disorder (items 79 and 80).				

The SNAP-IV-C Rating Scale is a revision of the Swanson, Nolan, and Pelham (SNAP) questionnaire (Swanson et al., 1983). The items from the *DSM-IV* (1994) criteria for ADHD are included for the two subsets of symptoms: inattention (items # 1–9) and hyperactivity/impulsivity (items # 11–19). Also, items are included from the *DSM-IV* criteria for oppositional defiant disorder (items # 21–28) since it often is present in children with ADHD. Items have been added to summarize the inattention domain (# 10) and the hyperactivity/impulsivity domain (# 20) of ADHD. Two other items were added: an item from *DSM-III-R* (# 29) that was not included in the *DSM-IV* list for ODD, and an item to summarize the ODD domain (# 30).

The 4-point response is scored 0–3 (Not at all = 0, Just a little = 1, Quite a bit = 2, and Very much = 3). Subscale scores for the ADHD and ODD subscales on the SNAP-IV are calculated by summing the scores on the items in the specific subset (e.g., inattention) and dividing by the number of items in the subset (e.g., 9). The score for any subset is expressed as the average rating-per-item. The 5% cut-off scores for teachers and parents are provided. Compare the average rating per item score to the cut-off score to determine if the score falls within the top 5% of extreme scores.

In addition to the *DSM-IV items* for ADHD and ODD, the SNAP-IV-C contains items from the Conners' Index Questionnaire (Conners, 1968) and the IOWA Conners' Questionnaire (Loney and Milich, 1985). The IOWA was developed using divergent validity to separate items which measure inattention/over

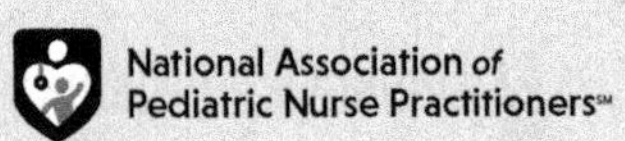

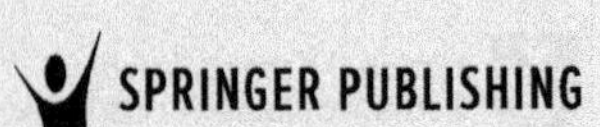

activity (I/O—items # 4, 8, 11, 31, 32) from those items which measure aggression/defiance (A/D—items # 21, 23, 29, 34, 35). The Conners' Index (items # 4, 8, 11, 21, 32, 33, 36, 37, 38, 39) was developed by selecting the items which loaded highest on the multiple factors of the Conners' Questionnaire, and thus represents a general index of childhood problems.

Finally, the SNAP-IV-C includes the 10 items (# 81–90) of the Swanson, Kotkin, Agler, MyInn, and Pelham (SKAMP) Rating Scale. These items are classroom manifestations of inattention, hyperactivity, and impulsivity (i.e., getting started, staying on task, interactions with others, completing work, and shifting activities). The SKAMP may be used to estimate severity of impairment in the classroom.

REFERENCE

Bussing, R., Fernandez, M., Harwood, M., Hou, W., Garvan, C. W., Eyberg, S. M., & Swanson, J. M. (2008). Parent and teacher SNAP-IV ratings of attention deficit hyperactivity disorder symptoms: Psychometric properties and normative ratings from a school district sample. *Assessment, 15*(3), 317–328. https://doi.org/10.1177/1073191107313888

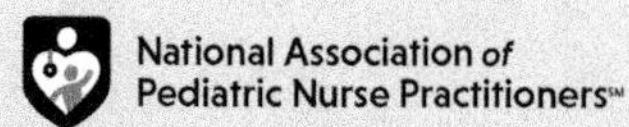

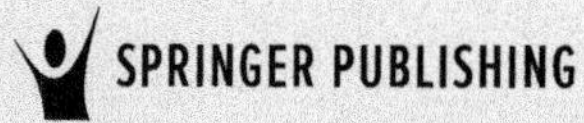

Information for Parents About Attention Deficit Hyperactivity Disorder (ADHD)

WHAT IS ADHD?

ADHD is the name of a group of behaviors found in many children and adults. People with ADHD have trouble paying attention in school, at home, or at work. They may be much more active and/or impulsive than what is usual for their age. These behaviors contribute to significant problems in relationships, learning, and behavior. For this reason, children with ADHD are sometimes seen as being "difficult" or as having behavior problems. ADHD is common, affecting 4% to 12% of school-age children. It is more common in boys than in girls.

WHAT ARE THE SYMPTOMS OF ADHD?

The child with ADHD who is inattentive will have six or more of the following symptoms:

- Difficulty following instructions.
- Difficulty keeping attention on work or play activities at school and at home.
- Loses things needed for activities at school and at home.
- Appears not to listen.
- Doesn't pay close attention to details.
- Seems disorganized.
- Has trouble with tasks that require planning ahead.
- Forgets things.
- Is easily distracted.

The child with ADHD who is hyperactive/impulsive will have at least 6 of the following symptoms:

- Runs or climbs inappropriately.
- Is fidgety.
- Can't play quietly.
- Blurts out answers.
- Interrupts people.
- Can't stay in seat.
- Talks too much.
- Is always on the go.
- Has trouble waiting his or her turn.

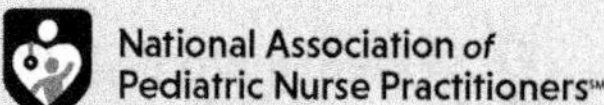

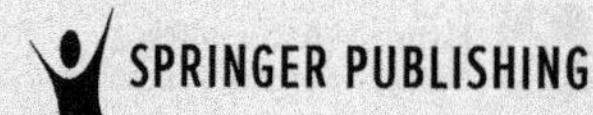

WHAT CAUSES ADHD?

Children with ADHD do not make enough chemicals in key areas in the brain that are responsible for organizing thought. Without enough of these chemicals, the organizing centers of the brain don't work well. This causes the symptoms in children with ADHD. Often there is a family history of ADHD. Things that ***don't*** cause ADHD: poor parenting (although a disorganized home life and school environment can make symptoms worse); too much or too little sugar, aspartame, food additives or colorings; lack of vitamins; food allergies or other allergies; fluorescent lights; video games; or too much TV.

WHAT CAN I DO TO HELP MY CHILD WITH ADHD?

A team effort, with parents, teachers, and doctors working together, is the best way to help your child. Children with ADHD tend to need more structure and clearer expectations. Families may benefit from talking with a specialist in managing ADHD-related behavior and learning problems. Medicine also helps many children. Talk with your doctor or nurse practitioner about treatments he/she recommends.

WHAT MEDICINES ARE USED TO TREAT ADHD?

Some of the medicines for ADHD are methylphenidate, dextroamphetamine, atomoxetine guanfacine, or clonidine. These medicines improve attention/concentration and decrease impulsive and overactive behaviors.

WHAT CAN I DO AT HOME TO HELP MY CHILD?

Children with ADHD may be challenging to parent. They may have trouble understanding directions. Children with ADHD are often in a constant state of activity. This can be challenging. You may need to change your home life a bit to help your child. Here are some things you can do to help:

- **Make a schedule.** Set specific times for waking up, eating, playing, doing homework, doing chores, watching TV or playing video games, and going to bed. Post the schedule where your child will always see it. Explain any changes to the routine in advance.
- **Make simple house rules.** It's important to explain what will happen when the rules are obeyed and when they are broken.
- **Make sure your directions are understood.** Get your child's attention and look directly into his or her eyes. Then tell your child in a clear, calm voice specifically what you want. Keep directions simple and short. Ask your child to repeat the directions back to you.
- **Reward good behavior.** Congratulate your child when he/she completes each step of a task.
- **Make sure your child is well supervised.** Because they are impulsive, children with ADHD may need more adult supervision than other children their age.
- **Watch your child around his or her friends.** It's sometimes hard for children with ADHD to learn social skills. Reward good play behaviors.

This handout may be distributed to families.
From Melnyk, B. M., & Lusk, P. (2022). *A Practical Guide to Child and Adolescent Mental Health Screening, Evidence-Based Assessment, Intervention, and Health Promotion* (3rd ed.).

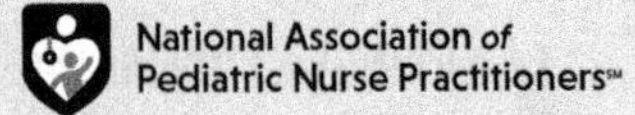

SPRINGER PUBLISHING

- **Set a homework routine.** Pick a regular place for homework, away from distractions such as other people, TV, and video games. Break homework time into small parts and allocate frequent breaks.
- **Focus on effort, not grades.** Reward your child when he or she tries to finish schoolwork, not just for good grades. You can give extra rewards for earning better grades.
- **Talk with your child's teachers.** Find out how your child is doing at school—in class, at playtime, at lunchtime. Ask for daily or weekly progress notes from the teacher.

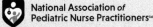

SPRINGER PUBLISHING

Information for Children and Teens About Attention Deficit Hyperactivity Disorder (ADHD)

"You're not paying attention." "Don't you know where you put your lunch money?" "Stop fidgeting!" "Don't interrupt." Can you imagine what it would be like to hear people talk to you this way every single day? If you can imagine it, or if it sounds just like what you're used to hearing, then you know what it's like to have attention deficit hyperactivity disorder or ADHD for short.

Children and teens who have ADHD are not "bad," "lazy," or "stupid." They have a behavior disorder, which means they may have problems paying attention or have trouble sitting still in their seats. They can also act on impulse—this means doing things without thinking about them first. Children and teens with ADHD may spend a lot of time in the principal's office. They also might change their friends a lot.

WHO GETS ADHD?

On average, five out of 100 children and youth have ADHD. That means that if your school has 500 students, 25 may have ADHD—that's like one whole class! Children and teens who have ADHD usually start having problems before they are 7 years old. Sometimes the problems begin when they start going to school. Boys have ADHD more often than girls, but no one knows why.

In fact, no one is sure why anyone has ADHD, although scientists think that it probably has to do with different levels of brain activity. No one gets ADHD on purpose, so it isn't ever anyone's fault. And ADHD isn't contagious—you can't catch it from someone like the flu. Someone might have a bigger chance of developing ADHD if one of his or her relatives already has ADHD.

WHAT IS ADHD?

ADHD stands for attention deficit hyperactivity disorder. ADHD is a disorder that affects the brain. It causes people to behave differently from others. People with ADHD have problems in one or two major ways. The first is that they may have trouble focusing on tasks or subjects. The second is that they may act on impulse (without thinking), which can lead to negative consequences. That's why ADHD gets a bad rap.

SYMPTOMS AND SIGNS OF ADHD

The first type of ADHD includes problems with paying attention, staying organized, remembering things, problems completing work at school or home, difficulty following instructions, losing or forgetting things (e.g., homework). This type used to be called attention deficit disorder, or ADD.

The second type involves hyperactivity and impulsivity and includes fidgeting, feelings of restlessness, difficulty awaiting your turn, and interrupting others.

The third type, which is the most common, involves a combination of the other two types. If you have ADHD, you may not be aware that you are behaving in a way that's different from others; you're just doing what comes naturally. But, you might notice that it's hard for you to pay attention. You might

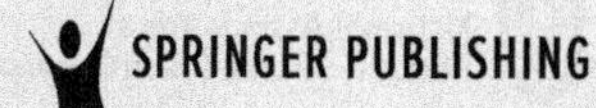

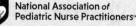

feel bored or frustrated in class. You may have a hard time getting started on assignments and finishing your work. Homework may take you much longer to complete.

ADHD can affect social situations, too. For example, you might react to someone by just saying what's on your mind—what comes naturally—and then you may get the feeling that you've shocked or offended the person or don't understand why people get mad at you. Some of the symptoms of ADHD can be difficult to deal with and can make a teen experience many different emotions. The more you understand about ADHD, the more involved you can be in your own treatment.

WHAT MEDICINES ARE USED TO TREAT ADHD?

Some medicines used to treat ADHD are called psychostimulants. They can help people with ADHD to focus their attention better on things.

SCHOOL TIPS FOR HELPING YOURSELF WITH ADHD

If you have a study hall available to you during one class period or after school, use it and take advantage of a quiet time to study and complete homework.

Take notes during class. This can help to keep you focused on the material being taught.

Use your assignment book to keep lists of things to do. Don't make lists on scraps of paper—you may end up losing them or forgetting about them. Get into the habit of completing a list of things to do each evening for what you want to accomplish the next day.

Talk to your teachers about your ADHD and how it affects your work. Ask for their assistance in areas you are experiencing problems. They will be more willing to help if they understand that you are trying to overcome these problems rather than making excuses.

Sit in front of the classroom. This will help you to focus on the lesson and will enable you to pay attention and will minimize distractions.

Be prepared. If you are constantly going to class unprepared, buy a box of pens and keep them in your locker. Buy several small pocket-size notebooks. Each morning, if you find you don't have a pen and paper, use a small pocket-size notebook, and take a pen from your locker.

If you end up each day at home without the books needed to complete your assignments, use different methods to remember which books to bring home. Ask the school about bringing home an extra set of books. You will not need to carry your books back and forth and will never forget your books at home or school.

Find a partner to help you. Find someone you trust and work well with to help you stay focused during the day. Have a special signal they can give you if they see you have lost your focus.

Clean out your locker every Friday. Get into the habit of bringing home all loose papers in your locker each Friday. When you get home, you can sort through to see what you need and organize the papers. Having a clean locker will help you to stay organized and be prepared.

Believe in yourself and your abilities. You can succeed in what you do.

Check out this helpful website for children, teens, and adults with ADHD: National Resource Center for ADHD, available at www.chadd.org.

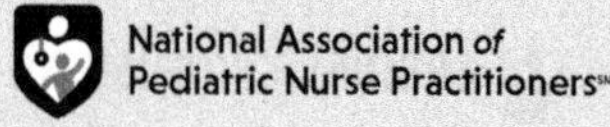

SPRINGER PUBLISHING

Internet Resources

American Academy of Child and Adolescent Psychiatry

www.aacap.org

This website is an excellent source of information on the assessment and treatment of child and adolescent mental health disorders. Handouts for use with families (i.e., *Facts for Families*) are available on a multitude of problems, including ADHD.

American Academy of Pediatrics (AAP)

www.aap.org

This website has excellent information for healthcare providers and parents on a variety of mental health topics, including ADHD. The AAP worked with the National Initiative for Children's Healthcare Quality to develop an evidence-based ADHD toolkit to assist practitioners in providing comprehensive care for children with this disorder.

Children and Adults with Attention-Deficit/Hyperactivity Disorder (CHADD)

www.chadd.org

This national nonprofit organization was founded in 1987 in response to the frustration and sense of isolation experienced by parents and their children with ADHD.

National Association of Pediatric Nurse Practitioners (NAPNAP)

https://www.napnap.org/behavioral-and-mental-health-resources/

NAPNAP has created an excellent resource that will help teens and families answer common questions about attention deficit hyperactivity disorder (ADHD).

National Institute of Mental Health

www.nimh.gov

This outstanding website has multiple educational handouts on a variety of mental health disorders, including ADHD, and links to informative website.

National Resource Center on ADHD

http://www.help4ADHD.org/

This resource center is a program of CHADD, funded through a cooperative agreement with the Centers for Disease Control and Prevention.

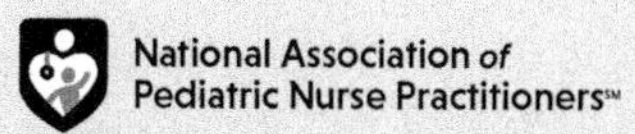

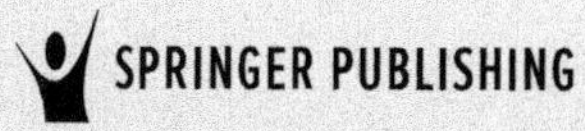

Vanderbilt Assessment Scale: *ADHD Toolkit* Parent-Informant Form

CLINICIAN TOOLS

Child's name: ______________________________ Parent's name: ____________________________

Date: __________________________ DOB: _______________________________Age: __________

Directions: Each rating should be considered in the context of what is appropriate for the age of your child. When completing this form, please think about your child's behaviors in the past 6 months.

This evaluation is based on a time when your child: ❑ Was on medication ❑ Was not on medication ❑ Not sure

Behavior	Never (0)	Occasionally (1)	Often (2)	Very Often (3)
1. Does not pay attention to details or makes mistakes that seem careless with, for example, homework	❑	❑	❑	❑
2. Has difficulty keeping attention on what needs to be done	❑	❑	❑	❑
3. Does not seem to listen when spoken to directly	❑	❑	❑	❑
4. Does not follow through on instructions and does not finish activities (not because of refusal or lack of comprehension)	❑	❑	❑	❑
5. Has difficulty organizing tasks and activities	❑	❑	❑	❑
6. Avoids, dislikes, or does not want to start tasks that require ongoing mental effort	❑	❑	❑	❑
7. Loses things necessary for tasks or activities (eg, toys, assignments, pencils, books)	❑	❑	❑	❑
8. Is easily distracted by noises or other stimuli	❑	❑	❑	❑
9. Is forgetful in daily activities	❑	❑	❑	❑

For Office Use Only 2s & 3s _____ /9

Behavior	Never (0)	Occasionally (1)	Often (2)	Very Often (3)
10. Fidgets with or taps hands or feet or squirms in seat	❑	❑	❑	❑
11. Leaves seat when remaining seated is expected	❑	❑	❑	❑
12. Runs about or climbs too much when remaining seated is expected	❑	❑	❑	❑
13. Has difficulty playing or beginning quiet play games	❑	❑	❑	❑
14. Is on the go or often acts as if "driven by a motor"	❑	❑	❑	❑
15. Talks too much	❑	❑	❑	❑
16. Blurts out answers before questions have been completed	❑	❑	❑	❑
17. Has difficulty waiting his or her turn	❑	❑	❑	❑
18. Interrupts or intrudes into others' conversations or activities or both	❑	❑	❑	❑

For Office Use Only 2s & 3s _____ /9

National Association of Pediatric Nurse Practitioners™

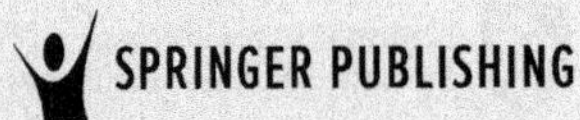

Behavior	Never (0)	Occasionally (1)	Often (2)	Very Often (3)
19. Loses temper	❑	❑	❑	❑
20. Is touchy or easily annoyed	❑	❑	❑	❑
21. Is angry or resentful	❑	❑	❑	❑
22. Argues with authority figures or adults	❑	❑	❑	❑
23. Actively defies or refuses to adhere to requests or rules	❑	❑	❑	❑
24. Deliberately annoys people	❑	❑	❑	❑
25. Blames others for his or her mistakes or misbehaviors	❑	❑	❑	❑
26. Is spiteful and wants to get even	❑	❑	❑	❑

For Office Use Only 2s & 3s _____ /8

Behavior	Never (0)	Occasionally (1)	Often (2)	Very Often (3)
27. Bullies, threatens, or intimidates others	❑	❑	❑	❑
28. Starts physical fights	❑	❑	❑	❑
29. Has used a weapon that can cause serious harm (eg, bat, knife, brick, gun)	❑	❑	❑	❑
30. Has been physically cruel to people	❑	❑	❑	❑
31. Has been physically cruel to animals	❑	❑	❑	❑
32. Has stolen while confronting the person	❑	❑	❑	❑
33. Has forced someone into sexual activity	❑	❑	❑	❑
34. Has deliberately set fires to cause damage	❑	❑	❑	❑
35. Deliberately destroys others' property	❑	❑	❑	❑
36. Has broken into someone else's home, business, or car	❑	❑	❑	❑
37. Lies to get out of trouble, to obtain goods or favors, or to avoidobligations (ie, cons others)	❑	❑	❑	❑
38. Has stolen items of value	❑	❑	❑	❑
39. Has stayed out at night without permission beginningbefore age 13	❑	❑	❑	❑
40. Has run away from home twice or once for an extended period	❑	❑	❑	❑
41. Is often truant from school (skips school)	❑	❑	❑	❑

For Office Use Only 2s & 3s _____ /15

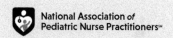

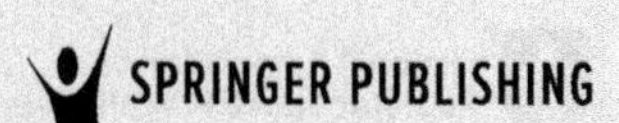

Behavior	Never (0)	Occasionally (1)	Often (2)	Very Often (3)
42. Is fearful, anxious, or worried	❑	❑	❑	❑
43. Is afraid to try new things for fear of making mistakes	❑	❑	❑	❑
44. Feels worthless or inferior	❑	❑	❑	❑
45. Blames self for problems or feels guilty	❑	❑	❑	❑
46. Feels lonely, unwanted, or unloved; often says that no one loveshim or her	❑	❑	❑	❑
47. Is sad, unhappy, or depressed	❑	❑	❑	❑
48. Is self-conscious or easily embarrassed	❑	❑	❑	❑

For Office Use Only 2s & 3s _____ /7

Academic and Social Performance	Excellent (1)	Above Average (2)	Average (3)	Somewhat of a Problem (4)	Problematic (5)
49. Overall school performance	❑	❑	❑	❑	❑
50. Reading	❑	❑	❑	❑	❑
51. Writing	❑	❑	❑	❑	❑
52. Mathematics	❑	❑	❑	❑	❑
53. Relationship with parents	❑	❑	❑	❑	❑
54. Relationship with siblings	❑	❑	❑	❑	❑
55. Relationship with peers	❑	❑	❑	❑	❑
56. Participation in organized activities (eg, teams)	❑	❑	❑	❑	❑

For Office Use Only 4s _____ /8

For Office Use Only 5s _____ /8

How old was your child when you first noticed the behaviors?

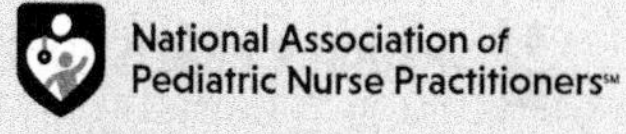

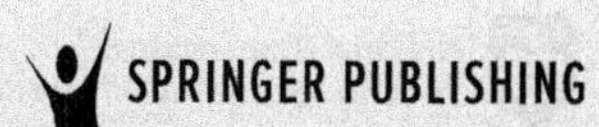

Tic behaviors: To the best of your knowledge, please indicate if your child displays the following behaviors:

1. **Motor tics:** Rapid, repetitive movements such as eye blinking, grimacing, nose twitching, head jerks, shoulder shrugs, arm jerks, body jerks, and rapid kicks.

   ❑ No tics present.

   ❑ Yes, they occur nearly every day but go unnoticed by most people.

   ❑ Yes, noticeable tics occur nearly every day.

2. **Phonic (vocal) tics:** Repetitive noises including, but not limited to, throat clearing, coughing, whistling, sniffing, snorting, screeching, barking, grunting, and repetition of words or short phrases.

   ❑ No tics present.

   ❑ Yes, they occur nearly every day but go unnoticed by most people.

   ❑ Yes, noticeable tics occur nearly every day.

3. If **YES** to 1 or 2, do these tics interfere with your child's activities (eg, reading, writing, walking, talking, eating)?

   ❑ No ❑ Yes

Previous diagnosis and treatment: Please answer the following questions to the best of your knowledge:

1.	Has your child been diagnosed as having ADHD or ADD?	❑ No	❑ Yes
2.	Is he or she on medication for ADHD or ADD?	❑ No	❑ Yes
3.	Has your child been diagnosed as having a tic disorder or Tourette syndrome?	❑ No	❑ Yes
4.	Is he or she on medication for a tic disorder or Tourette disorder?	❑ No	❑ Yes

Adapted from the Vanderbilt rating scales developed by Mark L. Wolraich, MD.

For Office Use Only

Total number of questions scored 2 or 3 in questions 1–9: 0

Total number of questions scored 2 or 3 in questions 10–18: 0

Total number of questions scored 2 or 3 in questions 19–26: 0

Total number of questions scored 2 or 3 in questions 27–41: 0

Total number of questions scored 2 or 3 in questions 42–48: 0

Total number of questions scored 4 in questions 49–56: 0

Total number of questions scored 5 in questions 49–56: 0

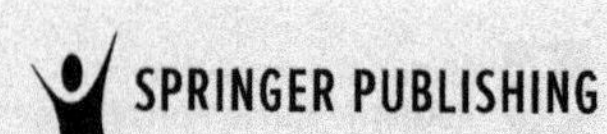

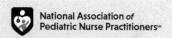

The recommendations in this resource do not indicate an exclusive course of treatment or serve as a standard of medical care. Variations, taking into account individual circumstances, may be appropriate. Original resource included as part of *Caring for Children With ADHD: A Practical Resource Toolkit for Clinicians*, 3rd Edition.

Inclusion in this resource does not imply an endorsement by the American Academy of Pediatrics (AAP). The AAP is not responsible for the content of the resources mentioned in this resource. Website addresses are as current as possible but may change at any time.

The American Academy of Pediatrics (AAP) does not review or endorse any modifications made to this resource and in no event shall the AAP be liable for any such changes.

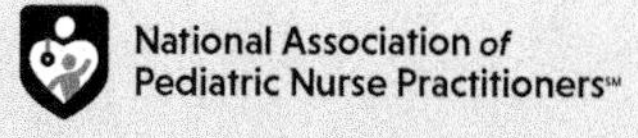

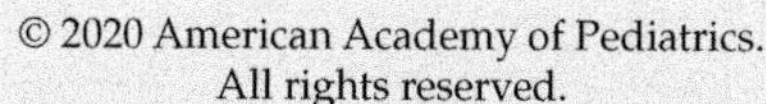

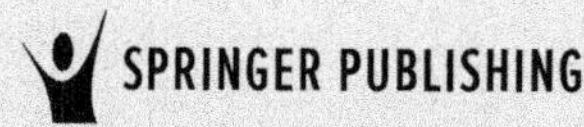

CHAPTER 6

Mary Lynn Dell, John V. Campo, and Pamela Lusk

Evidence-Based Assessment and Management of Somatoform Disorders

FAST FACTS

- This *Diagnostic and Statistical Manual of Mental Disorders, Fifth Edition (DSM-5)* group of disorders replaces the somatoform disorders category in previous versions of the *DSM*. This change is intended to simplify and lessen confusion compared to previous editions.
- These disorders often first present in general medical or non-psychiatric settings.
- Diagnostic criteria apply across the life span, so it is important to consider the child or adolescent's developmental level during assessment and diagnosis.
- These disorders may or may not overlap or be comorbid with other medical disorders, such as irritable bowel syndrome, abdominal pain, fibromyalgia, headaches, or chronic pain.
- These disorders may or may not overlap or be comorbid with other psychiatric disorders that may have physiological symptoms such as anxiety and depressive disorders.
- *Somatization* is a key concept. It refers to the subjective experience of physical symptoms for which clear pathology or injury is lacking or not diagnosable by standard-of-care methods, or when level or distress or disability exceeds what is typically associated with clinical findings.
- Due to complexities in the diagnosis of somatoform disorders historically, the term *medically unexplained symptoms* (MUSs) often has been used to describe features of the somatic symptom disorders (SSDs).
- Studies report MUSs range between 2% and 20% of children in various community and pediatric clinic settings.
- SSDs are associated with high healthcare costs and expenditures (Malas et al., 2017).
- Management of youth with SSDs can be associated with a high level of provider and family frustration (Ibeziako et al., 2019; Malas et al., 2017).
- Very minimal data exist currently regarding new *DSM-5* SSDs in children and adolescents.

FOUR DISORDERS PARTICULARLY RELEVANT TO CHILDREN AND ADOLESCENTS

Somatic symptom disorder (SSD):

- A combination of distressing, sometimes multiple symptoms, to which the patient responds in excessive or maladaptive ways, resulting in significant disruption of daily life or impairment in functioning.

- Involves two of the following: (1) persistent, disproportionate worries about the medical seriousness of symptoms; (2) excessive anxiety about the symptoms; and (3) excessive time and energy spent concerned with the symptoms or health issues.
- Presence of one or more somatic symptoms that are distressing or result in significant disruption of daily life.
- Persistently high levels of anxiety about symptoms or one's health.
- Excessive thoughts, feelings, or behaviors related to the somatic symptoms.
- Symptoms are persistent (usually greater than 6 months).
- Somatic symptoms can predominantly involve pain.

Other specified somatic symptom and related disorder:

- Presence of somatic symptoms that cause significant distress or impairment but do not meet full criteria for another category or somatic symptom and related disorders.
- May be used when symptoms are brief (less than 6 months) or just below diagnostic criteria.
- One or more somatic symptoms that the youth experiences as distressing or that interfere significantly with daily life.

Illness anxiety disorder:

- Preoccupation with having a serious illness (greater than 6 months); focused on underlying medical diagnosis.
- If a medical condition or strong family history is present, worry is out of proportion to the likelihood of severe illness; somatic symptoms are mild.
- High levels of anxiety about one's health.
- Can be care seeking or care avoiding (avoidance of necessary healthcare).
    - Excessive engagement in health-related behavior (e.g., repeatedly checking body for signs of illness).

Conversion disorder (functional neurological symptom disorder):

- Presence of one or more symptoms of altered voluntary motor or sensory function that results in significant distress or impairment (or cause loss of consciousness).
- Evaluation suggests that symptoms are incompatible with recognized medical conditions.
- Symptoms are not due to general medical conditions, substances, or cultural phenomena.
- There may be a relevant psychological stressor, but not required.
- Common symptoms include gait disturbances, tremors, shaking, jerking; weakness, numbness, tingling (often inconsistent with dermatomal patterns); vision or hearing deficits.
- Psychodynamic explanations have emphasized primary and secondary gain.

RISK FACTORS (BAUM & CAMPO, 2015)

- Family members with somatization symptoms (modeling)
- Genetics
- School stresses
- Difficulty with transitions
- Limited coping mechanisms

- Family stresses
- High achieving families
- Parental overprotection
- Emotional and physical abuse or neglect
- Sexual abuse
- Trauma
- Psychiatric comorbidities

COMMON PRESENTING COMPLAINTS

- Headache
- Abdominal pain
- Nausea, vomiting
- Fatigue
- Muscle aches and soreness
- Back pain
- Blurry vision
- Diarrhea
- Dyspnea
- Vocal cord dysfunction

SCREENING

- Thorough clinical history, with close attention to current stressors.
- Children's somatization inventory: 35 items.
- Functional disability inventory: 15 items, emphasizes past 2 weeks, school attendance.

ASSESSMENT

- Thorough medical and psychiatric histories.
- Thorough physical examination.
- Appropriate laboratory, imaging, and other diagnostic testing, always balancing thoroughness with possible unintended harm from medical procedures.
- Inquire about symptom models in relatives and significant others.
- Inquire about academic history.
- Inquire about peer relationships.
- Review early childhood education and other early experiences when separated from caregiver.
- Be alert to possible secondary gains.

MANAGEMENT

- Acknowledge symptoms, patient experience, and family concerns.
- Review past evaluations and treatment.
- Understand timing, context, and characteristics of symptoms.

- Investigate fears related to symptoms.
- Avoid unnecessary tests.
- Often require multidisciplinary care from several types of healthcare professionals.
- Emphasize collaboration and shared goals among patient, family, and caregivers
- Reassure patients and families that these symptoms are not fatal.
- Address anxiety directly.
- Cognitive behavioral interventions, successful for abdominal pain, has addressed school absences and pain complaints.
- Emphasize coping and minimizing sick role behaviors.
- Behavioral and operant interventions to reinforce healthy, adaptive behaviors and decrease incentives and reinforcements for maladaptive behaviors.
- Parent training in basic behavioral and operant interventions is very helpful, often essential.
- Biofeedback, hypnosis, guided imagery, and relaxation techniques can be helpful. Imagery and relaxation are especially advantageous because patients can be taught to administer themselves.
- Family therapy—reinforce healthy attitudes and behaviors, cope with symptoms, address underlying conflicts.
- Communication with other professionals: medical, psychological, school, clergy, others.
- Treat comorbid psychiatric disorders aggressively.
- Pharmacological interventions (refer to Table 6.1).
- Monitor treatment outcomes, with particular attention to goals of school attendance, and healthy, fulfilling interpersonal, family, academic, and psychosocial functioning.

Facilitate the development of a treatment plan that addresses physical pain, stress reduction, and reduction of stigma while fostering hope that the child will improve. Goals should be developed collaboratively with family, so that the management is meaningful to child and family (Baum & Campo, 2015, p. 661).

Table 6.1. Pharmacological Interventions in Somatic Symptom and Related Disorders (SSDs)

- No randomized controlled trials of psychoactive medications in pediatric SSDs.
- Use of psychoactive medications primarily based on case reports or extrapolated from adult populations with medical and psychiatric diagnoses.
- Psychopharmacologic treatment most appropriately considered in the presence of comorbid anxiety or depression, especially when non-medication treatments have not been helpful.

  Examples:

  1. Recurrent abdominal pain: May start citalopram or fluoxetine at low dose (10 mg per day), increase to therapeutic dose of 20 mg daily over the next week, with maximum dose of 40 mg daily after 4 weeks.
  2. Low dose benzodiazepines may be helpful short-term if symptoms accompanied by severe anxiety, for instance, clonazepam 0.25 mg at bedtime gradually increased to maximum of 0.5 mg twice daily, or lorazepam 0.5 mg three times a day, gradually increased to 1.0 mg three times a day.
- If medications are used, obtain informed consent, carefully explaining side effects, FDA Black Box warnings for antidepressants and suicidality for those 24 years of age and under. Also, monitor for serotonin syndrome if the child is on more than one serotonergic agent, regardless of drug class.

In general, the prognosis for children presenting with MUSs is favorable; proper recognition and intervention are essential. Family support and care coordination can reduce child and family frustration, lead to improved outcomes, and be a more rewarding experience for the provider (Baum & Campo, 2015, p. 663).

REFERENCES

Baum, R., & Campo, J. (2015). Medically unexplained symptoms, Chapter 54. In H. Adam & J. M. Foy (Eds.), *Signs & symptoms in pediatrics* (pp. 657–664). American Academy of Pediatrics.

Ibeziako, P., Brahmghatt, K., Chapman, A., De Souza, C., Giles, L., Gooden, S., Latif, F., Malas, N., Namerow, L., Russell, R., Steinbuchel, M., Pao, M., & Piloplys, S. (2019). Developing a clinical pathway for somatic symptom and related disorders in pediatric hospital settings. *Hospital Pediatrics*, *9*, 147. https://doi.org/10.1542/hpeds.2018-0205

Malas, N., Ortiz-Aguayo, R., Giles, L., & Ibeziako, P. (2017). Pediatric somatic symptom disorders. *Current Psychiatry Reports*, *19*, 11. https://doi.org/10.1007/s11920-017-0760-3

SUGGESTED ADDITIONAL READINGS

American Academy of Child and Adolescent Psychiatry. (2017). *Physical symptoms of emotional distress: Somatic symptom and related disorders*. https://www.aacap.org/AACAP/AACAP/Families_and_Youth/Facts_for_Families/FFF-Guide/Physical_Symptoms_of_Emotional_Distress-Somatic_Symptoms_and_Related_Disorders-124.aspx

American Psychiatric Association. (2000). *Diagnostic and statistical manual of mental disorders, fourth edition, text revision (DSM-IV-TR)*.

American Psychiatric Association. (2011). DSM-V somatic symptom disorders, draft.

Campo, J. V. (2008). Disorders primarily seen in general medical settings. In R. L. Findling (Ed.), *Clinical manual of child and adolescent psychopharmacology* (pp. 375–423). American Psychiatric Publishing, Inc.

Campo, J. V., Fridge, J., Ehmann, M., Altman, S., Lucas, A., Birmaher, B., Di Lorenzo, C., Iyengar, S., Brent, D. A. (2004). Recurrent abdominal pain, anxiety, and depression in primary care. *Pediatrics*, *113*, 817–824. https://doi.org/10.1542/peds.113.4.817

Campo, J. V., & Fritz, G. (2001). A management model for pediatric somatization. *Psychosomatics*, *42*, 467–476. https://doi.org/10.1176/appi.psy.42.6.467

Dell, M. L., & Campo, J. V. (2011). Somatoform disorders in children and adolescents. *Psychiatric Clinics of North America*, *34*, 643–660. https://doi.org/10.1016/j.psc.2011.05.012

Fritz, G. K., Fritsch, S., & Hagino, O. (1997). Somatization disorders in children and adolescents: A review of the past 10 years. *Journal of the American Academy of Child and Adolescent Psychiatry*, *36*, 1329–1338. https://doi.org/10.1097/00004583-199710000-00014

Looper, K. J., & Kirmayer, L. J. (2002). Behavioral medicine approaches to somatoform disorders. *Journal of Consulting and Clinical Psychology*, *70*, 810–827. https://doi.org/10.1037/0022-006X.70.3.810

Sanders, M. R., Shepherd, R. W., Cleghorn, G., & Woolford, H. (1994). The treatment of recurrent abdominal pain in children: A controlled comparison of cognitive-behavioral family intervention and standard pediatric care. *Journal of Consulting and Clinical Psychology*, *62*, 306–314. https://doi.org/10.1037/0022-006X.62.2.306

Schulman, J. L. (1988). Use of a coping approach in the management of children with conversion reactions. *Journal of the American Academy of Child and Adolescent Psychiatry*, *27*, 785–788. https://doi.org/10.1097/00004583-198811000-00021

Stone, J., LaFrance, W. C., Levenson, J. L., & Sharpe, M. (2010). Issues for *DSM-5:* Conversion disorder. *American Journal of Psychiatry*, *167*, 626–627. https://doi.org/10.1176/appi.ajp.2010.09101440

Walker, L. S., Garber, J., & Greene, J. W. (1993). Psychosocial correlates of recurrent childhood pain: A comparison of pediatric patients with recurrent abdominal pain, organic illness, and psychiatric disorders. *Journal of Abnormal Psychology*, *102*, 248–258. https://doi.org/10.1037/0021-843X.102.2.248

Walker, L. S., & Greene, J. W. (1991). The functional disability inventory: Measuring a neglected dimension of child health status. *Journal of Pediatric Psychology*, *16*, 39–58. https://doi.org/10.1093/jpepsy/16.1.39

Witek, M. W., Rojas V., Alonso, C., Minami, H., & Silva, R. R. (2005). Review of benzodiazepine use in children and adolescents. *Psychiatric Quarterly*, *76*, 283–296. https://doi.org/10.1007/s11126-005-2982-5

Wood, B. L. (2001). Physically manifested illness in children and adolescents: A biobehavioral family approach. *Child and Adolescent Psychiatric Clinics of North America*, *10*, 543–562. https://doi.org/10.1016/S1056-4993(18)30045-2

Somatic Symptom Disorders Parent/ Caregiver Information

WHAT IS A SOMATIC SYMPTOM DISORDER?

Somatic symptom disorders (SSDs) are conditions in which individuals experience physical symptoms that are not fully explained by the presence of a general medical condition after standard-of-care evaluations and diagnostic tests. In some patients, there may be a known medical condition or injury, but the amount of distress, worry about the condition, and disturbance in daily life are greater than what medical professionals and parents/caregivers would expect given the actual severity of the medical condition or injury.

ARE THE SYMPTOMS REAL?

Most definitely, yes! The symptoms your child is experiencing, whether abdominal pain, headache, muscle weakness or tingling, are very real, but *medically unexplained.* Telling your loved one that their symptoms are not real, or that they are "faking" or "making it up" just because the medical workup cannot explain the cause almost never helps the symptoms go away.

WHAT SYMPTOMS ARE MOST COMMONLY INVOLVED?

Children and adolescents with this disorder may experience headaches, abdominal pain, nausea, vomiting, bloating, fatigue, muscle aches and soreness, back pain, diarrhea, vocal cord or voice problems, numbness, tingling, blurry vision, inability to walk or move a limb, and other issues. People of all ages have occasional aches and pains that come and go without an obvious explanation. In this instance, however, the severity of the symptoms intrudes on and disrupts functioning in daily life at home, school, and in other activities.

WHAT OTHER PROBLEMS ARE SEEN WITH THESE DISORDERS?

Sometimes disabling somatic symptoms may begin after a physical illness, infection, or injury. Examples include prolonged abdominal pain after a viral illness has cleared up, or numbness or tingling of the leg after being kicked in soccer practice. The somatic symptoms seem to "take on a life of their own" after the initial problem should have healed or resolved. Youth with SSDs also have higher rates of depression and anxiety than general pediatric populations.

ARE THERE OTHER RISK FACTORS?

Physical and emotional abuse or neglect and sexual abuse are known risk factors for medically MUS. Also, having other family members or significant others with unexplained medical symptoms may predispose a child to symptom expression, particularly during stressful life events.

HOW SERIOUS IS THIS?

SSDs are not fatal, but they can be serious if they interfere with a child's normal growth and development, including learning and academic achievement, peer and family relationships. Occasionally a child may be harmed if concerns about illness lead to prolonged physical inactivity and loss of healthy

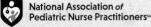

SPRINGER PUBLISHING

muscle tone. Children may also be harmed if clinicians order unnecessary tests, procedures, and treatments. Consequently, it is critical to avoid the temptation to request unnecessary medical testing or treatments that put the child at risk for complications and adverse effects.

HOW IS THE DIAGNOSIS MADE?

There is no single test or procedure for SSDs. The diagnosis is made from a thorough clinical history, physical examination, and laboratory, imaging, and diagnostic tests appropriate for the concerns and problems the child is experiencing. Children should also be assessed for depression, anxiety, and the possibility of abuse or other traumatic experiences.

HOW ARE SOMATIC TREATMENT DISORDERS TREATED OR MANAGED?

There is no single quick and easy procedure or medication for this. Treatment is based primarily on accumulated clinical wisdom and experience.

First of all, children and families should be assured that appropriate medical monitoring will be done for new or changing symptoms. In the meantime, many types of healthcare professionals may be involved in your child's care, including pediatric subspecialists, psychiatrists, nurses, physical and occupational therapists, teachers, and others. Families and the treatment team should establish and collaborate to achieve shared goals.

Specific treatment modalities often helpful include:

- **Cognitive behavioral therapy and skills building**: A particular type or school of therapy helpful in addressing stresses and behaviors that may be exacerbating the symptoms, as well accompanying symptoms of depression and anxiety; encouraging a "rehabilitative" mindset that emphasizes the child's fundamental strengths and relative health is often critical.
- **Behavioral therapies and parent training**: Assists parents with addressing illness behaviors and reinforcing healthy habits at home.
- **Family therapy**: Helps the patient and the entire family deal with the effects of the illness on everyone, as well as factors at home that might be contributing to the symptoms.
- Many children and adolescents benefit from relaxation techniques, guided imagery, biofeedback, and hypnosis for symptom management.
- Psychotropic medications for accompanying depression, anxiety, or other psychiatric disorders can sometimes be very helpful.
- Communication with significant others in the youth's life is essential, including teachers, counselors, primary care doctors, therapists, clergy, and coaches.

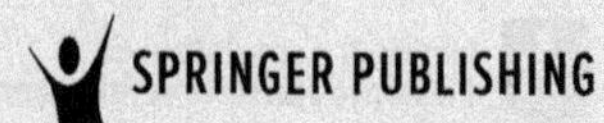

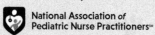

Resources for Somatoform Disorders

THE AMERICAN PSYCHOSOMATIC SOCIETY

www.psychosomatic.org/about/index.cfm

The mission of the American Psychosomatic Society is to promote and advance the scientific understanding and multidisciplinary integration of biological, psychological, behavioral, and social factors in human health and disease, and to foster the dissemination and application of this understanding in education and healthcare.

AMERICAN ACADEMY OF CHILD AND ADOLESCENT PSYCHIATRY (AACAP)

www.aacap.org

This website contains information about research, legislative activities, and meetings regarding child and adolescent mental health; policy statements; clinical practice guidelines; and a directory of child and adolescent psychiatrists. It also offers a set of FACT SHEETS for families in English, Spanish, and several other languages on a variety of topics that include ADHD, bullying, depression, and suicide.

This is an excellent handout for families are physical symptoms of emotional distress and somatic symptom and related disorders.

www.aacap.org/AACAP/AACAP/Families_and_Youth/Facts_for_Families/FFF-Guide/Physical_Symptoms_of_Emotional_Distress-Somatic_Symptoms_and_Related_Disorders-124.aspx

THE REACH INSTITUTE

www.thereachinstitute.org

The REACH Institute is dedicated to improving the mental health of American children and adolescents with emotional and behavioral challenges. It provides workshops for healthcare providers that teach the best evidence-based therapies, from psychotherapy to pharmacology, to improve the mental health of children and teens. Excellent resources at the website are available for healthcare providers, agencies, and families.

COPE (CREATING OPPORTUNITIES FOR PERSONAL EMPOWERMENT) FOR CHILDREN, ADOLESCENTS AND YOUNG ADULTS

www.COPE2Thrive.com

The COPE Program is an evidence-based, seven-session manualized cognitive behavioral skills building intervention program, based on the 12 key components of cognitive behavior therapy (CBT). Over 20 studies have supported the program's efficacy in decreasing anxiety, stress, and depression as well as improving healthy behaviors. Developmentally appropriate versions of COPE are available for 7- to 11-year-old children, 12- to 17-year-olds, and 18- to 24-year-olds. The program can be delivered in individual, small group, classroom, or virtual formats. Healthcare providers delivering the program in primary care receive reimbursement with the 99214 CPT code. An on-line interactive version is available for adolescents. A workshop that can be completed on-line is required prior to delivering the COPE programs.

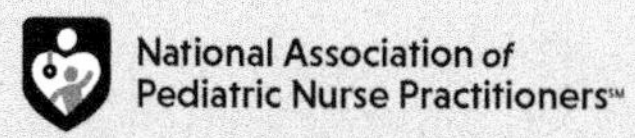

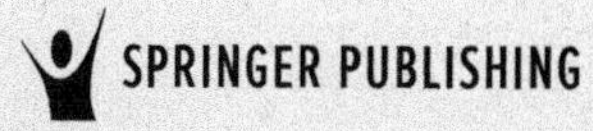

CHAPTER 7

Pamela Lusk

Evidence-Based Assessment and Management of Disruptive Behaviors

Fast Facts

- All children are oppositional from time to time, particularly when tired, hungry, stressed, or upset. They may argue, talk back, disobey, and defy parents, teachers, and other adults in authority.
- Openly uncooperative and angry/hostile behavior becomes a concern when it is so frequent and consistent that it stands out when compared to other children of the same age and developmental level and when it affects the child's home, school, and social life (AACAP—2019 Facts for Families).
- The child with disruptive behaviors may have attention deficit hyperactivity disorder (ADHD) or the "externalizing behaviors" (i.e., acting out behaviors) may be the symptoms of anxiety or depression. They may meet *Diagnostic and Statistical Manual of Mental Disorders, Fifth Edition* (*DSM-5*) criteria for a trauma and stressor related disorder, such as adjustment disorder with disturbance of emotions and conduct or that child may meet criteria for a *DSM-5* disruptive, impulse-control, and conduct disorder, such as oppositional defiant disorder or conduct disorder.
- Symptoms of ADHD that present as disruptive behaviors include impulsivity, not following directions, intruding in others' activities, and not listening. These behaviors cause difficulties at home, school, and social situations.
- The first rule out diagnosis will be ADHD if there is a possibility that the child's behaviors may meet the criteria for the disorder. Screening with the Vanderbilt Parent Assessment Scale or Vanderbilt Teacher Assessment Scale can be started in the office. These scales also have oppositional defiant subscales.
- In addition to the significant overlap between ADHD and oppositional defiant (ODD), the two conditions are often comorbid. Current evidence-based guidelines for treating ODD recommend treating the ADHD symptoms first as the best initial approach.
- Children with disruptive behavior disorders have difficulty with: (a) flexibility; (b) frustration tolerance; and (c) problem-solving.
- Oppositional behavior is sometimes used by the child to manage anxiety in the face of overwhelming demands. Irritable, antagonistic behaviors in youth are commonly found in anxiety disorders and depression.
- Children are barometers of family and environmental stress. When a child who has been functioning well presents with disruptive behaviors, a thorough exploration of what is going on in that child's life is warranted. They may meet acute stress disorder or adjustment disorder criteria.

- Additional appointments can be scheduled to leverage the positive relationship the child has with the primary care provider (PCP) to explore the child's worries (e.g., the possibility of family distress, loss of a job by parent, uncertainty and instability about where the family lives, abuse—physical or sexual—to that child or someone they care about, neglect due to parent illness/substance use, bullying/aggressive peers at school).
- In outpatient health settings, a good plan of care can begin with engaging the child and family in care by recognizing and reinforcing strengths of the child and family, avoiding taking sides, and acknowledging the legitimacy of feelings and reminding the family that strong feelings often occur in families and when people care about each other (Wissow, 2015).
- The plan also includes psychoeducation re: differences in children's temperament, families evolving circumstances, and challenges and other factors that can contribute to difficulties with behavioral regulation.
- "Usually, what parents are hoping to hear is a combination of reassurances that behavior will improve over time and concrete plans that will work toward improvement in the short term" (Wissow, 2015)
- Parenting factors can play a significant role in problem behaviors. There may be incentive for the behavior (e.g., gaining attention from the parent).
- Parents can be encouraged to ignore some behaviors (prioritize), focus on positive interactions and prevention strategies (when they identify the situations where the child has more difficulty maintaining good self-control), provide advance notice (age appropriate) of what will be expected of them and discuss and give opportunity to make choices about participating, and provide consistent, calm consequences for misbehavior.
- Finding a way for children to make reparation for a negative behavior (cleaning up a mess they made during a tantrum) can provide helpful corrective experience and the child then earns praise.
- Sometimes it is the provider that identifies a behavior, such as talking back to authority as a significant problem. Physicians and nurse practitioners are more comfortable initiating a conversation about their observations of a child's behavioral, emotional, or developmental issues with a parent they have known over a period of time.
- One indication of oppositional defiant disorder is when the child is consistently oppositional or challenging in the office with the provider and staff.
- Some parents hold overly permissive, child-centered views of parenting. Following the long tradition of anticipatory guidance, parents are reminded that firm discipline combined with love is an important part of parenting. Discipline is a way of teaching a child how to live comfortably and successfully in a world that will make requests, have rules, and have expectations.
- Parents will bring their concerns about their child to the trusted expert—the pediatric provider; however, there are barriers to parent disclosure about disruptive behaviors. These include cultural beliefs and norms about normal and abnormal behavior, stigma, family conflict or dysfunction, being uninsured or underinsured, or not knowing where to go for mental health services.
- The pediatric practitioner can help parents "reframe" their understanding of the well-child visit as not only physical, but also a place where behavioral and emotional concerns are assessed. An office equipped with prepared screening tools, handouts, books, audio and video resources for families reinforces this message.
- Oppositional defiant disorder is found in 3% to 4% of children whose disruptive behaviors persist over months or years, occur across many situations, and result in pronounced impairment in their functioning in home, school, and peer settings. These children's

anger is usually directed at authority figures. These children show extreme levels of argumentativeness, disobedience, stubbornness, negativity, and provocation of others.

- The more serious symptoms of conduct disorder, also included in *DSM-5* disruptive, impulse-control, and conduct disorder will be covered in the next section. Conduct disorder focuses largely on poorly controlled behaviors that violate the rights of others.
- Aggressive children underutilize pertinent social cues, misattribute hostile intent to peers, and generate fewer solutions to problems.
- An evidence-based approach to the child with disruptive behavior is empathy for the child and parents, and a reminder that *children do well if they can* (collaborative problem-solving approach, explosive child).
- Children with behavioral problems and irritable, fussy temperaments are at higher risk to be abused. Abuse may be triggered by the child's oppositional behaviors.
- Hope is instilled when the provider puts in place a plan to work with that child so they can acquire coping skills and learn to behave in ways that are more successful at home, school, and in the community (Greene, 2014).
- As an active intervention, the provider along with the parents and child at the time of the visit can identify *one* problem to start working on first and put that plan into place immediately. Often, because the parents are so overwhelmed, the provider will need to elicit the child's input and make the decision as the expert/authority for the first target behavior.
- Brief, simple interventions have an enduring effect on families' abilities to problem solve.
- The PCP has a major role in preventive mental health strategies: Early interventions with problem behaviors may eliminate the progression of more serious and persistent mental health concerns.
- Intensity of problems from early symptoms to oppositional defiant disorder and conduct disorder frequently follows the path below:

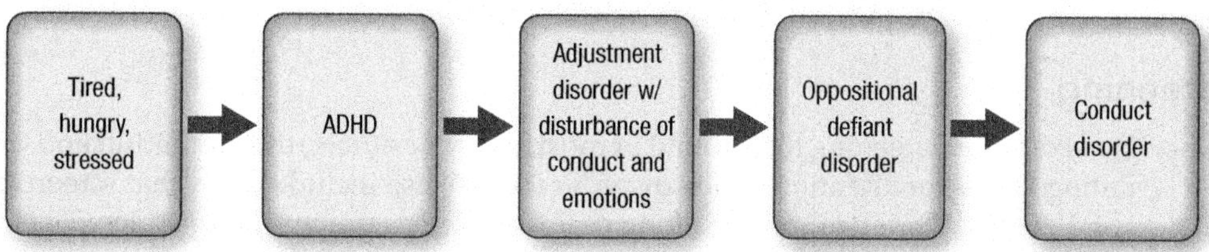

Risk Factors

- Disruptive behaviors can occur in a variety of conditions such as ADHD, anxiety, depressive and psychotic disorders.
- There are complex combinations of risk factors: biologic, psychologic, and social factors.
- The disruptive, impulse-control, and conduct disorders all tend to be more common in males than in females. These disorders tend to have first onset in childhood or adolescence.
- Biologic factors may include family clustering of similar disorders, genetic predisposition, and comorbid conditions, such as ADHD. Disruptive or oppositional behaviors are common in children with language disorders (receptive disorders in particular), cognitive deficits, delays in development with limited problem-solving skills, and other neuropsychologic deficits.

- Psychologic factors may include temperament, goodness of fit with family, school, and/or neighborhood. Parenting can be a significant factor; that is, parenting style, parenting inconsistency.
- Social factors may include stress related to the parent–child relationship, childcare experiences, and acute stressors in the family or environment, history of abuse, and exposure to parental discord or family violence.
- It is helpful to consider the particular child's risk/protective factor ratio.

Common Presenting Complaints

- Parents, appearing weary from their child's irritable, angry, externalizing behaviors, may present to the primary care or pediatric office with instructions from the school (or childcare provider) to "Get your child evaluated and treated for his problem behaviors or because he cannot continue to attend here!"
- Parents may describe previous good functioning, but now the child is irritable, does not seem to listen, storms around angrily, and seems preoccupied with his own thoughts.
- The child may arrive at the appointment with downcast eyes and a tense, if not angry, countenance. They may avoid eye contact, refuse to speak, or speak with a defiant, uncooperative attitude.
- The child may talk back to the provider, and present as "the boss" in interactions with family and healthcare team. They may be verbally oppositional and argumentative.
- The parent may say, "I can't do anything with him now." "He won't do anything I tell him to do." "He is always throwing temper fits."
- The child's behaviors may be so loud and disruptive in the waiting and exam rooms that it is clear why the referral for evaluation has been made.
- The ODD child is often overly sensitive to authority and the slightest perception of provocation will fuel their avoidant, defiant, or oppositional behavior. The pediatric clinician will need to be straightforward with a caring, concerned, matter-of-fact approach, aware that the goal for the clinician is "To not give in, and not give up" (The Psychiatric Interview of Children & Adolescents, Cepeda, 2010)

Screening

Two common screening tools found in most pediatric offices, the Vanderbilt and Conners' Assessment/Rating Scales for attention deficit disorder (ADD) also include items that screen for oppositional/defiant disorder. There are teacher rating scales as well as parent rating scales. These scales are presented in the section on ADHD along with the online links to obtain them. The KySS Worries Questionnaire (also in this manual) can be very helpful in identifying that child's stressors.

Assessment

When addressing problematic or disruptive behaviors, the differential starts with the child's history and physical exam, and interview of the child and parents. The teacher and parent's completed screening tools (Vanderbilt or Conners') also provide valuable information for the clinician as the assessment proceeds.

A good beginning assessment/diagnostic guide for the child with aggression is from the T-MAY toolkit (available online TMAY.org). Parents and teachers can keep a journal of this information.

The use of the "BOLDER" mnemonic is helpful in the assessment:

B—Behavior: In what ways does the child exhibit aggression?

O—Onset: When does it happen? What triggers it, and why?

L—Location: Where do the symptoms occur—home/school?

D—Duration: How long does it last?

E—Exacerbating factors: What makes it worse?

R—Relief: What makes it better?

**RISK ASSESSMENT: Whenever a young person is seen who has extreme impulsive anger, a risk assessment needs to be conducted. Often we ask parents, "Do you feel safe with this young person?" and we ask the youth, "Do you feel you can keep yourself safe from hurting yourself or hurting others?"

A psychiatry consult or evaluation in the emergency department by a mental health crisis team can always be arranged if the PCP assesses the situation to be acute and requiring immediate psychiatric evaluation and treatment.

The following questions to assess *risk* are from The REACH Institute, Action Signs for Helping Kids program:

Do you have:

Involvement in many fights, using a weapon, or wanting to badly hurt others?

Severe out of control behavior that can hurt yourself or others?

It is always good to ask the family about a crisis plan. What would they do if the situation became unsafe? Who would they call? Where would they go for immediate help? Having a well thought out crisis plan allows them to react quickly in the event of a crisis.

Used with permission: The REACH Institute and T-MAY Steering Committee, www.thereachinstitute.org/tmay-static.html

DSM-5 Diagnoses for Disruptive Behaviors

The diagnosis related to disruptive disorders fall on a continuum from ADHD (which needs to be ruled out first) to adjustment disorders. If those criteria are not met, then consider the behaviors as symptoms of oppositional defiant disorder and disruptive disorder not otherwise specified (NOS) or the more serious conduct disorder. This section will focus on adjustment disorders, oppositional defiant disorder, and disruptive disorder NOS. ADHD is covered in a previous section, and conduct disorders will be covered in the next section.

In *DSM-5*, *adjustment disorders with disturbance of conduct and emotions* are found in the section on *trauma and stressor related disorders.*

In *DSM-5*, *oppositional defiant disorder and disruptive disorder NOS* are found in the section on *disruptive, impulse control, and conduct disorders.*

Specific diagnostic criteria for each disorder will be presented as each is discussed.

Adjustment Disorders

Always consider adjustment disorder (a trauma and stressor-related disorder) first while the workup is in progress. You can always add that a diagnosis is "provisional."

Children's behaviors often represent distress in their home or environment.

When bad things happen, most people get upset. Adjustment disorder is diagnosed when the magnitude of the distress (e.g., alterations in mood, anxiety, conduct) exceeds what would normally be expected. Whenever there is a significant stress, children and teens can respond with externalizing symptoms—anger, impulsivity, and disruptive conduct.

Adjustment disorder is in the trauma and stress section of the *DSM-5*, and so are acute stress disorder and posttraumatic stress disorder (PTSD)—all three of these disorders involve emotional and behavioral symptoms in response to an identifiable stressor. Stressors may be single events, recurrent or continuous; stressors may affect a single person, an entire family, or a larger group or community (as with disasters). Some stressors accompany specific developmental events (such as starting middle school). Individuals from disadvantaged life circumstances experience a high rate of stressors and may be at increased risk for adjustment disorders. In adjustment disorder the stressor can be of any severity rather than the severity and type required of acute stress disorder and PTSD. There are timing and symptom differences between adjustment disorder and acute stress disorder and PTSD. Adjustment disorders can be diagnosed immediately and persist up to 6 months after exposure to the traumatic event. Acute stress disorder and PTSD are covered in Section 3: the anxiety disorders section of this guide.

The prevalence of adjustment disorder has been reported to be between 2% and 8% in community samples of children and adolescents. Boys and girls are equally likely to receive this diagnosis.

ASSESSMENT/DIAGNOSIS BASED ON THE *DSM-5*

Adjustment Disorder

- Severe emotional or behavioral symptoms that have developed as a reaction to an identified stressor in the last 3 months.
- The symptoms seen are more severe than the level of the specific stressor or they cause significant difficulty in the day-to-day functioning of the child or adolescent.
- These symptoms should not be a part of a normal grief process and do not continue 6 months after the stressor has completed.

Acute Stress Disorder

- Severe distress caused acutely after a severe trauma, usually within 1 month, with the symptoms lasting for at least 3 days.
- The child or adolescent should have nine or more symptoms that can include irritability, intrusive thoughts, avoiding anything associated with the trauma, low mood, nightmares, negative thoughts, and guilt.
- If the person has had an exposure to actual or threatened death, serious injury, or sexual violation by directly experiencing the traumatic event, witnessing the event, or learning that a traumatic event occurred to a close family member or close friend then they may meet criteria for *acute stress disorder for 3 days to a month after trauma exposure.*

Posttraumatic Stress Disorder

- Symptoms-based categories in which the child or adolescent will see negative changes in awareness and mood.
- The patient must meet all three categories to achieve the diagnosis along with the symptoms being present for 1 month. The patient also must have significant stress in their level of functioning in day-to-day life.
  - Intrusive recollections (flashbacks, nightmares)
  - Avoidance/numbing symptoms (withdrawal from activities, isolating)
  - Hyperarousal (hypervigilance)

If the person has had an exposure to actual or threatened death, serious injury, or sexual violation by directly experiencing the traumatic event, witnessing the event, or learning that a traumatic event occurred to a close family member or close friend then they may meet criteria for *acute stress disorder for 3 days to a month after trauma exposure.*

If the child behaviors cannot be accounted for as adjustment disorder with mixed disturbance of emotion and conduct, or adjustment disorder with disturbance of conduct, then the next differential diagnosis to be considered will be oppositional defiant disorder from the *DSM-5* section disruptive, impulse-control, and conduct disorders.

In the *DSM-5*, disruptive, impulse-control, and conduct disorders are the conditions involving problems in the self-control of emotions (anger and irritation) and behaviors (argumentativeness and defiance). Intermittent explosive disorder is also in this section, as is conduct disorder, which will be discussed in another section of this guide.

The disruptive, impulse-control, and conduct disorders all tend to be more common in males than in females. These disorders tend to have first onset in childhood or adolescence. Conduct disorder (which now has a childhood onset or adolescent onset clarifier) or intermittent explosive disorder represent patterns of serious disruptive behaviors over time and generally clinicians hold off on assigning these diagnoses in younger patients. Intermittent explosive disorder can include verbal aggression as well as nondestructive, noninjurious behaviors. This must occur after the age of 6 years. The aggressive outbursts are impulsive and anger based.

There is a developmental relationship between oppositional defiant disorder and conduct disorder in that most cases of conduct disorder previously would have met criteria for ODD, at least in cases in which conduct disorder emerges prior to adolescence. However, most children with ODD do not eventually develop conduct disorder. Furthermore, children with ODD are at risk for eventually developing other problems besides conduct disorder, including anxiety and depressive disorders (*DSM-5*).

Oppositional Defiant Disorder

Children with ODD show extreme levels of argumentativeness, disobedience, stubbornness, negativity, and provocation of others. While such behavior can be true of most children at some point of their lives, this diagnosis is warranted only for the few children (3%–4%) whose symptoms persist over months or years, occur across many situations, and result in pronounced impairment in their functioning in home, school, and peer settings (TheREACHInstitute.org/). ODD is a milder form and sometimes a precursor to conduct disorder. In contrast to children with conduct disorder, the behavior of children with ODD does not involve serious violations of others' rights. It does, however, impair the child's family, academic, and social functioning (TheREACHInstitute.org/).

ASSESSMENT/DIAGNOSIS BASED ON THE *DSM-5*

Oppositional Defiant Disorder

A pattern of angry/irritable mood, argumentative/defiant behavior, or vindictiveness lasting at least 6 months as evidenced by at least four symptoms from any of the following categories and exhibited during interaction with at least one individual *who is not a sibling*.

Angry/irritable mood which can include often loses temper, is often touchy or easily annoyed and/or often angry and resentful.

Argumentative/defiant behavior which can include often arguing with authority figures or, for children and adolescents, with adults; often actively defies or refuses to comply with requests from authority figures or with rules; deliberately annoys others and/or often blames others for his or her mistakes or misbehavior.

Vindictiveness which can include having been spiteful or vindictive at least twice within the past 6 months. Persistence and frequency of these behaviors should be used to distinguish a behavior that is within normal limits from behavior that is symptomatic. For children younger than 5 years, the behavior should occur on most days for a period of at least 6 months. For individuals 5 years or older, the behavior should occur at least once per week for at least 6 months, frequency and intensity of the behaviors are outside a range that is normative for the individual's developmental level, gender, and culture.

Evidence-Based Management

An evidence-base update for psychosocial treatments for disruptive behaviors in *children* by Kaminski and Claussen (2017) reviewed 86 empirical papers covering 50 unique treatment protocols and, according to support criteria, classified treatments as well-established, probably efficacious, possibly efficacious, experimental, or questionable efficacy based on existing evidence. Often the evidence-based treatments for disruptive children intervene on maladaptive parenting and children's basic cognitive skills. For adolescents, parenting/family relations remain important but treatment often focuses on adolescents' more advanced cognitive skills, their peer relationships, and their school environment. McCart and Sheidow (2016) conducted an evidence-based update of psychosocial treatments for *adolescents* with disruptive behaviors.

For disruptive behaviors in children two multicomponent treatments that integrate strategies from family, behavioral, and cognitive behavioral treatments met criteria as well established: group parent behavior therapy and individual parent behavior therapy with child participation. Although treatment programs can be effectively used with different cultural groups, there is also evidence that cultural background affects the effectiveness of interventions such as parent training and needs to always be considered.

With adolescents two multicomponent treatments that integrate strategies from family, behavioral, and cognitive behavioral therapy (CBT) met criteria as well established. These two treatments, Multisystemic Therapy (MST) and Treatment Foster Care Oregon (TFCO), were delivered to justice-involved youth. MST also met criteria as probably efficacious delivered to disruptive youth who were not justice involved. MST is family based, and often involves home therapy teaching modules to parents to assist them in generating change. TFCO integrates cognitive behavioral interventions within the teen's environment. Both treatments also consider the other systems the child interacts with—peers, school, community.

These evidence-based treatment studies reinforce what we have known, that children and teens with disruptive behavior disorders require intensive treatment—therapeutic programs where family behavioral and CBT are integrated. Often these treatments are not available in the child/teen's community. Community Mental Health Centers are best equipped to meet the needs of these youth, having in-home therapists, family/parent therapists, as well as contacts for referral to higher levels of care.

Initial treatment and management planning include:

- Referral to specialty psychiatry services is always considered as an option, depending on patient presentation and availability of such specialists in the community, but in this guide we offer ways to start active intervention with the families—capitalizing on the trusting relationship the family has with the PCP.

From T-MAY:

PRESTO plan:

P—Partner with the family

R—Assess risk, identify professional reinforcements, and refer if need be

E—Educate the family on evidence-based practices and expectations of treatment

S—Ascertain support in the community

T—Track signs and symptoms with tools

O—Objectives and action plans are established with the family

- In obtaining information for both assessment and subsequent treatment, the success will require building a therapeutic alliance with the parents, and the child separately. Engagement with the child is often best achieved by empathizing with the child's anger and unhappiness. Focus on the problem at hand, and let the child know you are aware that he or she is hurting. Engage the child in problem-solving. Most youth realize their behavior is out of line.
- When the child exhibits problems with behavior, the plan of care will routinely include the parents, the child, and the school (or childcare provider setting). Parents may need to be informed that, in children, involving the teacher, parent, and healthcare providers is the best evidence-based care. The team approach—multimodal—is most effective and parents and the child need not feel embarrassed, as it is standard best practice.
- Initially, with signed consent of the parent or guardian, the PCP will want collateral information from the school regarding the child's behaviors there, and a coordination of care can begin—always keeping the parents and child informed and central to the communications back and forth.
- If the parents request, the PCP can write out a note that the child is being evaluated and followed by that provider. School officials likely will grant an extension for a deadline final decision about the child's continued attendance, and this will relieve some of the immediate family pressure.
- Sometimes it takes finesse for the PCP to be the leader/coordinator of the parent/child/teacher/healthcare provider/and specialty psychiatry (if involved) team—and keep everyone reminded that the "battle" is against the "problem behaviors" (not blame for each other) and all are on the same team—moving forward, fighting that battle together.
- Identify the child's strengths (and the family's) and praise the child's steps toward solving the problem.
- Pediatric healthcare providers have long recognized the important role of providing guidance to parents. PCPs already provide behavioral interventions in their practice. They have coached many parents through the steps of setting up a reward chart with stickers for a child with an identified problem behavior/habit.
- Most pediatric clinicians have an assortment of favorite behavioral strategies that they use in counseling parents about behavior management (checklists/monitoring, reward charts, special times, planned ignoring, time outs logical consequences, goal setting/target behaviors, positive and negative reinforcements).
- Parents are also reminded that the problem behaviors may escalate at first, as the child "tests" the new parenting approaches.
- Referral to family therapy is often recommended, as well as linking the family to community agencies that provide classes, support, and connections with families struggling with similar challenges.

According to the American Academy of Child and Adolescent Psychiatry, in the 2007 Practice Parameter for the assessment and treatment of children and adolescents with oppositional defiant disorder, the "treatment of ODD may be particularly problematic and often requires multimodal treatment, including psychosocial interventions and occasionally medication therapy."

Psychosocial Interventions

The two types of evidence-based treatments for youth with ODD are:

Individual approaches in the form of problem-solving skills training.

Individual approaches should be specific to problems encountered, behaviorally based, and as much as possible oriented to the development of problem-solving skills.

Examples of problem-solving, skills-building programs are:

Collaborative Problem-Solving: www.ccps.info/ and www.livesinthebalance.org/

Child Protective Services views the child's disruptive, explosive behavior as the child's inadequate and inappropriate attempt to solve a problem in his or her world. The child's particular means of "solving his problem" may not be satisfactory to the parent or teacher, but it is the only solution the child can figure out at this point. In collaborative problem-solving therapy (CPS), the parent's or teacher's role is to "figure out" what problem the child is struggling with, such as having a constitutionally short fuse, a need to be in control of what seems to be an unpredictable environment, and an inability to understand adults' requests. Once the parent understands the child's problem, their next role is helping the child find a solution, given the problem, and to "scaffold" (assist) the child to a next step in developing new skills and behaviors that help them solve the problem (Greene, 2014).

Creating Opportunities for Personal Empowerment (COPE) for Children and Adolescents is a seven-session evidence-based manualized cognitive behavioral skills building program, presented at length in the *depressive disorders* and *brief interventions* section of this manual. In the COPE program, there is a major emphasis on teaching the child self-regulation (i.e., how to positively control emotions). The young person learns strategies and skills to positively influence their thoughts, emotions, and behaviors. The homework in COPE provides opportunities for practice of these self-control skills in their home, school, and social environment.

Family Interventions in the Form of Parent Management Training

The best family interventions encompass training in effective disciplining and age-appropriate supervision. The main principles of evidence-based family interventions are:

- Reduce positive reinforcement of disruptive behavior
- Increase reinforcement of prosocial and compliant behavior. Positive reinforcements can vary, but parental attention is the priority. Punishment usually consists of time out and loss of rewards/privileges.
- Apply consequences and/or punishment for disruptive behavior.
- Make parental response predictable, contingent, and immediate.

The clinician may know of good parenting programs in their community.

Examples of recommended Parent Management Training programs are:

- Triple P: www.triplep.net/
- Incredible Years: www.incredibleyears.com/
- Parent empowerment program: www.thereachinstitute.org/pep.html

Medication

Many primary care/pediatric providers will consult with child psychiatric clinicians in initiating medication as an adjunct to psychosocial interventions.

According to the American Academy of Child and Adolescent Psychiatry (AACAP), medications may be helpful as adjuncts to psychosocial treatment for symptomatic treatment and to treat comorbid conditions. Medication should not be the sole intervention in ODD. The following are recommendations from AACAP Practice Parameters for children and teens with ODD.*

- Prescribing medications without enlisting the child's support or assent is unlikely to be successful, especially with adolescents.
- Pharmacologic agents for ODD are not well studied, but several agents have received support in double-blind, placebo-controlled studies of disruptive behavior.
- Medications such as stimulants, atomoxetine and guanfacine, used to treat ODD in the context of ADHD, may result in improvement of the oppositional behavior.
- Promise has been shown for mood stabilizers such as divalproex sodium and lithium carbonate, antipsychotics, and stimulants for the target behavior aggression.
- Regardless of diagnosis, atypical antipsychotics seem to be the most commonly prescribed medications for the treatment of acute and chronic maladaptive aggression.
- Typical and atypical antipsychotics are helpful in treating aggression after appropriate psychosocial interventions have been applied in the context of mental retardation and pervasive developmental disorders.

If comorbid conditions are present, then medication should be targeted to those specific symptoms as much as possible.

Consider adding an antipsychotic, taking into account the latest available evidence on efficacy and safety if severe aggression persists after an adequate trial of treatments for the underlying disorder.

Start low! Go slow! And stop slowly. Avoid abruptly stopping and/or switching to reduce risk of rebound. Slow switch using cross titration is the preferred method.

Use a recommended titration schedule and deliver an adequate medication trial before changing or adding medication.

Nonresponsiveness to a specific compound should lead to a trial of another class of medication instead of adding on medications (to avoid further clouding the case). If a trial of an atypical antipsychotic is not effective, then a trial of another atypical or switch to a mood stabilizer is recommended. Atypical antipsychotics should be prescribed in consultation and collaboration with a mental health provider.

Avoid using more than two psychotropic medications simultaneously.

SSRIs are not considered first line agents unless major depressive disorder or anxiety is diagnosed along with ODD.

Conduct side effect (AIMS) and metabolic assessments and laboratory tests that are clinically relevant, comprehensive, and based on established guidelines.

Provide accessible information to parents and families about identifying and managing side effects. Promote healthy lifestyle changes that may reduce the risk of physical adverse events and medication consequences.

See the T-MAY Pocket Guide at www.TheREACHInstitute.org/TMAY.html

*Practice Parameter for the Assessment and Treatment of Children and Adolescents with Oppositional Defiant Disorder is available at www.aacap.org

For comorbid ADHD and aggression/ODD—www.guideline.gov/content.aspx?id=15628&search=antipsychotics+in+primary+care

From the T-MAY Pocket Guide www.TheREACHInstitute.org/TMAY.html

The REACH Institute, Rutgers CERTs Reference Guide for Primary Care Clinicians and Mental Health Specialist for medication guidelines: "Psychotropic agents, particularly second-generation antipsychotics and mood stabilizers are increasingly given to youth on an outpatient basis for treatment for overt aggression . . . despite troubling side effects and a lack of supportive empirical evidence of their effects on adolescents and children" Medications are nicely presented in the T-MAY Reference Guide in a very clear chart (anticonvulsants, and the atypical antipsychotics—dosages, indications, side effects).

The following charts of antipsychotic medications and mood stabilizers: from the website www.medicaid.gov

www.medicaid.gov/medicaid/prescription-drugs/drug-utilization-review/antipsychotic-medication-use-children/index.html

A Review of State Medicaid Approaches on Child Antipsychotic Monitoring Programs 2016: https://www.medicaid.gov/medicaid-chip-program-information/by-topics/prescription-drugs/downloads/state-medicaid-dur-summaries.pdf

The U.S. Food and Drug Administration (FDA) has no approved indications for aggressions in children and adolescents apart from irritability associated aggression in children with autism. In other populations, recent federally supported evidence-based reviews suggest efficacy for some psychotherapeutic agents (Wissow, 2015).

The second-generation antipsychotics on the following list (asenapine, lurasidone, olanzapine, quetiapine, risperidone, and paliperidone) and the third-generation antipsychotic (aripiprazole) and lithium, mood stabilizer are approved for treatment of youth with psychosis (all but asenapine); mania in bipolar disorder (all but paliperidone and lurasidone); and irritability in autism (risperidone and aripiprazole).

However, these medications are most commonly used off label (outside FDA indications) in youth to treat behavioral problems, especially aggression that can cause harm to self or others.

In primary care pediatric practice, mostly risperidone and aripiprazole are prescribed (the specialists in behavioral/developmental pediatrics and psychiatric/mental health practice are more familiar with the other second-generation antipsychotic (SGA) and mood stabilizers use in children and adolescents (Riddle, 2019).

Guanfacine also is used in pediatric/primary care practice for impulsivity and inattentiveness as an adjunct to ADHD medications or alone.

Atypical Antipsychotics

Drug (Generic)	Drug (Brand)[b]	Initial Dosage	Literature-Based Maximum Dosage	FDA-Approved Maximum Dosage for Children and Adolescents	Schedule	Patient Monitoring Parameters	Black Box Warning	Warnings and Precautions
aripiprazole	Abilify	2 mg/day	Children: 15 mg/day Adolescents: 30 mg/day	Approved for treatment of bipolar mania or mixed episodes (age 10–17 years) and schizophrenia (13–17 years): 30 mg/day Approved for treatment of irritability associated with autistic disorder (age 6–17 years): 15 mg/day	Once daily	Fasting plasma glucose level or hemoglobin A1c: at baseline, at 3 months, then every 6 months. Lipid screening: (total cholesterol, low- and high-density lipoprotein [LDL and HDL] cholesterol, and triglycerides): baseline, at 3 months, then every 6 months. CBC: as indicated by guidelines approved by the FDA in the product labeling. Pregnancy test: as clinically indicated. Blood pressure, pulse rate, height, weight, and BMI measurement: when a new antipsychotic is initiated and at every visit. Sexual function inquiry: inquire yearly for evidence of galactorrhea/gynecomastia, menstrual disturbance, libido disturbance or erectile/ejaculatory disturbances in males (priapism has been reported with iloperidone, risperidone and ziprasidone). This inquiry should be done at each visit (quarterly for inpatients) for the first 12 months after starting an antipsychotic or until the medication dose is stable and then yearly.	Not approved for depression under age 18. Increased the risk of suicidal thinking and behavior in short-term studies in children and adolescents with major depressive disorder and other psychiatric disorders.	Neuroleptic malignant syndrome Tardive dyskinesia Hyperglycemia and diabetes mellitus Weight gain Dyslipidemia Orthostatic hypotension Leukopenia, neutropenia, and agranulocytosis Lowers seizure threshold Cognitive and motor impairment Hyperthermia Dysphagia Hyperprolactinemia (except not reported with aripiprazole, clozapine, and asenapine) Extrapyramidal side effects

(*continued*)

Atypical Antipsychotics (*continued*)

Drug (Generic)	Drug (Brand)[b]	Initial Dosage	Literature-Based Maximum Dosage	FDA-Approved Maximum Dosage for Children and Adolescents	Schedule	Patient Monitoring Parameters	Black Box Warning	Warnings and Precautions
quetiapine[a]	Seroquel	Age ≤9 years: 12.5–25 mg/day Age 10–17 years: 50 mg/day	Age ≤9 years: 400 mg/day Age 10–17 years: 800 mg/day	Approved for treatment of bipolar mania (age 10–17 years): 600 mg/day Approved for treatment of schizophrenia (13–17 years): 800 mg/day	Two to three times daily	EPS evaluation (examination for rigidity, tremor, akathisia): before initiation of any antipsychotic medication, then weekly for the first 2 weeks after initiating treatment with a new antipsychotic or until the dose has been stabilized and weekly for 2 weeks after a dose increase. Tardive dyskinesia evaluation: every 12 months. For high-risk patients (including the elderly), every 6 months. Vision questionnaire: ask whether the patient has experienced a change in vision and should specifically ask about distance vision and blurry vision yearly. (Cataracts have been reported for quetiapine) EKG: baseline and as clinically indicated (QTc prolongationreported for asenapine, clozapine, iloperidone, paliperidone, quetiapine, and ziprasidone)		
	Seroquel XR (brand only)							
olanzapine[a]	Zyprexa	Age <6 years: 1.25 mg/day Age 6–12 years: 2.5 mg/day Age ≥13 years: 2.5–5 mg/day	Children: 12.5 mg/day Adolescents: 20 mg/day	Approved for treatment of bipolar mania or mixed episodes and schizophrenia (age 13–17 years): 20 mg/day	Once daily		None related to youth	

(*continued*)

Atypical Antipsychotics (*continued*)

Drug (Generic)	Drug (Brand)[b]	Initial Dosage	Literature-Based Maximum Dosage	FDA-Approved Maximum Dosage for Children and Adolescents	Schedule	Patient Monitoring Parameters	Black Box Warning	Warnings and Precautions
risperidone[a]	Risperdal	Children: <20 kg: 0.25 mg/day >20 kg: 0.5 mg/day Adolescents: 0.5 mg/day	Children: 3 mg/day Adolescents: 6 mg/day	Approved for treatment of schizophrenia (age 13–17 years) and bipolar mania or mixed Episodes (age 10–17 years): 6 mg/day Approved for treatment of irritability associated with autistic disorder (age 5–16 years): 3 mg/day	Once or twice daily		None related to youth	
clozapine[a]	Clozaril Fazaclo (oral disintegrating tablet)	Children: 6.25–12.5 mg/day Adolescents: 6.25–25 mg/day	Children: 150–300 mg/day Adolescents: 600 mg/day Target serum clozapine level of 350 ng/mL for optimal efficacy	Not approved for children and adolescents	Once or twice daily		Risk of life-threatening agranulocytosis Seizures Myocarditis Other adverse cardiovascular and respiratory effects	
asenapine (sublingual)	Saphris	Insufficient evidence	Insufficient evidence	Not approved for children and adolescents	Insufficient evidence; nothing by mouth for 10 minutes after sublingual administration		None related to youth	

(*continued*)

Atypical Antipsychotics (*continued*)

Drug (Generic)	Drug (Brand)[b]	Initial Dosage	Literature-Based Maximum Dosage	FDA-Approved Maximum Dosage for Children and Adolescents	Schedule	Patient Monitoring Parameters	Black Box Warning	Warnings and Precautions
iloperidone	Fanapt	Insufficient evidence	Insufficient evidence	Not approved for children and adolescents	Insufficient evidence		None related to youth	
paliperidone	Invega	Children: Insufficient evidence Adolescents: 3 mg/day	Children: Insufficient evidence Adolescents: Weight < 51 kg: 6 mg/day Weight ≥ 51 kg: 12 mg/day	Approved for treatment of schizophrenia (age 12–17 years): Weight < 51 kg: 6 mg/day Weight ≥ 51 kg: 12 mg/day	Once daily		None related to youth	
ziprasidone[a]	Geodon	Bipolar disorder (age 10–17 years): 20 mg/day Tourette's disorder: 5 mg/day	Bipolar disorder Weight ≤ 45 kg: 80 mg/day Weight > 45 kg: 160 mg/day Tourette's disorder: 40 mg/day	Not approved for children and adolescents	Insufficient evidence; take with ≥500 calorie meal		None related to youth	
lurasidone	latuda	Insufficient evidence	Insufficient evidence	Not approved for children and adolescents	Insufficient evidence; take with >350 calorie meal		None related to youth	

[a]Generic available; [b]XR, extended-release.

ADHD Medications

- The stimulants and nonstimulant ADHD medications are covered in detail in that section.
- Treat comorbid diagnoses such as ADHD. High level of evidence studies has suggested improvement in conduct disorder symptoms with treatment with psychostimulants in aggression improvement.
- Guanfacine for impulsivity/inattentiveness: For youth with impaired impulse control and inattentiveness due to toxic stress, instead of stimulants there has been reported success with nonstimulants:
    - Guanfacine is a nonstimulant that was originally developed to treat high blood pressure but also is used for ADHD. Guanfacine targets specific circuits in the prefrontal cortex where adrenaline and noradrenaline exert their action, improving impulsiveness and concentration, even in situations of high stress. Guanfacine can be helpful for poor impulse and frustration control (Riddle, 2019, pp. 94–100).
    - Guanfacine is not FDA approved for use in youth younger than 6 years.
    - Extended release (ER) guanfacine (generic and Intuniv) is FDA approved for ADHD in children and adolescents ages 6 years and older. Initial dose is 1 mg. Max daily dose is 4 mg. Duration of ER guanfacine is up to 24 hours—once daily dosing. It should not be taken with a high fat meal; regular checks of blood pressure and heart rate are recommended. Can be used alone or in combination with a stimulant.

Mood Stabilizers

Drug (Generic)	Drug (Brand)	Initial Dosage	Target Dosage Range	Literature-Based Maximum Dosage	FDA-Approved Maximum Dosage for Children and Adolescents	Schedule	Baseline Monitoring	Black Box Warning	Warnings and Precautions
carbamazepine*	Carbatrol(ER)	Age <6 years: 10–20 mg/kg/day	Age <6 years: 35 mg/kg/day Ages 6–12 years: 400–800 mg/day Age >12 years: 800– 1200 mg/day	Age <6 years: 35 mg/kg/day Ages 6–12 years: 800 mg/day Age 12–15 years: 1000 mg/day Age > 15 years: 1200 mg/day	Approved for treatment of seizure disorders in all ages Age <6 years: 35 mg/kg/day Age 6–15 years: 1000 mg/day Age > 15 years: 1200 mg/day	Twice daily	HLA-B*1502 Allele (risk of SJS) Pregnancy test CBC Electrolytes	Stevens-Johnson Syndrome Aplastic Anemia/granulocytosis	Stevens-Johnson syndrome Aplastic anemia Suicidality Teratogenicity Neutropenia Hyponatremia Induces metabolism of itself and some other drugs Decreased efficacy of oral contraceptives Withdrawal seizures
	Tegretol	Age 6–12 years: 10 mg/kg/day or 200 mg/day Age >12 years: 400 mg/day				Two to four times daily			

(*continued*)

Mood Stabilizers (*continued*)

Drug (Generic)	Drug (Brand)	Initial Dosage	Target Dosage Range	Literature-Based Maximum Dosage	FDA-Approved Maximum Dosage for Children and Adolescents	Schedule	Baseline Monitoring	Black Box Warning	Warnings and Precautions
	TegretolXR					Twice daily			
divalproex sodium*	Depakote	10–15 mg/kg/day	30–60 mg/kg/day	Serum level: 125 μg/mL, or 60 mg/kg/day	Approved for treatment of seizure Disorders (age ≥10 years) Maximum dose based upon serum level: 50–100 μg/mL, or 60 mg/kg/day	One to three times daily	Chemistry panel CBC (with platelets) LFTs Pregnancy test	Hepatotoxicity Teratogenicity Pancreatitis	Hepatotoxicity Pancreatitis Urea cycle disorders Teratogenicity Suicidal ideation Thrombocytopenia Hyperammonemia Multi-organ hypersensitivity reaction Withdrawal seizures Polycystic ovaries Neutropenia

(*continued*)

Mood Stabilizers (*continued*)

Drug (Generic)	Drug (Brand)	Initial Dosage	Target Dosage Range	Literature-Based Maximum Dosage	FDA-Approved Maximum Dosage for Children and Adolescents	Schedule	Baseline Monitoring	Black Box Warning	Warnings and Precautions
lithium*	Eskalith	Children: Lesser of 15–20 mg/kg/day or 150 mg twice per day Adolescents: Lesser of 15–20 mg/day or 300 mg twice per day	Dose adjustment based upon serum level Serum level: 0.6–1.2 mEq/L	Serum level: 1.2 mEq/L, or 1800 mg	Maximum dose based upon serum level: 1.2 mEq/L	One to four times daily	Chemistry panel CBC (with platelets) Serum creatinine LFTs Pregnancy test ECG Blood for lithium serum levels should be drawn 10–12 hours after the last dose.	Toxicity above therapeutic serum levels	Toxicity above therapeutic serum levels Chronic renal function impairment Special risk patients: those with significant renal or cardiovascular disease, severe debilitation, dehydration, or sodium depletion · Polyuria Tremor Diarrhea Nausea Hypothyroidism Teratogenicity
	Eskalith CR								
	Lithobid (ER)								

(*continued*)

Mood Stabilizers (*continued*)

Drug (Generic)	Drug (Brand)	Initial Dosage	Target Dosage Range	Literature-Based Maximum Dosage	FDA-Approved Maximum Dosage for Children and Adolescents	Schedule	Baseline Monitoring	Black Box Warning	Warnings and Precautions
lamotrigine*	Lamictal	Children: 2–5 mg/day Adolescents: 25 mg/day (increase by 25 mg every 2 weeks)	Children Monotherapy: 4.5–7.5 mg/kg/day With valproate: 1–3 mg/kg/day With valproate and EIAEDs: 1–5 mg/kg/day With EIAEDs: 5–15 mg/kg/day Adolescents Monotherapy: 225–375 mg/day With valproate: 100–200 mg/day With Valproate and EIAEDs: 100–400 mg/day With EIAEDs: 300–500 mg/day		Approved for adjunctive therapy for Seizure disorders: Age 2–12: 400 mg/day Age >12: 500 mg/day Safety and effectiveness for treatment of bipolar disorder in patients younger than 18 years has not been established	Once or twice daily		Serious rashes including Stevens-Johnson syndrome	Dermatologic reactions Potential Stevens-Johnson syndrome Multi-organ hypersensitivity reactions and organ failure Blood dyscrasias Suicidal ideation Aseptic meningitis Concomitant use with oral contraceptives increases lamotrigine clearance Withdrawal seizures

(*continued*)

Mood Stabilizers (*continued*)

Drug (Generic)	Drug (Brand)	Initial Dosage	Target Dosage Range	Literature-Based Maximum Dosage	FDA-Approved Maximum Dosage for Children and Adolescents	Schedule	Baseline Monitoring	Black Box Warning	Warnings and Precautions
oxcarbazepine*	Trileptal	8–10 mg/kg/day	Monotherapy (based on weight): 20–24.9 kg: 600–900 mg/day 25–34.9 kg: 900–1200 mg/day 35–44.9 kg: 900–1500 mg/day 45–49.9 kg: 1200–1500 mg/day 50–59.9 kg: 1200–1800 mg/day 60–69.9 kg: 1200–2100 mg/day ≥70 kg: 1500–2100 mg/day	Children: 60 mg/kg/day or 1500 mg/day Adolescents: 60 mg/kg/day or 2100 mg/day	Therapy in (age ≥ 2 years): 60 mg/kg/day or 1800 mg/day	Twice daily	CBC Electrolytes Pregnancy test		Hyponatremia Anaphylactic reactions and angioedema Patients with a past history of hypersensitivity reaction to carbamazepine Serious dermatologic reactions Withdrawal seizures Cognitive/neuro-psychiatric adverse events Multiorgan hypersensitivity Hematologic events

RESOURCES FOR PROVIDERS

American Psychiatric Association. (2013). *Diagnostic and statistical manual of mental disorders* (5th ed.). www.dsm5.org

T-MAY (*Treatment of Maladaptive Aggression in Youth) Rutgers CERTs Pocket Reference Guide for Primary Care Clinicians and Mental Health Specialists.* (2010). Center for Education and Research on Mental Health Therapeutics (CERTs) Rutgers University, The REACH Institute, University of Texas at Austin College of Pharmacy, New York State Office of Mental Health, California Department of Mental Health ACH.

Hans Steiner, M. D., Lisa Remsing, M. D., & The Work Group on Quality Issues. (2007). Practice parameters for the assessment and treatment of children and adolescents with oppositional defiant disorder. *Journal of the American Academy of Child & Adolescent Psychiatry, 46*(1).

The REACH Institute www.thereachinstitute.org/behavior therapy, www.TheREACHInstitute.org/behavioral-therapy.html

Greene, R. W. (2014). *The explosive child: A new approach for understanding and parenting easily frustrated, "chronically inflexible" children (Revised 4th edition).* HarperCollins.

R. W. Greene's website with resources for his collaborative problem-solving (cps) www.livesinthebalance.org/; this website has an extensive Q & A section for parents, and even audio lectures by Dr. Greene. It is factual and positive.

Another website with information on collaborative problem-solving is www.TheREACHInstitute.org/cps.html

Parent Empowerment Training - www.TheREACHInstitute.org/pep.html

Cepeda, C. (2010). *Clinical manual for the psychiatric interview of children and adolescents.* American Psychiatric Publishing, Inc.

RESOURCES FOR FAMILIES

AACAP (*American Academy of Child and Adolescent Psychiatry Campaign for America's Kids* website—nformation pages: Facts for Families. Children with ODD, "Facts for Families," No. 72 (3/11).

www.aacap.org/cs/root/facts_for_families/facts_for_families_numerical_list

Greene www.explosivechild.com and www.livesinthebalance.org/ This is a most helpful website, which has very helpful information and links for parents and healthcare providers. These sites focus on the collaborative problem-solving approach.

Oppositional Defiant Disorder Resource Center link: www.aacap.org/cs/ODD.Resource_Center

https://www.aacap.org/AACAP/Families_and_Youth/Facts_for_Families/Layout/FFF_Guide-01.aspx

Incredible Years Program: www.incredibleyears.com

COPE—Creating Opportunities for Personal Empowerment, a manualized seven-session evidence-based cognitive-behavioral skills building program for children, adolescents, and young adults by Bernadette Melnyk. To obtain the COPE program, contact cope.melnyk@gmail.com

CHILDREN'S BOOKS

When Sophie Gets Angry — Really, Really Angry…

Written and illustrated by Molly Bang

When Sophie's sister swipes her stuffed animal, she feels ready to explode "like a volcano." Vibrant illustrations depict Sophie kicking, screaming, and even roaring. But then the color palette of the illustrations changes as Sophie cries a little and lets the outdoors comfort her. "This book normalizes anger and shows that it doesn't last forever," says an expert from the Child Mind Institute. Ages 4 to 8. Published by Scholastic Paperbacks.

Tease Monster: A Book About Teasing vs. Bullying

Written by Julia Cook, illustrated by Anita DuFalla

Particularly good for an anxious or literal child, this rhyming book helps distinguish between teasing and bullying. "There are two types of teasing: the nice and the mean," Cook writes. "You think that everyone's against you, but it's not like it seems." Readers will learn strategies for responding to both good-natured teasing and bullying. Ages 5 to 10. Published by Boys Town Press.

Warp Speed

Written by Lisa Yee

In a fast-paced chapter book that will appeal to reluctant readers, Marley thinks seventh grade will be boring until he draws attention from the school bully. Digger pushes Marley down in the hallway, and the drama unfolds. "It's a very relatable story for kids who feel like outsiders," says an expert at the Child Mind Institute. Bonus: If your child is a fan of Star Wars, there are loads of references. Ages 8 to 12. Published by Arthur A. Levine Books.

APP Daniel Tiger for Parents DTParents

Greene, R. (2014). *The explosive child: A new approach for understanding and parenting easily frustrated, chronically inflexible children.*

Book by Dr. Greene promotes a "collaborative problem-solving approach." That approach has been incorporated into this resource page for parents. There is an excellent website for you to check out this approach to see if it fits with your family values/preferences.

www.livesinthebalance.org/

The research evidence to support "collaborative problem-solving" can be found on this website: www.explosivechild.com

Fact sheet: Children with Oppositional Defiant Disorder
www.aacap.org/cs/root/facts_for_families/children_with_odd

REFERENCES

Cepeda, C. (2010). *Clinical manual for the psychiatric interview of children and adolescents*. American Psychiatric Publishing, Inc.

Greene, R. W. (2014). *The explosive child: A new approach for understanding and parenting easily frustrated, "chronically inflexible" children* (Rev. 4th ed.). HarperCollins.

https://www.aacap.org/AACAP/Families_and_Youth/Facts_for_Families/FFF-Guide/Children-With-Oppositional-Defiant-Disorder-072.aspx

https://www.aacap.org/AACAP/Families_and_Youth/Facts_for_Families/Layout/FFF_Guide-01.aspx

Hirsch, G. S. (2018). Dosing and monitoring: Children and adolescents. *Psychopharmacology Bulletin, 48*(2), 34–92.

Kaminski, J., & Claussen, A. (2017). Evidence-based update for psychosocial treatments for disruptive behaviors in children. *Journal of Clinical Child & Adolescent Psychology, 46*(4), 477–499. https://doi.org/10.1080/15374416.2017.1310044

McCart, M., & Sheidow, A. (2016). Evidence-based psychosocial treatments for adolescents with disruptive behavior. *Journal of Clinical Child and Adolescent Psychology, 45*(5), 529–563. https://doi.org/10.1080/15374416.2016.1146990

Melnyk, B. M. (2004). *COPE–Creating Opportunities for Personal Empowerment for children, adolescents and young adults*. COPE2Thrive, LLC.

A Review of State Medicaid Approaches on Child Antipsychotic Monitoring Programs. (2016). https://www.medicaid.gov/medicaid-chip-program-information/by-topics/prescription-drugs/downloads/state-medicaid-dur-summaries.pdf

Riddle, M.A., (2019). Pediatric Psychopharmacology for Primary Care. 2nd edition. American Academy of Pediatrics. ISBN: 978-1-61002-199-9

The Reach Institute. www.thereachinstitute.org/

Steiner, H., Remsing, L., & The Work Group on Quality Issues. (2007). Practice parameters for the assessment and treatment of children and adolescents with oppositional defiant disorder. *Journal of the American Academy of Child & Adolescent Psychiatry, 46*(1), 126–141. https://doi.org/10.1097/01.chi.0000246060.62706.af

T-MAY (Treatment of Maladaptive Aggression in Youth) Rutgers CERTs pocket reference guide for primary care clinicians and mental health specialists. (2010). Center for Education and Research on Mental Health Therapeutics (CERTs) Rutgers University, The REACH Institute, University of Texas at Austin College of Pharmacy, New York State Office of Mental Health, California Department of Mental Health.

Wissow, L. (2015). Disruptive behavior and aggression, Chapter 16. In H. Adam & J. Foym (Eds.), *Signs and symptoms in pediatrics*. American Academy of Pediatrics.

Information for Parents About Behavior Problems in Children and Teens

- Pediatric providers recognize how difficult your role as parent is with this challenging child. You still may want to remind us about how exhausting it is to have a child with behavior issues.
- Please write down and tell us about every positive step that is being made as you parent your child.
- Always build on your child's particular positives; give your child praise and positive reinforcement when he or she shows flexibility or cooperation.
- Your child's problems are "loud" problems—they stand out for all to notice (as opposed to anxiety, which is more of a private child problem). You may be bombarded by others in your community telling you about your child's behaviors.
- The journey of working with a child who has problem or disruptive behaviors can be frustrating, draining, and isolating. This website connects you to a vast array of resources and links that can help you better understand challenging children: www.livesinthebalance.org/
- We want you to be well informed so you can teach others what you know. Your child's behaviors get "louder" and more obvious to others when they don't have the skills to deal with the demands being placed on them.
- Your child's difficulties are complicated, and may have come with the child. Maybe it is in their hard wiring—their brain anatomy and connections. Maybe it is in subtle temperament qualities; maybe it is compounded with traumatic experience. Maybe your style of parenting is perfect for one type of child but not such a "good fit" with this child's strong personality traits. Another significant factor is family stress, and family distress, including socioeconomic status.
- Whatever the combination of factors, there is no blame; rather, there is assurance that your child can learn to be more flexible, and can learn problem-solving skills, and can get better at tolerating frustration.
- Recognize that, as Dr. Greene writes in the *Explosive Child*—***children do well if they can.***
- Your child longs for your approval, so provide it when your child does something positive.
- Because your child has some very real challenges with their "wiring" and temperament, possibly genetics and early developmental stress, it is very likely that your child has trouble with (a) flexibility, (b) frustration tolerance, and (c) problem-solving (from *The Explosive Child* by Ross W. Greene, 2014), just as other children lag behind in acquiring academic or athletic skills).

- Some of the skills children similar to yours (with problem behaviors) have trouble with include:
  - Difficulty handling transitions—shifting from one mind-set task to another,
  - Difficulty reflecting on multiple thoughts or ideas simultaneously (disorganized),
  - Difficulty considering a range of solutions to a problem,
  - Difficulty considering the likely outcomes or consequences of actions (impulsive),
  - Difficulty expressing concerns, needs, or thoughts in words,
  - Difficulty managing emotional response to frustration in order to think rationally, and
  - Chronic irritability and/or anxiety significantly impede capacity for problem-solving.
- One of the biggest favors you can do for an explosive child is to identify the lagging skills that are setting the stage for his or her challenging behavior so that you and others understand what is getting in his or her way. Also, identify what problems may be causing explosive episodes and what helps to calm your child down. You and the teacher can keep a journal of these observations.
- Build in some extra minutes for the child to comply with your request. Your child may have trouble "switching gears" and moving to the new activity. Don't add time for their time out for every minute they stall on the way. That is the way they are wired; that is, they are slower to process a change in activity.
- Take a break or time out if you are about to make the conflict with your child worse. This is good modeling for the child of using self-control strategies.
- The best parenting style is a warm and involved guiding approach—providing discipline. Being consistent and firm, yet loving, is the best approach.
- Build on the positives of your individual child (an example would be the COPE exercise in the Child Handout—where you and your child list three positive things particular to your child, and you display those prominently and bring those up regularly and add to them).
- Dr. Greene writes, "Good parenting means being responsive to the hand you were dealt."
- Your child likely had developmental "lags" or challenges in these areas:
  - Difficulty seeing the "grays": concrete, literal, black and white thinking,
  - Difficulty deviating from rules or routine,
  - Difficulty handling unpredictability, ambiguity, uncertainty, or novelty,
  - Difficulty shifting from original idea or solution, or
  - Difficulty taking into account situational factors that would suggest the need to adjust a plan.
- Pick your battles. Prioritize the tasks you want the child to do, or habits you want to develop.
- Avoid power struggles. The child with ODD has trouble avoiding power struggles so you may have to go the "extra mile" to avoid getting into the battle of wills.

- Set up reasonable, age-appropriate limits with consequences that can be enforced consistently. Review these with an expert you trust, such as your pediatrician or nurse practitioner. Once these are set, feel confident they are what are best for the child, and stick consistently with your limits and consequences.
- All "adults" that are authorities in your child's life should also know your rules and also consistently enforce them. If the other parent disagrees, then there must be a plan made that all of the important adults in that child's life can consistently enforce.
- Your child has difficulty sorting out what to do if rules are not black and white.

  Because of this difficulty—the adults caring for and parenting this child will have to be super consistent *in consistently enforcing the rules.*
- Sticking to your expectations is very important. If you eventually give up your resolve and give in, the child will learn to persist until you give in.
- Remember that the problem behaviors may escalate, get worse at first, as the child "tests" the new parenting approaches.
- Parents will need to make special efforts to care for themselves. The strong willed, explosive child consumes so much of the parent's time and energy, it is easy to become exhausted physically and mentally. Maintain interests other than your child and ODD.
- Parents can seek out supports from other parents who are raising challenging children. When you receive regular calls from the school or childcare setting with complaints about your child's behavior, you need sounding boards. You need people around you who support your heroic efforts in parenting this child.
- Remember, much of the intense effort you are putting into your child is directly focused on making sure that other people will want to be around them. You have a good parenting goal.
- Please know that your healthcare provider knows and applauds how much time and energy you are investing—to make the tiny steps that seem undetectable but, in fact, are the necessary steps for your child's march toward success.

The *Explosive Child* book by Dr. Greene promotes a "collaborative problem-solving approach." That approach has been incorporated into this resource page for parents. There is an excellent website for you to check out this approach to see if it fits with your family values/preferences.

www.livesinthebalance.org/

The research evidence to support "collaborative problem-solving" can be found on this website: www.explosivechild.com

Fact sheet: Children with Oppositional Defiant Disorder
https://www.aacap.org/AACAP/Families_and_Youth/Facts_for_Families/FFF-Guide/Children-With-Oppositional-Defiant-Disorder-072.aspx

REFERENCE

Greene, R. W. (2014). *The explosive child: A new approach for understanding and parenting easily frustrated, "chronically inflexible" children* (Rev. 4th ed.). HarperCollins.

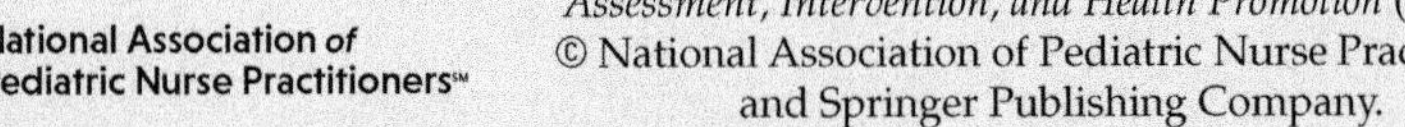

SPRINGER PUBLISHING

Handouts for Children to Help Them Cope and Behave in Positive Ways

Your doctor/nurse practitioner, parents/guardians, and you are all on the same team, helping you to deal with things that you find hard to do. As a team, we want to help you deal with things and behaviors at home and school that tend to get you in trouble. We are on your side. The other team is the problem behaviors. We know what behaviors will help you to be accepted by others at school and other places you go, and we are going to work with you so that you can learn behaviors that are positive. We may have to all take tiny steps, but with one step at a time, we will get there to watch you succeed.

Here are two handouts that will help you to feel more positive about you and deal with things that you find hard. It is a good idea to work on these with your parents, teacher, doctor, or nurse practitioner.

POSITIVE THINGS ABOUT ME

(From: *COPE for Children*, copyright by Bernadette Melnyk)

Positive self-talk helps you to fill your mind with positive thoughts. Thinking positive thoughts will help you to feel better and behave in positive ways.

Here are some examples:

- I am a good friend.
- I am really good with my dog.
- I am good at running.
- I really like to go to the park with my family.
- I can keep in control of my anger when my little brother bothers me.

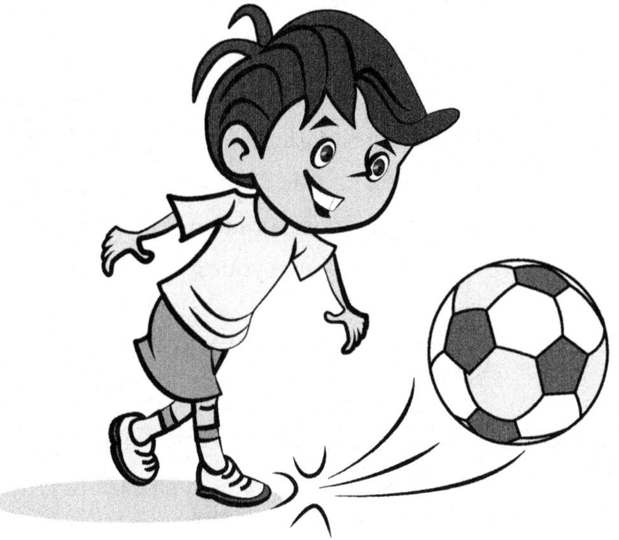

Let's write out your own positive self-talk statements.

List three positive things about you.

Place this paper where you can see it, and say these positive things about you out loud at least 10 times every morning and every night. Keep adding to the list as you and your parents notice more positive things about you.

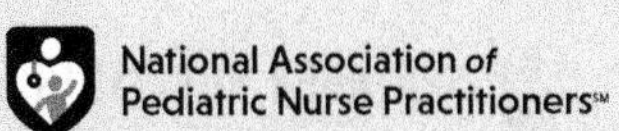

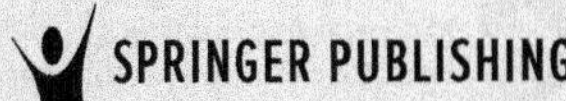

STRONG FEELINGS—ANGER, HURT, FEAR, SADNESS

(From: *COPE for Children*, copyright 2004 by Bernadette Melnyk)

Children, like adults, have times when they feel hurt, sad, fear, or anger. These are all normal feelings. All people feel angry, sad, or afraid sometimes.

These can be very strong feelings, but we can control how we COPE with these feelings in positive ways.

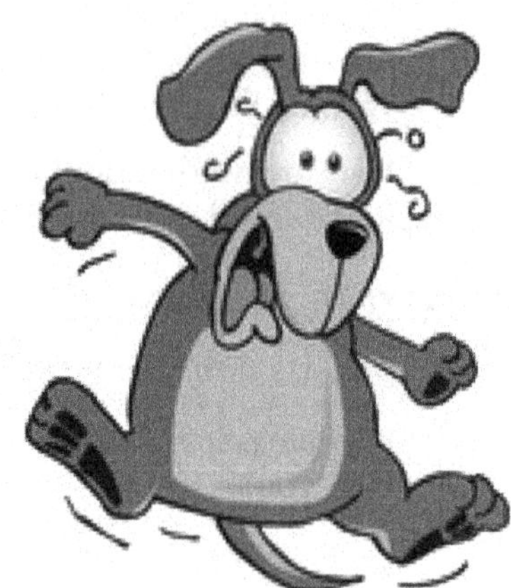

- Our bodies might signal strong feelings by:
- A hot face
- Tense muscles
- A fast heartbeat
- Fast or loud breathing
- Feeling like exploding with my hands, feet, or mouth
- Sweating
- Restlessness (feeling like you have to keep moving)
- Headaches
- Stomachaches
- Trouble thinking clearly

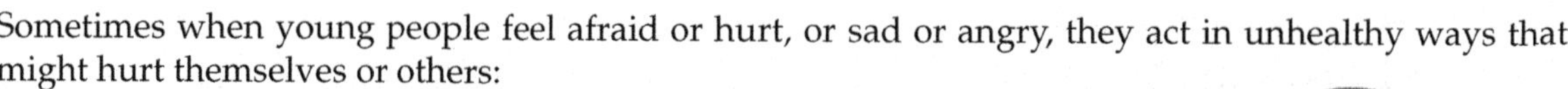

Sometimes when young people feel afraid or hurt, or sad or angry, they act in unhealthy ways that might hurt themselves or others:

- Fighting with parents or friends
- Hitting, kicking, screaming, or using mean words
- Getting bad grades or not doing homework
- Tearing up things, or hitting walls
- Not showering or taking care of your body
- Staying alone in your room too much

Name things you do when you have strong feelings (fear, sadness, or anger).

TAKING CONTROL OF YOUR ANGER (STRONG FEELINGS)

Let's list some positive things you can do when you are feeling angry, sad, or afraid, that don't hurt you and don't hurt other people.

Here are some ways children COPE and take control of their strong feelings in a positive way:

- Talking about how you feel
- Exercise/playing outside
- Going to family or friends for help

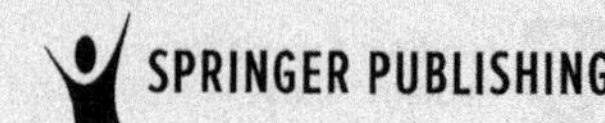

- Counting to 10 or saying the ABCs
- Walking away and deep breathing
- Thinking of a time when you did something great
- Writing your thoughts and feelings down
- Using positive self-talk (saying your positive self-statements)
- Doing something that you enjoy (like reading or drawing)

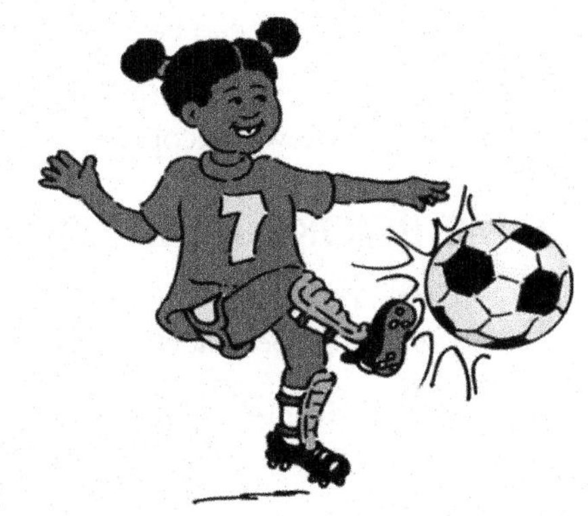

Which of these do you do?

Which sound like new ideas you can practice doing to deal with your feelings in positive ways?

Draw a picture of a time when you had strong feelings—were sad, hurt, afraid, or angry.

You can decide to make healthy choices about your feelings—it is under your control. At first, it may be hard to make good choices. But, with practice, it will get easier over time. (It will feel good to be in control!)

Let's write down a plan. When I feel angry, sad, or afraid,

I will: ____

____

I can talk to: ____

(Adapted with permission from *COPE for Children*, copyright by Bernadette Melnyk)

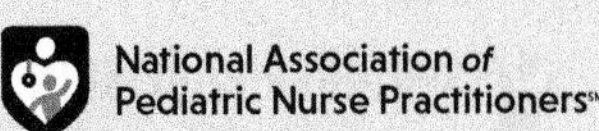

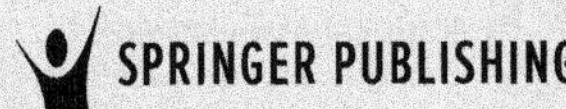

This handout can be copied and disseminated for patient use only without permission.

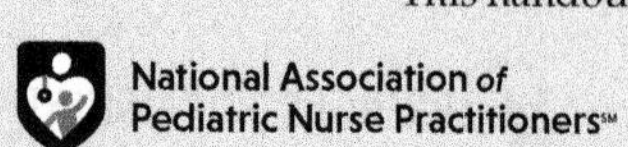

For more information on COPE and the complete COPE Programs for Children, Teens and Young Adults see www.cope2thrive.com.

SOME BOOKS THAT YOU MIGHT LIKE TO READ

Cook, J. (2011). *I just don't like the sound of no! My story about accepting no for an answer and disagreeing the right way! (Best me I can be)*. Boys Town Press.

Meiners, C. (2010). *Cool down and work through anger: Learning to get along*. Free Spirit Publishing.

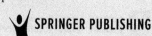

CHAPTER 8

Richard E. Kreipe and Emily Payton

Evidence-Based Assessment and Management of Eating Disorders

INTRODUCTION

Eating disorders in children and adolescents are increasingly recognized as potentially serious threats to normal growth and development in the first two decades of life, requiring a biopsychosocial approach, rather than one focused exclusively on associated mental health issues, such as anxiety or depression. Increasingly being considered "brain disorders," optimal mental health outcomes for pediatric age patients may require initial emphasis on restoration of nutrition and physiologic stability to support family-based cognitive behavioral treatment. Early recognition and treatment improve outcomes.

Fast Facts

- Once limited to a single eating disorder—anorexia nervosa—in the initial version of the *Diagnostic and Statistical Manual of Mental Disorders (DSM)*, decades later the current *DSM-5* (APA, 2013) includes six diagnoses related to dysfunctional feeding or eating patterns affecting children and adolescents.
- A biological basis for eating disorders is being defined as sophisticated technology focused on brain function that has enabled the identification of altered brain pathways and circuitry, and the processing of sensory input in a variety of eating disorders, resulting in eating disorders being considered as "brain disorders."
- A biological basis for eating disorders is being defined. Sophisticated technology focused on brain function has identified altered brain pathways, circuitry, and processing of sensory input in a variety of eating disorders, resulting in them being considered as "brain disorders."
- Eating disorders associated with body image disturbance tend to emerge during adolescence, between 11 and 19 years of age, related to normal developmental tasks related to transformative changes of puberty, identity formation, establishing autonomy, and maturation of brain pathways.
- Although predominantly affecting teenage females, eating disorders associated with body image disturbance are distributed widely across populations; they are increasingly found in young children, adults, and males, including those with gender dysphoria, and all racial, ethnic, and cultural groups.
- Eating disorders are complex conditions, requiring attention to biological, psychological, and social factors, not only for the pediatric patient, but also for her/his family by ensuring adequate nutrition to optimize biological functions (including brain development), as well as attention to underlying issues such as anxiety, depression, obsessive/compulsive traits, and trauma that may be relevant (Seetharaman & Fields, 2020).

- Although a common central feature of eating disorders is disturbance in how an affected person experiences body shape or weight (negative body image) leading to dysfunctional eating habits fueled by a drive for thinness or avoidance of obesity, new to the *DSM-5* is avoidant/restrictive food intake disorder (ARFID), which is *not* associated with body image disturbance (Lock & Agras, 2019).

Disordered Eating Patterns

- Pica: Characterized by persistent eating of non-nutritive, non-food substances that is not expected developmentally (e.g., infants put things in their mouth while exploring their environment) and that is neither culturally nor socially normative, nor associated body image problems. Commonly associated with intellectual developmental disorder, autism spectrum disorder, schizophrenia, or obsessive-compulsive disorder. Pica is only diagnosed separately if it warrants specific clinical attention in treatment. Depending on what is being ingested, consideration should be given to blood or imaging tests to identify potential complications from poisoning or gastrointestinal perforation or obstruction.
- Rumination Disorder (RD): Characterized by repeated spontaneous regurgitation of food that may be re-chewed, re-swallowed or spit-out and not due to any associated gastrointestinal condition or problem with body image. Thus, RD is not related to eating per se, but to what happens to food after it is eaten. Infants with RD often have associated intellectual developmental disorder and typically arch their backs and head while making sucking movements with their tongue, and often appear hungry between episodes of regurgitation. Older children and adolescents, on the other hand, recognize the social stigma and physical discomfort of regurgitation and tend to disguise the event by covering their mouth with a hand or by coughing. Unfortunately, the diagnosis of RD is often not considered when older patients are evaluated for episodic regurgitation, often having ineffective medical therapy and/or surgical procedures, rather than begin taught and using physical measures such as diaphragmatic breathing which have the strongest evidence base for effectiveness.
- Avoidant/Restrictive Food Intake Disorder (ARFID): Characterized by a pattern of limiting food intake based on its neurosensory qualities (e.g., color, appearance, smell, taste, consistency, mouth feel, or other difficult-to-describe features), adverse response to eating (e.g., choking, nausea, vomiting, or other physical symptoms—either experienced or anticipated), or merely lack of interest in eating. ARFID is *not* associated with fear of gaining weight or a distorted body image; affected individuals may be distressed by their weight loss or thinness. Compared to other eating disorders, patients with ARFID are more likely to be male and younger, may have a longer duration of illness prior to diagnosis, and be severely undernourished. Understanding that symptoms experienced in ARFID are related to brain processing issues (similar to autism) when presented with certain foods, or as a negative conditioned response based on events that have happened or are anticipated, without labeling them "behavioral" or "parenting" problems, helps guide treatment.
- Anorexia Nervosa (AN): Characterized by a strong drive for thinness (to either lose weight or limit weight gain) leading to behaviors intended to restrict caloric intake (especially of foods considered "fattening") through eliminating or restricting meals while also increasing intake of no- or low-calorie drinks and food. Behaviors intended to reduce or eliminate the effects of ingested calories (most commonly exercise, but also induced vomiting, or laxative use) have the potential to become difficult to change once established as habits. Although prolonged dietary restriction can be associated with depression, the most common trait associated with the emergence and maintenance of AN is anxiety. Obsessive-compulsiveness, perfectionism and harm-avoidance also commonly occur in

patients with AN. Combined reduced intake and increased output of calories can result in dramatic weight loss and death. Early recognition and multi-modal treatment improve outcome, but adequate nutrition is central to recover, leading to the adage, Food IS Medicine with respect to AN.

- Bulimia Nervosa (BN): Characterized by ingestion of large amounts of food over a short period of time (binge eating), without a sense of control over the eating, resulting in feelings of shame, guilt, depression and/or anxiety that quickly trigger self-punitive compensatory behaviors (most commonly inducing vomiting or laxative use, but also exercise) intended to reduce the effects of having "binged," even if the amount of food was relatively small, but consisted of "forbidden" food. Almost half of adolescents with BN have a period of severely restricted caloric intake (anorexia nervosa) prior to their bulimic, potentially addictive, patterns emerging. Depression, substance abuse, novelty-seeking, and a history of trauma (including sexual) are commonly associated with BN, each complicating treatment. Although body weight and appearance are not as dramatically affected in BN compared to AN, medical complications and psychological morbidity may be high in BN.
- Binge-Eating Disorder (BED): Although similar to BN with respect to uncontrolled binge eating, in BED there are no compensatory behaviors to rid the body of the calories. Although more common in adults, BED in the pediatric age group is associated with high rates of obesity, substance use, anxiety, depression, and social impairment, and may be the most common eating disorder in adolescents, especially among adolescent males.

SCREENING QUESTIONS (ELSTER, 2021)

Questions for Parents

- Are you concerned about your child's weight or eating habits?
- Does your child make negative comments about weight or shape, or needing to lose weight?

Questions for the Younger Adolescent

- Do you spend a lot of time thinking about ways to be skinny or lose weight?
- Do you do things to lose weight (e.g., skip meals, take pills, starve yourself, and vomit)?
- Do you work, play, or exercise to make you sweat or breathe hard at least three times a week?

Questions for the Middle to Older Adolescent

- Are you satisfied with your eating habits?
- Do you ever eat in secret?
- Do you spend a lot of time thinking about ways to be thin?
- In the past year, have you tried to lose weight or control your weight by vomiting, taking diet pills or laxatives, or starving yourself?
- Do you exercise or participate in sports activities that make you sweat and breathe hard for 20 minutes or more at a time at least three times during the week?

TARGETED PHYSICAL EXAMINATION

- Body Weight: Because prior to being weighed, patients with AN may drink water or hide heavy objects on their body or in their underwear, it is important for clinicians to be able to perform a physical examination that includes measuring urine specific gravity (diluted with water loading), body temperature (hypothermia with low lean body mass), orthostatic change in pulse and blood pressure (from supine to sitting to standing), and peripheral circulation (cold, cyanotic hands, and feet with slow capillary refill). Thus, body weight should be measured with a patient wearing only a hospital gown to allow a physical examination that may reveal changes associated with unrecognized weight loss, noted below.

- Central and Peripheral Cardiovascular System: Significantly reduced lean body mass can be associated with central autonomic nervous system imbalance manifested by a slow pulse when supine which increases on sitting and further increases on standing, sometimes more than 30 beats per minute, often with dizziness. Such orthostatic change in pulse is more sensitive to physical deconditioning than drop in blood pressure. In addition to those centrally mediated changes, blood flow to the hands and feet is often reduced, resulting in cold, blue hands and feet with slow capillary refill, similar to that seen in patients with shock.
- Skin: In addition to the peripheral circulatory changes, the skin of the lower extremities may show edema with inadequate caloric intake, generally related more to capillary fragility than protein deficiency. Also, the skin should be examined for evidence of cutting or other self-injury.
- Oral: Swelling of the parotid and submandibular salivary glands can occur with recurrent binge eating and vomiting in BN. Recurrent vomiting can also result in dental enamel erosion due to stomach acid etching the teeth, usually worst on the inner surfaces of the lower teeth. Oral examination should also include testing for the gag reflex because repeated stimulation of the pharynx to induce vomiting can cause the loss of that protective response.

TARGETED MENTAL HEALTH EVALUATION

- Strength-Based Positive Youth Development (PYD) Approach: Although children and adolescents with eating disorders tend to have comorbid mental health disorders (most commonly anxiety but also depression, obsessive-compulsive disorder, and post-traumatic stress disorder) requiring thorough and ongoing evaluation and treatment, a biopsychosocial approach, informed by the principles of positive youth development (PYD) that builds on strengths and developmental assets rather than focusing on psychopathology, is recommended with respect to mental health treatment (Ginsburg & Ramirez-McClain, 2020).
- Family History: Family history is especially relevant in the evaluation of children and adolescents with eating disorders. Because anxiety tends to be heritable, if a parent has a history of an eating disorder, anxiety, or depression, there is often self-incrimination, or blaming by the other parent, for having "caused" or "given" the eating disorder to the child. Fathers of children who develop AN often voice the advice: "just eat." In our experience when those fathers learn about the details of AN, they can be much more supportive of the patient and the patient's mother.
- Trauma History: Although a history of trauma (physical, emotional, and/or sexual abuse) is not necessarily more common in patients with eating disorders, clinical experience suggests that recovery from the eating disorder may be more difficult and prolonged if there is such a history. Inquiring routinely about various types of trauma indicates to patients that this is a topic open to discussion, while it may have been suppressed by the patient, family, or both.

LABORATORY TESTS (BASED ON HISTORY AND PHYSICAL EXAMINATION)

- Serum electrolytes (metabolic alkalosis with low K^+ and high CO_2 with significant vomiting).
- Renal function tests (high BUN in presence of low protein intake with dehydration).
- CBC (neutropenia associated with marginated WBCs with starvation).
- Liver function tests (mildly elevated liver enzymes, but not to hepatitis levels).

- EKG (sinus bradycardia with low voltage with low weight).
- Thyroid function tests (significantly low weight associated with low T_3 and high ***reverse*** T_3).

MANAGEMENT OF AVOIDANT/RESTRICTIVE FOOD INTAKE DISORDER

- The treatment of any underlying medical condition or complication in ARFID should proceed along with a family-based cognitive behavioral approach adapted to the underlying neurobiological problem (fear of aversive consequences of the process of eating, or sensory features of foods, or lack of interest).
- Depending on dominant symptoms, pediatric patients with ARFID may be seen by subspecialists unfamiliar with the diagnosis, delaying comprehensive treatment as isolated medical treatment is pursued.
- The medical care of patients with ARFID may require the use of liquid nutrition and naso-gastric tube feedings to restore nutrition and weight, similar to severe restrictive anorexia nervosa.
- A multi-disciplinary team may be required if a patient as cooccurring neurocognitive disorder such as autism spectrum disorder.

MANAGEMENT OF ANOREXIA NERVOSA

- Depending on the degree of under-nutrition, initial treatment for AN requires restoration of caloric intake and lean body mass to optimize brain metabolism and physical health upon which mental health treatment can succeed (Hornberger et al., 2021).
- Parents have a central role in family-based treatment models, which have been shown to be the most effective in helping individuals recover from AN.
- Because food is the most important "medicine" in the initial phase of treatment, anxiety and depression commonly found on presentation may resolve with weight restoration and initiating family-based treatment, with parents ensuring adequate nutritional intake by their child. Selective serotonin reuptake inhibitors (SSRIs) may be added later in treatment if anxiety, depression, or both persist following restoration of physical health.
- Nutritional counseling by a registered dietitian (RD) familiar with common issues related to eating and drinking for patients with an eating disorder is important, especially for those with common ingrained beliefs and practices that result in conflict at home.
- Some patients with AN may require hospitalization if weight loss is extreme or health is poor (e.g., if pulse is low, or differential between supine and standing pulse is high), or inadequate nutritional intake cannot be interrupted in intensive outpatient therapy.
- Adolescents with severe weight loss may have decreased gastric volume and motility, necessitating eating smaller amounts of food frequently, often starting with nutritionally complete and easily digested liquid feeding, which is emptied more quickly from the stomach. This also allows the same nutrition to be delivered by nasogastric tube, possibly by continuous slow feeding, if the patient is unable to drink it.
- Refeeding syndrome is a potentially fatal condition associated with rapid increase in caloric intake following prolonged weight loss, causing hormonal and metabolic changes, the most serious of which is low blood potassium levels, affecting muscle contractility, especially potentially fatal heart rhythms.
- Mindfulness (purposely paying attention to the present with non-judgmental awareness) has a role in the treatment of AN, and emerging evidence that mindfulness-based interventions can promote enhanced interoceptive awareness and self-regulation (Schuman-Olver et al., 2020).

MANAGEMENT OF BULIMIA NERVOSA

- The primary treatment target in BN is to reduce binge-eating and compensatory behaviors; reducing binge eating may itself reduce the associated vomiting, laxative use, or exercise.
- SSRIs should be added to structured eating habits and mental health measures relatively early in treatment, but dosage may need to be increased to two to three times that usually effective in simple anxiety or depression.
- Restoring and maintaining structured nutritional balance is central to the success of counseling by a trained mental health provider; the simple act of eating a nutritionally balanced breakfast and lunch after a binge-purge the night before may reduce physical hunger that triggers a binge later in the day.
- Counseling is directed at the patient's self-image overall and the profound shame, guilt and embarrassment related to the vicious cycle of both uncontrollable binge eating and compensatory "purging" behaviors.
- Occasionally, some adolescents need to be admitted to the hospital if their fluid loss is extreme and/or health is threatened (e.g., if heart rate becomes too irregular or if blood pressure becomes too low).
- Sometimes intermediately intensive partial hospitalization programs are required to interrupt the harmful dieting–binge eating–purging cycle that affects individuals.

MANAGEMENT OF BINGE-EATING DISORDER

- Lacking a scientific evidence base for treatment of BED in pediatric patients, CBT and FBT are reasonable management approaches, given their effectiveness in BN, in addition to addressing comorbid conditions such as anxiety, depression, substance abuse, or trauma (Bohon, 2019).
- Although lisdexamphetamine is a stimulant approved for use in patients 6 years old to treat ADHD, it is only approved for use in treating adults, not younger patients, with BED.

KEY FEATURES OF *DSM-5* DIAGNOTIC CRITERIA

Pica

- Pica is characterized by persistent eating of non-nutritive, non-food substances over a period of at least 1 month.
- The eating of non-nutritive substances is inappropriate to developmental level.
- Even if the eating behavior is in the context of another mental disorder (intellectual disability, autism, schizophrenia), it is severe enough to warrant clinical attention.

Coding: ICD-10-CM codes for pica are (F98.3) in children and (F50.8) in adults.

Rumination Disorder

- RD is characterized by repeated regurgitation of food over a period of at least 1 month, not attributable to an associated gastrointestinal or other medical condition (e.g., gastroesophageal reflux, pyloric stenosis).
- Regurgitated food may be re-chewed, re-swallowed, or spit out.
- The eating disturbance does not occur only during the course of another eating disorder (AN, BN, ARFID).
- Even if the eating behavior is in the context of another mental disorder (intellectual disability, neurodevelopmental disorder) it is severe enough to warrant clinical attention.

Coding: ICD-10-CM code for rumination disorder is F98.21.

Anorexia Nervosa

- AN is characterized by restrictions of caloric intake relative to energy requirements, with significantly low body weight (less than minimally normal) in the context of age, sex, developmental trajectory, and physical health.
- There are fears of gaining weight and/or becoming fat.
- There is a disturbed evaluation of one's body weight/shape, and negative self-image.
- There is lack of insight regarding the seriousness of the current low body weight.

Subtype Coding: ICD-10-CM coding has two subtypes based on restrictive eating without or with binge/purge behaviors.

(F50.01) Restricting type: In the last 3 months, there has not been recurrent episodes of binge eating or purging behavior (i.e., self-induced vomiting or the misuse of laxatives, diuretics, or enemas). Weight loss is primarily from dieting, fasting, and/or excessive exercise.

(F50.02) Binge-eating/purging type: In the last 3 months, there has been recurrent episodes of binge eating or purging behavior (i.e., self-induced vomiting or the misuse of laxatives, diuretics, or enemas).

Severity: ICD-10-CM coding includes four levels of severity based on adult BMI (kg/m^2) levels (mild: BMI ≥17; moderate: BMI 16-16.99; severe: BMI 15-15.99; extreme: BMI ≤15). In pediatric cases, the level of severity may be increased to reflect clinical symptoms, functional disability, and/or need for supervision regardless of BMI.

Avoidant/Restrictive Food Intake Disorder

- Restrictive eating/feeding disturbance (e.g., apparent lack of interest in eating or food; avoidance based on sensory characteristics of food; concern about aversive consequences of eating) is characterized by persistent failure to meet nutritional and/or energy needs due to one or more of:
  1. Significant weight loss (failure to gain expected weight or faltering growth).
  2. Significant nutritional deficiency.
  3. Dependence on enteral feeding or oral nutrition supplements.
  4. Symptoms interfere with psychosocial functioning.
- Restrictive food intake is not associated with AN or BN, and there is no disturbed body image.
- The restrictive eating disturbance is not due to a medical condition and if associated with another condition or disorder the severity of the food restriction/ avoidance is severe enough to warrant clinical attention.

Coding: ICD-10-CM code for ARFID is F50.8.

Bulimia Nervosa

A. BN is characterized by recurrent episodes of binge eating. An episode of binge eating includes both:
   1. Eating, in a defined period of time (e.g., within any 2-hour period), an amount of food that is much larger than others would consume in that period of time under similar circumstances, AND
   2. A sense of lack of control during the binge eating (e.g., a feeling that one cannot stop eating or control what or the amount one eats).

- In addition to the binging episodes there are behaviors to prevent weight gain, such as self-induced vomiting; misuse of laxatives, diuretics, or other medications; fasting; or excessive exercise occurring at least once a week for 3 months.

- There is negative body image; self-evaluation is based on body shape and weight.
- The bulimia, binge eating, does not occur only during episodes of AN.

Coding: ICD-10-CM code for BN is rumination disorder is F50.2.

Severity: Specify current severity level, based on the average frequency of compensatory behaviors each week (mild: 1–3 episodes/week; moderate: 4–7 episodes/week; severe: 8–13 episodes/week; extreme: 14 or more episodes/week). Severity is increased if there is significant functional disability.

Binge-Eating Disorder

- BED is characterized by recurrent binges that involve both:
  1. Eating, in a discrete period of time (e.g., within any 2-hour period)), an amount of food that is much larger than others would consume in that period of time under similar circumstances, and
  2. A sense of lack of control during the binge eating (e.g., a feeling that one cannot stop eating or control what or the amount one eats).
- The binge eating occurs at least once a week for 3 months and is associated with marked distress.
- The binge-eating episodes are associated with three (or more) of the following:
  1. Eats more rapidly than normal.
  2. Eats until feeling uncomfortably full.
  3. Eats large amounts of food even though not physically hungry.
  4. Eats alone due to embarrassment of how much one is eating.
  5. After binging, feels disgusted, depressed, or guilty.
- The binge eating does not occur during the course of AN or BN and does not include the behaviors to prevent weight gain seen in BN, such as self-induced vomiting; misuse of laxatives, diuretics, or other medications; fasting; or excessive exercise.

Coding: ICD-10-CM code for BED is F50.8.

Severity: Specify current severity based on the frequency of episodes of binge eating each week (mild: 1–3; moderate: 4–7; severe: 8–13; extreme: 14 or more). Severity level is increased with disruption of functioning.

INTERNET RESOURCES

American Academy of Child and Adolescent Psychiatry (AACAP)

www.aacap.org/AACAP/resources_for_primary_care/information_for_patients_and_their_families/home.aspx

This AAACAP website is an excellent source of information on the assessment and treatment of child and adolescent mental health disorders. Handouts for use with families (i.e., *Facts for Families*, at link above) are available on a multitude of problems, including eating disorders.

American Academy of Pediatrics (AAP)

www.aap.org

This website contains information for both healthcare providers and parents, including excellent clinical practice guidelines and handouts, and a review on eating disorders in children and adolescents published in 2021 (pediatrics.aappublications.org/content/147/1/e2020040279). *Bright Futures*, a national health promotion and prevention initiative, is another AAP resource (brightfutures.aap.org/) with educational and clinical materials.

Centers for Disease Control and Prevention (CDC)

www.cdc.gov

The CDC website contains the latest information for healthcare professionals and the public on many topics, including childhood overweight and obesity (www.cdc.gov/obesity/childhood/)

National Eating Disorders Association (NEDA)

www.nationaleatingdisorders.org/

NEDA is the largest nonprofit organization dedicated to supporting individuals and families affected by eating disorders. It supports individuals and families affected by eating disorders, and serves as a catalyst for prevention, cures, and access to quality care.

Academy for Eating Disorders (AED)

www.aedweb.org

AED is global professional association committed to leadership in eating disorders research, education, treatment, and prevention. This website contains a great deal of practical information for both professionals and the lay public, including an Expert by Experience Committee to fully integrate the perspective, wisdom, and knowledge of patients and caregivers into AED programs and services.

Families Empowered and Supporting Treatment for Eating Disorders (F.E.A.S.T.)

www.feast-ed.org

F.E.A.S.T. is an international non-profit organization of, and for, caregivers of loved ones suffering from eating disorders, with a mission to support caregivers by providing information and mutual support, promoting evidence-based treatment, and advocating for research and education to reduce the suffering associated with eating disorders. It offers a series of guides that address issues from the family point-of-view (www.feast-ed.org/family-guide-series).

REFERENCES

American Psychiatric Association. (2013). *Diagnostic and statistical manual of mental disorders* (5th ed.). Author.

Bohon, C. (2019). Binge eating disorder in children and adolescents. *Child and Adolescent Psychiatric Clinics of North America*, *28*(4), 549. https://doi.org/10.1016/j.chc.2019.05.003

Elster, A. (2021). Guidelines for adolescent preventive services. In M. M. Torchia (Ed.), *UpToDate*. www.uptodate.com/contents/guidelines-for-adolescent-preventive-services

Ginsburg, K. R., & Ramirez-McClain, Z. B. (2020). *Reaching teens: Strength-based, trauma-sensitive, resilience-building communication strategies rooted in positive youth development* (2nd ed.). American Academy of Pediatrics.

Hornberger, L, L., Lane, M. A., & AAP. The Committee on Adolescence. (2021). Identification and management of eating disorders in children and adolescents. *Pediatrics*, *147*(1), e2020040279. https://doi.org/10.1542/peds.2020-040279

Lock, J., & Agras, W. S. (2019). Eating and feeding disorders. In L. W. Roberts (Ed.), *The American Psychiatric Association Publishing textbook of psychiatry* (7th ed., pp. 497–516). American Psychiatric Association Publishing.

Schuman-Olver, Z., Trombka, M., Lovas, D. A., Brewer, J. A., Vago, D. R., Gawande, R., Dunne, J. P., Lazar, S. W., Loucks, E. B., & Fulwiler, C. (2020). Mindfulness and behavior change. *Harvard Review of Psychiatry*, *28*(6), 371–394. https://doi.org/10.1097/HRP.0000000000000277

Seetharaman, S., & Fields, E. L. (2020). Avoidant/restrictive food intake disorder. *Pediatrics in Review*, *41*, 613. https://doi.org/10.1542/pir.2019-0133

Information for Parents About Anorexia Nervosa in Children or Teens

WHAT IS ANOREXIA NERVOSA?

Anorexia nervosa is a complex health problem that occurs most commonly in pre-teens or adolescents and is associated with a distorted body image (feeling or fearing overweight, even when underweight) and a strong drive for thinness. This combination causes people with this illness to try to gain a sense of control in their life by restricting the intake of food or beverages, and to exercise often to burn calories. Eating may be considered a sign of weakness or lack of self-control, but the relentless, rigid habits meant to reduce body weight or limit weight gain have serious, but unintended, medical, psychological, and social consequences. Many symptoms that patients with anorexia nervosa have are related to their brain being undernourished and their body attempting to conserve energy (calories). Thus, restoring nutrition to "feed the brain" becomes an important first treatment step.

WHAT ARE SOME THINGS RELATED TO ANOREXIA NERVOSA THAT PARENTS MAY NOTICE?

- Restriction of caloric intake resulting in loss of weight or failure to gain weight as expected.
- Food rituals, such as cutting food into tiny pieces, hiding food for later discarding, or eating slowly.
- Extreme irritability and emotional instability.
- Having a variety of excuses for not eating related to schedule, time, other commitments, and so forth.
- Wearing layers of baggy clothes to hide appearance and for warmth.
- Social withdrawal and isolation, especially to eat alone.
- Frequent body checks, such as weighing, looking in mirror, or pinching skin folds.
- Exercise to burn calories, not for fun or enjoyment, but being driven to do so.
- Loss of menstrual periods in females.
- Hair loss on scalp, or growth of fine hair on face or body.
- Feeling tired, lacking energy and feeling cold.
- Reporting eating a meal, or an amount of food, that was discarded or not eaten

HOW CAN ANOREXIA NERVOSA AFFECT SOMEONE'S HEALTH? (EVERY ORGAN IS AFFECTED, BUT NOTABLY...)

- **Heart**: Low and irregular heart beat; poor circulation causing cold, blue hands and feet.
- **Bones**: Bone growth can be slowed and bone density reduced, increasing the risk of fracture.
- **Metabolism**: Malnutrition slows all metabolism, including activity in the sex glands.

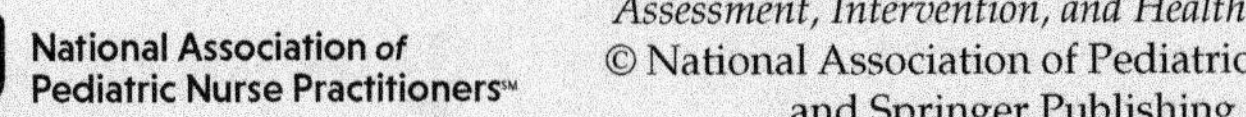

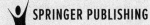

SPRINGER PUBLISHING

- **Gastrointestinal**: Muscle activity slows, causing feelings of fullness after eating and constipation.
- **Nervous system**: The brain is about 60% fat; attempts to reduce fat eaten or in the body has significant effects on brain function that are often not recognized until nutrition is restored.

WHAT CAUSES ANOREXIA NERVOSA?

There is no single cause for anorexia nervosa. Because pathways and circuits related to rewards and threats in the brain appear to respond differently to food and eating in people with anorexia nervosa, it is now considered a "brain disorder," but with many biological, psychological, and social factors that may both trigger and maintain the illness. Parents do *not* cause anorexia nervosa and should not be blamed for it occurring in their daughter or son, although traits with genetic linkages like worrying (anxiety) or sadness (depression) or perfectionism (obsessive-compulsiveness) that are commonly associated with this disorder tend to run in families. Likewise, anorexia nervosa is not merely a "choice."

Anorexia nervosa most commonly develops between 12 and 21 years of age, in individuals facing normal developmental transitions related to adolescence (puberty, identity, independence, and thinking about the future), but without effective coping skills to deal with these issue. They may have difficulty in social relationships or problems making friends, having been bullied or excluded, and weight is something that can be controlled. Comments about weight or appearance by a family member or friend may trigger dieting and exercise with weight loss becoming out-of-control as the desire to be thinner is constantly present. Or, focusing on controlling weight may reduce the stress of emotional tensions in the family. Perfectionism and worrying about the future are common traits in teens with anorexia nervosa, but they never consider themselves to be "good enough" and find it difficult to stay "in the moment." Setting unrealistically high and impossible-to-achieve standards for themselves, they may have feelings of failure and inadequacy, despite being viewed by others as successful and accomplished.

HOW IS ANOREXIA NERVOSA TREATED?

Treatment for anorexia nervosa needs to focus on the biological, psychological, and social factors related to the illness emerging and persisting, but initially should ensure adequate nutritional intake to restore brain function and physical health upon which mental health treatment can succeed. Cognitive behavioral therapy (CBT) in the context of family-based treatment (FBT) models have the best record of effectiveness and long-term recovery from anorexia nervosa in children and teens. In FBT, parents initially assume responsibility for their daughter or son having adequate nutritional intake over the course of the day, gradually turning that over to their child as she/he demonstrates the ability to do so on her/his own. This effort often results in significant conflicts, the resolution of which is the focus of the FBT. Thus, rather than avoiding conflict, FBT focuses on resolution of conflict. Later in recovery, CBT becomes the dominant approach as patients demonstrates the ability to feed themselves adequately.

Medications, such as antidepressants or anti-anxiety medications, may be used alongside intensive counseling, but food remains the most important "medicine" in the initial phase of treatment. Nutritional counseling by a trained specialist is often helpful, especially if the patient is focused on "healthy eating," which is often full of misconceptions regarding nutrition. With significant weight

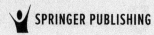

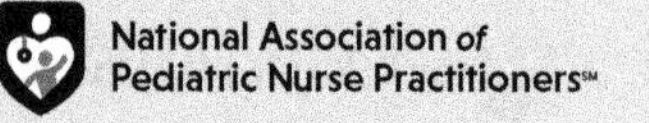

loss, restoring nutrition may require frequent small meals or liquid supplements. The latter may need to be given via a tube passed through the nose into the stomach. Although tube-feeding can be done as an outpatient, the need for it to ensure adequate nutrition may suggest the need to be admitted to the hospital for more intensive treatment. Hospitalization also may be required if the individual shows signs of medical instability, such as fainting, low temperature or pulse, heart rhythm problems, or if inadequate nutritional intake cannot be interrupted in intensive outpatient treatment.

Anorexia does not develop quickly and treatment may take months to years. However, the evidence from comprehensive treatment programs that address the biological, psychological and social needs of a young person with anorexia nervosa demonstrates that it is reasonable to expect full recovery and a productive life. Although relapse is possible, especially at times of transition or with high levels of stress, interrupting symptoms with self-care skills learned in treatment, return to normal life can occur.

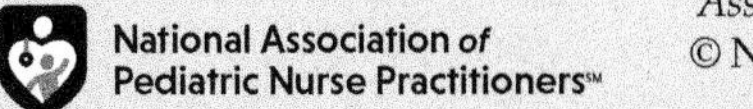

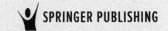

SPRINGER PUBLISHING

Information for Parents About Avoidant/Restrictive Food Intake Disorder

AVOIDANT/RESTRICTIVE FOOD INTAKE DISORDER (ARFID)

Persons with ARFID avoid or restrict eating due to an anticipated negative sensory experience related to the color, texture, consistency, taste, or smell of food, or fearing a bad reaction to eating something, such as choking, gagging, or vomiting, often having experienced such reaction in the past. A few young people with ARFID simply are not interested in eating. Although sometimes called "picky eating," like other eating disorders, it can have serious effects on physical and mental health or socialization. Unlike other eating disorders, however, there is *no* associated negative body image or desire to lose weight; in fact, low weight or being unable to eat can be quite bothersome to individuals with ARFID.

WHAT ARE SOME THINGS RELATED TO AVOIDANT/RESTRICTIVE FOOD INTAKE DISORDER THAT PARENTS MAY NOTICE?

- Avoiding or refusing to eat food based on its appearance, color, taste, smell, texture, or consistency.
- Avoiding or refusing to eat based on fear of choking, gagging, or vomiting.
- Weight loss or failure to gain weight as expected based on limited food intake.
- Worrying about the consequences of eating, as well as not eating.
- Anxiety about disappointing others based on unusual food habits.

HOW CAN AVOIDANT/RESTRICTIVE FOOD INTAKE DISORDER AFFECT SOMEONE'S HEALTH?

For most children and adolescents, eating occurs several times a day and tends to be a highly social activity. Although there is no associated body image disturbance or drive for thinness as occurs in anorexia nervosa, depending on the extent of the avoidance or restriction of food intake with ARFID, the loss of weight or failure to gain weight deserves similar attention. Often associated with underlying anxiety, young people with ARFID may feel distress at struggling with eating, or with the restricted social interactions with peers or family when unable to eat with them. Sometimes the self-directed distress is magnified if there is a perception that the AFRID patterns also cause disappointment in one's parents or peers. Heightened levels of anxiety make eating more difficult, not easier. Thus, ARFID can affect both physical and mental health.

WHAT CAUSES AVOIDANT/RESTRICTIVE FOOD INTAKE DISORDER?

The causes of ARFID are poorly understood, but a central feature is a disturbance in the individual's overall lived experience of eating. The overall experience of how food looks, smells, tastes, and/or feels in the mouth of a boy may be unpleasant to the point of his refusing to even consider eating it. This overlaps with some of the neurosensory symptoms related to eating experienced by individual

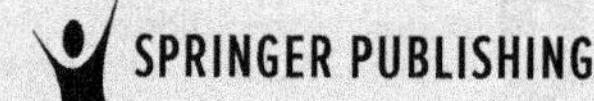

on the autism spectrum. On the other hand, after choking on a potato chip, a girl with ARFID may refuse to eat anything for fear that her throat will "close up" again. Finally, for some individuals there is no past or anticipated negative association with eating, merely lack of interest in eating. The sensory issues in ARFID can be subtle, such as not being able to eat any peas that have touched mashed potatoes on the plate, or exquisite, such as differentiating between different brands of ketchup, but being able to eat only one of them.

HOW IS AVOIDANT/RESTRICTIVE FOOD INTAKE DISORDER TREATED?

Similar to other eating disorders in young people, CBT in the context of FBT seems to be most effective. However, it needs to be guided by an understanding of the underlying biological traits that triggered the eating patterns in the first place, helping to avoid problems, but eventually became dysfunctional habits. A four-stage treatment program over 20 to 30 sessions has been developed involving: (1) learning about ARFID and making changes in eating, (2) continuing changes and setting goals to increase variety and volume of food, (3) exposure to feared elements of food, starting with very small amounts and then advancing, and (4) preventing relapse by continuing to practice the skills that were learned.

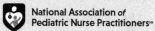

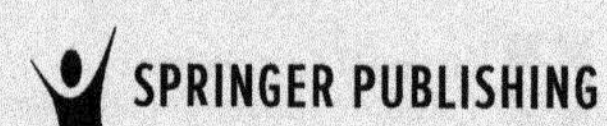

Information for Parents About Bulimia Nervosa in Children and Teens

WHAT IS BULIMIA NERVOSA?

Bulimia nervosa is an eating disorder that tends to occur in older adolescents, sometimes after having previously restricted intake and lost weight with anorexia nervosa. It involves repeated episodes of eating large quantities of food in a short time (binge eating), often containing high-calorie "forbidden foods," with binges quickly followed by feelings of shame, guilt, or sadness that trigger compensatory behaviors to "purge" the body of the binge. Mostly commonly these behaviors include inducing vomiting, taking laxatives, or compulsively exercising. In severe cases, the binge-purge cycle may be repeated more than once a day. With strong addictive and compulsive features, the binge-purge cycle can create havoc with daily routines, including stealing food for the binges, and then shame or guilt from attempting to hide the evidence of binge eating and/or purging.

WHAT ARE SOME THINGS THAT PARENTS MAY NOTICE IN THEIR CHILD WITH BULIMIA NERVOSA?

- Eating large amounts of food quickly, followed by going to the bathroom (to purge or exercise).
- Heavy use of laxatives or diuretics, or being asked to purchase them for their child.
- Large amounts of food "missing" from refrigerator or pantry.
- Highly irregular eating patterns, with fasting the day after a binge/purge event.
- Large weight fluctuations.
- Puffy cheeks due to enlarged salivary glands at the angles and underside of the jaw.
- Use of alcohol or other drugs.
- Thrill-seeking behaviors without much concern about consequences.
- Erosion of dental enamel, leading to weaking or loss of teeth or cavities.
- Uncontrollable regurgitation of food from the stomach into the throat and back of the mouth.
- Abdominal pain and bloating.

WHAT CAUSES BULIMIA NERVOSA?

Eating disorders are called "brain circuit disorders" because of the way in which the brain of affected individuals responds to food and eating, and distorts their own body image: What is positive for most people is extremely threatening or overly rewarding for those with an eating disorder. Worry, stress, or feeling angry, lonely, or abandoned are common triggers to binge eating. Dieting and missing meals as a form of weight control may trigger food cravings and overeating. Sometimes bulimia can develop as a complication of some physical or emotional trauma (such as unwanted sexual behavior) or upsetting event, such as family breakdown, or the death of a loved one or friend. Other risk factors for the development of bulimia include poor self-esteem, extreme anxiety, and a highly sensitive nature, or a family history of substance abuse.

This handout may be distributed to families.

From Melnyk, B. M., & Lusk, P. (2022). *A Practical Guide to Child and Adolescent Mental Health Screening, Evidence-Based Assessment, Intervention, and Health Promotion* (3rd ed.).

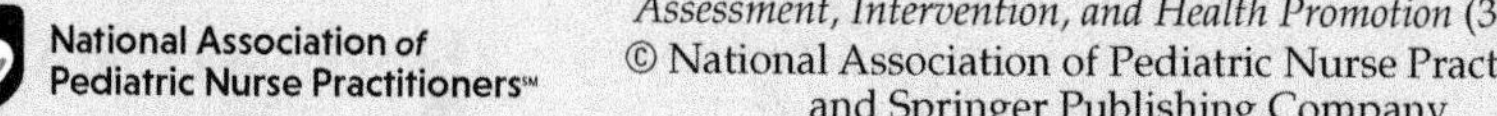

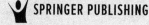

SPRINGER PUBLISHING

HOW IS BULIMIA NERVOSA TREATED?

As with anorexia nervosa, restoring nutritional balance and maintaining structured dietary intake is central to the success of counseling by a trained mental health provider using cognitive behavioral therapy (CBT) with elements of family-based treatment. However, unlike anorexia nervosa, in bulimia nervosa the intake and output of nutrition is chaotic, and the focus needs to be on reducing both the binge eating and the purging behaviors. In addition to nutritionally balanced meals distributed across the day to avoid binge eating followed by purging, selective serotonin reuptake inhibitors (SSRIs) are also an important element of treatment. Although SSRIs are medicines to combat anxiety, depression, or both, even if they do not have symptoms of anxiety or depression, individuals with bulimia nervosa benefit from taking SSRIs and similar medications. Therapy focuses on understanding the complex emotions that trigger binge eating and purging, as well as how normalizing eating itself can break the vicious binge-purge cycle. For some teens, especially those who have experienced trauma, dialectical behavior therapy (DBT) may be helpful to manage unregulated emotional reactions and behaviors with serious consequences. Those with bulimia nervosa and severe fluid and electrolyte imbalance may need to be hospitalized to both restore balance and interrupt the binge-purge cycle. Intensive outpatient treatment may help to interrupt harmful dieting-binge eating-purging cycles that can entrap individuals.

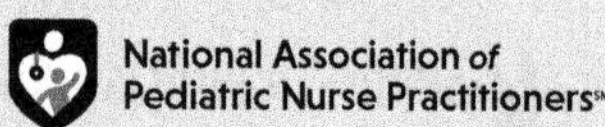

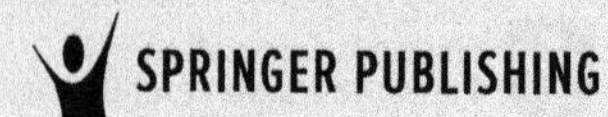

CHAPTER 9

Vicki M. Knapp, Deborah A. Napolitano, and Holly E. Brown

Evidence-Based Assessment and Management of Autism and Pervasive Developmental Disorder

AUTISM SPECTRUM DISORDER (ASD)

Fast Facts

- The diagnostic category of ASD refers to a group of symptoms characterized by delays in the development of socialization and communication skills in addition to the presence of restrictive and repetitive behaviors.
- Parents may note symptoms as early as infancy, although the typical age of onset is before 3 years of age, but the social aspects of the disorder (diagnosis) might not show until social opportunities are available (e.g., school).
- Symptoms may include problems with using and understanding language; difficulty relating to people, objects, and events; unusual play with toys and other objects; difficulty with changes in routine or familiar surroundings; and repetitive body movements or behavior patterns.
- One of the early indicators of a possible ASD is a child's lack of responsiveness to their name or other social communication. It is important to rule out any hearing deficits.
- Some children do not speak at all, others speak in limited phrases or conversations, and some have relatively normal language development. Repetitive play skills and limited social skills are generally evident.
- Unusual responses to sensory information, such as loud noises and lights, also are common.
- Individuals with a diagnosis of ASD should also have an accompanying level of severity rating ranging from one (lower level of support needed) to three (high level of support needed).
- Children with ASD vary widely in abilities, intelligence, and behaviors.
- The diagnostic criteria support and allow for some characterization of these associated symptoms (e.g., ASD with or without accompanying intellectual impairment).
- Primary care providers play an integral role in screening for an ASD and, therefore, are the first line of defense in detecting symptoms associated with ASDs.
- The earlier an accurate diagnosis can be made, the earlier treatment can begin, which may have significant educational and developmental benefits to the child.
- The primary care provider is often the medical professional most trusted by the parents. Their opinion and information may be held with a great deal of trust and respect, so it is incumbent upon those individuals to have accurate and sufficient information to help guide the parents toward the next steps on what will likely be a life-long journey.

Therefore, questions being asked by parents are important and not to be dismissed or overlooked by primary care practitioners. That said, this is a topic that also can strike fear in a parent who has begun to imagine their child's future almost as soon as they know they will be parents. This is a sensitive topic and should be carefully addressed with accurate and reliable information about autism.

- It is critical to also provide families with anticipatory guidance about what to expect in terms of further evaluation, treatment, and resources once an ASD diagnosis is suspected.
- Information about ASD has become quite easy to obtain. Unfortunately, for many reasons, there is a great deal of information out there that would not meet a best practice or "evidence-based litmus test." Controversies abound and are often promulgated by parents trying to find the next best treatment, practitioners who think they have hit upon the next best thing, or in some cases people who are looking to make a lot of money.
- The best place to quickly find information is the internet. Unfortunately, it is also the best place to quickly find misinformation or become connected to groups who promote treatments that may sound great but are ineffective at best and harmful at worst.
- One reliable resource for pediatric providers can be found at the American Academy of Pediatrics: www.aap.org/en-us/advocacy-and-policy/aap-health-initiatives/Pages/autism-initiatives.aspx#:~:text=Autism%20resources%20for%20parents%2C%20families,parenting%20website%2CHealthyChildren.org.&text=According%20to%20the%20Centers%20for,autism%20spectrum%20disorder%20(ASD).
- Additional resources can be obtained from the National Institute of Neurological Disorders and Stroke: www.ninds.nih.gov/Disorders/All-Disorders/Autism-Spectrum-Disorder-Information-Page

Some Key Points to Consider

- ASD is a neurodevelopmental disorder.
- The prevalence of ASD is currently reported as: 1:54 children (Maenner et al., 2020).
- ASD is 4.3 times more common in boys (Maenner et al., 2020).
- The prevalence of ASD is lower in Hispanic children compared to Black and White children. Black and Hispanic children were identified later than White children and were more likely to have a cooccurring diagnosed intellectual disability (Maenner et al., 2020).
- The etiology of ASD is not well understood but there is clearly a genetic link as evidenced by occurrence among siblings and the research increasingly demonstrating gene-related mutations and structural variations (Abrahams & Geschwind, 2008; Taylor et al., 2020).

Autism Spectrum Disorder

ASD is characterized by deficits in social communication and interaction, and the presence of repetitive or rigid behaviors. To qualify for a diagnosis of ASD according to the *Diagnostic and Statistical Manual of Mental Disorders, Fifth Edition (DSM-5)*, an individual must display characteristics of each of the three social communication and interaction areas and two of the four repetitive or rigid behaviors or interest areas. Characteristics of ASD must be present in the early developmental period, yet unlike the previous diagnostic criteria, an age is not specified. Children with an ASD may have intellectual disabilities or challenges that make testing intelligence and development difficult. Others with an ASD may score well on standardized testing but struggle with abstract concepts, subtle social cues, and concepts and language variations (e.g., slang).

According to the *DSM-5*, a diagnosis of an ASD should be accompanied by a specified level of severity ranging from 1 (lower level of support needed) to 3 (high level of support needed; APA, 2013). An ASD diagnosis should also include specification about whether an intellectual disability, language impairment, or catatonia is present, as well as whether any known medical, genetic, or environmental events influenced the individual's development (APA, 2013).

When the *DSM-5* (APA, 2013) was published, it resulted in a significant change in the characterization of autism and related diagnoses. Notably, what was previously characterized as the "Pervasive Developmental Disorders," of which autistic disorder was a part, was mostly collectively considered to be ASD. ASD is the diagnosis that is comprehensive of what was previously known as Autistic Disorder, Asperger Syndrome, Pervasive Developmental Disorder—Not Otherwise Specified (PDD-NOS), and Childhood Disintegrative Disorder. Rett Syndrome was once considered a Pervasive Developmental Disorder; however, a clear genetic marker was discovered, and it is now considered to be a genetic neurological disorder (Schaefer & Mendelsohn, 2013).

Some individuals who identify as having Asperger syndrome do not approve of the new diagnostic categorization of ASD and have reported that their form "High Functioning Autism" (HFA) should not be categorized within ASD (Giles, 2014). One of the defining differences between Autistic Disorder and Asperger syndrome was typical language development and even early language development and/or reading skills. Another difference is that individuals with Asperger's do not present with intellectual or cognitive delays. The *DSM-5* is clear that individuals with previous diagnoses of Asperger syndrome should be given the diagnosis of ASD (APA, 2013). When possible, it is appropriate to ask the individual how they would like for their diagnosis to be discussed.

Descriptions of the disorders and categories previously diagnosed under the Pervasive Developmental Disorders from the *DSM-IV-TR* (APA, 2000) can be found at Healthy Children.org: www.healthychildren.org/English/health-issues/conditions/developmental-disabilities/Pages/Asperger-Syndrome.aspx

SCREENING FOR AUTISM SPECTRUM DISORDER

It is recommended by the American Academy of Pediatrics (AAP) that screenings for ASD be conducted at regular intervals. The AAP recommends that all children be screened for developmental delays and disabilities during regular well-child doctor visits at 9, 18, and 24 to 30 months with standardized screenings for ASD at 18 and 24 months (Hyman et al., 2020). Additional considerations for screenings should occur if there are risk factors present for developmental problems (e.g., low birth weight or a sibling is diagnosed with autism). There is a need for additional screening tools that are culturally sensitive and inclusive of variables including ethnicity and gender identity (Rea et al., 2019). There are specific screening tools that may be used in addition to some critical history-taking questions. The questions include:

- **a.** Does your child make eye contact?
- **b.** Does your child look to you to share their toys and activities?
- **c.** Does your child share their enjoyment with you?
- **d.** Does your child point to things they want to show you?
- **e.** Does your child respond to their name or other attempts to get their attention?
- **f.** Does your child repeat words or phrases over and over?
- **g.** Does your child have any repetitive movements or behaviors that are different than other same age children?
- **h.** Does your child have very specific interests (e.g., lining up toys, schedules, pre-occupation with wheels on a car)?

You will want to collect a basic medical history as outlined in Table 9.1.

Table 9.1. Medical History

1. **Birth history**: Were there any known risk factors for ASD such as:
   a. parental age,
   b. drug or alcohol use, and
   c. method of pregnancy.
2. **Developmental history**: Has the child developed typically and met his or her milestones (e.g., sitting and babbling at 6 months), beginning word use at 1 year, following two-step commands or using two or three word phrases by 24 months).
3. **Behavioral or medical history**: These might include sleep difficulties, gastrointestinal problems, intellectual disability, or neurological problems such as seizures.
4. **Family history**: Research has demonstrated that ASD is a genetic, neurological disorder. This is due to the numbers of twins diagnosed with the disorder and family members with associated diagnoses. Some questions to ask are:
   a. Is there a twin or sibling with an ASD?
   b. Is there a family history of ASD, intellectual disabilities, known genetic syndromes (e.g., Fragile X), metabolic disorders, or epilepsy?
   c. Do any family members appear socially awkward?

Source: Adapted from Mazefsky, C. A., Filipink, R., Lindsey, J., & Lubetsky, M. (2011). Medical evaluation and comorbid psychiatric disorders. In M. J. Lubetsky, B. L. Handen, & J. J. McGonigle (Eds.), *Autism spectrum disorders: Pittsburgh pocket psychiatry* (p. 44). Oxford Press.

MEDICAL CONDITIONS WITH NEUROLOGIC OVERLAP TO AUTISM SPECTRUM DISORDER

Hyman (2020) describes syndromes with specific genetic markers associated with syndromic ASD. These include Fragile X, tuberous sclerosis complex, Smith-Magenis syndrome, and Rett syndrome, neurofibromatosis 1, PTEN harmatoma tumor syndrome, Smith-Lemli-Opitz syndrome, and Timothy syndrome. These are often associated with higher rates of dysmorphic features, chromosomal abnormalities, and/or intellectual disability. Up to 20% of persons with previously diagnosed ASD may have one of these genetic markers or genetic lesions, making genetic testing an important recommendation for any child who receives a diagnosis of ASD.

Behavioral characteristics of all the associated syndromes are similar to those in non-syndromic ASD. Some key concerns with each syndrome include:

a. Fragile X. Individuals with Fragile X may have facial (e.g., protruding ears) and other physical differences (e.g., large hands). They also may have joint hyperextension, mitral valve prolapse, and 20% may have epilepsy. Fragile X is related to the gene *FMR1* (Hyman, 2020; Mazefsky et al., 2011).

b. Tuberous sclerosis complex (TSC). TSC is most often characterized by intellectual disabilities (ID) and benign tumors throughout the body (e.g., brain, heart, lungs, eyes). Additionally, up to 80% of individuals with TSC have a seizure disorder. TSC is related to the *TSC1* and *TSC2* genes (Hyman, 2020; Mazefsky et al., 2011).

c. Smith-Magenis. Individuals with Smith-Magenis often have intellectual disabilities. As with individuals with Fragile X, they also have some craniofacial abnormalities. These individuals may also have hearing loss and other sensory-related difficulties (e.g., ear infections, eye abnormalities). Smith-Magenis is related to the deletion of a small piece on chromosome 17 (Elsea & Girirajan, 2008; Smith et al., 2001/2019).

d. Rett syndrome. Girls are more likely to be diagnosed with Rett syndrome and it is often characterized by a period of near typical development followed by a loss of previously learned skills. They often display repetitive hand motions that may involve bringing the hands together near the chest and mouth areas. If Rett syndrome is suspected, practitioners should refer the patient for testing of the implicated gene: *MECP2* (Hyman, 2020; Schaefer & Mendelsohn, 2013).

e. Neurofibromatosis 1. Children with NF1 have many café-au-lait spots that may increase in size and number with age. This is related to the *NF1* gene (Hyman, 2020).

f. PTEN harmatoma tumor syndrome. Children have multiple benign tumor-like growths throughout the body (e.g., thyroid, breast, and endometrium). PTEN harmatoma tumor syndrome is related to the *PTEN* gene (Hyman, 2020).

g. Smith- Lemli-Opitz syndrome. Individuals with Smith-Lemli-Opitz syndrome present with facial (e.g., narrow forehead, low-set ears, and short nose) and other physical differences (e.g., microcephaly and cleft palate). Smith-Lemli-Opitz syndrome is related to the *DHCR7* gene (Hyman, 2020).

h. Timothy syndrome. Children with Timothy syndrome present with congenital heart defects, EKG Abnormalities, and frequent infections. Additionally, they may present facial (e.g., low-set ears, thin upper lip) and other physical differences (e.g., thin scalp hair, dental abnormalities). Timothy syndrome is related to the *CACNA1C* gene (Hyman, 2020).

SCREENING TOOLS FOR AUTISM SPECTRUM DISORDER

There are a variety of screening tools and checklists for the primary care professional to use in identifying whether further evaluation for an ASD is warranted. These tools have varying evidence of sensitivity and treatment validity (Livanis & Mouzakitis, 2010; Marlow et al., 2019), however, they all provide some information that helps the front-line professional identify whether additional screening and evaluation are necessary. This is critical as early intervention is the key to an effective treatment plan. Table 9.2 provides a description of some of the most used checklists, screening tools, and diagnostic instruments.

Table 9.2. Screening Tools for ASD

Name	Description	Ordering and Additional Information
Checklists		
Modified checklist of autism in toddlers—revised/follow-up (M-CHAT-R/F) The M-CHAT-R/F™	M-CHAT-R/F is 23-item questionnaire for parents and asks whether their child does or does not engage in specific behaviors including social approaching and gesturing. It also asks about walking and sensitivities. The M-CHAT-R/F is an updated and expanded version of the M-CHAT and contains additional questions to help the evaluator determine a more accurate rating.	M-CHAT-R/F: mchatscreen.com/mchat-rf/ M-CHAT: mchatscreen.com/m-chat/

(continued)

Table 9.2. Screening Tools for ASD (*continued*)

Name	Description	Ordering and Additional Information
Screening for autism in 2-year olds (STAT)	The STAT is an interactive measure designed for use with children from 24 through 35 months of age. It is a screening tool to be administered by community providers who have experience with ASD. There are 12 activities in which early social and communication behaviors are observed.	stat.vueinnovations.com/about
Social communication questionnaire (SCQ), previously called Autism Screening Questionnaire (ASQ)	Social communication questionnaire (SCQ) previously called Autism Screening Questionnaire (ASQ), is a brief instrument completed by a parent or primary caregiver. The SCQ evaluates communication skills and social functioning in children 4 or older, who may have autism or ASDs. The SCQ is available in both English and Spanish.	www.wpspublish.com/scq-social-communication-questionnaire
Communication and Symbolic Behavior Scales (CSBS)	The Communication and Symbolic Behavior Scales Developmental Profile Infant/Toddler Checklist is designed to measure the seven language predictors, including emotion/eye gaze, communication, gestures, sounds, words, understanding of words, and object use. It can be used as part of a routine developmental screening/well child visits for children as young as 6 months, through 24 months. The CSBS is to be completed by a parent or other familiar caregiver.	firstwords.fsu.edu/pdf/Checklist_Scoring_Cutoffs.pdf products.brookespublishing.com/CSBS-DP-Manual-P273.aspx
Rating Scales		
Childhood Autism Rating Scale 2 (CARS2):	The Childhood Autism Rating Scale (CARS) has been in use for many years. Based on direct observation, it yields a composite score to help differentiate autism from developmental disabilities. The tool can be used by clinicians, parents, and teachers. The CARS2 includes a rating scale to identify individuals with high functioning autism.	www.wpspublish.com/cars-2-childhood-autism-rating-scale-second-edition

(*continued*)

Table 9.2. Screening Tools for ASD (*continued*)

Name	Description	Ordering and Additional Information
Guilliam Autism Rating Scale-3 (GARS-3)	The GARS-3 is a norm-referenced instrument that assists teachers, parents, and clinicians in identifying and diagnosing ASD in individuals ages 3 through 22. Items were developed based on the *DSM-5*.	www.pearsonassessments.com/store/usassessments/en/Store/Professional-Assessments/Behavior/Gilliam-Autism-Rating-Scale-%7C-Third-Edition/p/100000802.html
Diagnostic Assessments		
Autism Diagnostic Interview—Revised (ADI-R)	The Autism Diagnostic Interview, Revised (ADI-R) is a structured interview used for diagnosing autism, planning treatment, and distinguishing autism from other developmental disorders. To administer the ADI-R the clinician must be trained. Levels of training are determined by the purpose of the assessment (diagnosis or research).	Purchase: www.wpspublish.com/adi-r-autism-diagnostic-interview-revised Training: psychiatry.weill.cornell.edu/education-training/adi-r
Autism Diagnostic Observation Schedule 2 (ADOS-2)	The ADOS-2 allows you to accurately assess and diagnose ASD in toddlers to adults. This is a standardized observational measure that requires specific training to implement.	ADOS-2 www.wpspublish.com/ados-2-autism-diagnostic-observation-schedule-second-edition

ASD, autism spectrum disorder.

MEDICAL CONDITIONS ASSOCIATED WITH AUTISM SPECTRUM DISORDER

Additional associated conditions include:

Individuals with ASD have an increased likelihood of developing associated medical conditions, including seizure disorders, sleep disorders, gastrointestinal (GI) disorders, feeding disorders, obesity, and catatonia (Hyman, 2020).

a. **Seizure disorder**: There is a 6.3% chance that a person with ASD will develop a seizure disorder. Often people with ASD who develop a seizure disorder begin having seizures in adolescence.

b. **Sleep disorder**: Between 50% and 80% of children with ASD have difficulty going to sleep and staying asleep.

c. **Gastrointestinal disorder**: Many individuals with ASD have GI symptoms which may include constipation, diarrhea, pain, and reflux. These symptoms may be related to feeding disorders, medication, or a tendency toward restricted behavior.

d. **Feeding disorders**: Many individuals with ASD have significant food preferences and aversions that can severely limit a balanced diet. A poor diet may lead to vitamin and mineral deficiencies, obesity, and lethargy.

e. **Obesity**: Individuals with ASD may be at greater risk for becoming obese than other individuals. Some medications that are prescribed may lead to obesity and healthy behaviors may be less preferred by people with ASD.

f. **Catatonia**: A diagnosis of an ASD should specify whether catatonia is present. Catatonia is a psychomotor syndrome in which individuals may display, in addition to other symptoms, stupor, mutism, and/or agitation (Walther et al., 2019).

g. **Endocrine diseases**, such as hypothyroidism tend to occur in individuals with ASD than in a typically developing population. In the case of endocrine diseases, the estimated prevalence of two or more forms in autism was 0.7%, approximately seven times greater than in the general population.

h. **Metabolic diseases**, such as homocystinuria, have been associated with ASDs. This indicates that metabolic testing should be considered when clinical symptoms are present, such as lethargy, seizures, and dysmorphic features (Manzi et al., 2008).

COMORBIDITIES IMPORTANT FOR CONSIDERATION WHEN ASSESSING AUTISM SPECTRUM DISORDER

There are many physical and psychiatric symptoms associated with ASD that may in fact be symptoms of other disabilities or disorders. In all cases it is important to determine the primary presenting problems in assessing for an ASD, a disorder or disability with similar features, or cooccurring disorders and disabilities.

Obsessive compulsive disorder (OCD) is the disorder most often associated with an ASD. This is due to an overlap in symptoms as well as a relationship between parents with OCD and children with an ASD. A diagnosis of OCD in an individual with an ASD can be difficult. Because of the overlap in symptoms (i.e., repetitive behaviors), it is very important to rule OCD out as the primary condition. In a study where children with ASD and children with OCD were compared children diagnosed with ASD and those with OCD were reported to display similar levels of sameness behavior and repetitive movements. While both groups were reported to have more compulsions than a typical population, children with OCD were more likely than those with ASD to display compulsions. One important distinction between the groups may be in the types of routines, compulsions, and other repetitive-like behaviors displayed. Persons with OCD tended to display more sophisticated or complex sets of behaviors than those with ASD.

Some other conditions that may warrant particular attention include:

a. Intellectual disabilities,

b. Learning disabilities,

c. Language and communication disorders,

d. Developmental delay,

e. Reactive attachment disorder,

f. Anxiety spectrum disorders (e.g., OCD),

g. ADHD,

h. Selective mutism,

i. Mood dysregulation,

j. Childhood onset schizophrenia, and

k. Disruptive behavior disorders.

Psychiatric comorbidities are of particular interest when evaluating individuals with ASDs as evidence has indicated comorbidity between ASD and psychiatric diagnoses may be quite common.

While there is debate about diagnosing comorbid disorders with overlapping symptoms to an ASD, research has demonstrated a high rate of psychiatric disorders present in individuals with an ASD. For example, Simonoff et al. (2008) found that for 112 individuals diagnosed with ASD, ranging in age from 10 to 14, 70% had at least one comorbid disorder, however anxiety was scored most often (29%), with Attention Deficit Hyperactivity Disorder (ADHD) and Oppositional Defiant Disorder (ODD) both at 28%. Similarly, Rosen et al. (2018) found that approximately 40% of children with ASD also have a comorbid anxiety disorder, up to 29% have a comorbid depressive disorder, under 2% have comorbid bipolar disorder, up to 30% have comorbid ADHD, and the occurrence of ASD and a comorbid diagnosis of schizophrenia or a psychotic disorder is extremely low (0%–0.3%). There is no agreement about the comobility of ASD and disruptive behavior disorders, but some studies have reported that around 25% of children might qualify for both diagnoses (Rosen, et al., 2018). It is unclear if the differences in comorbid disorders are due to the differing diagnosis or the differing ages of the participants, however these studies and others confirm the high prevalence of comorbid symptoms.

Identifying a comorbid psychiatric diagnosis is particularly difficult due to the lack of measures specifically designed to detect these disorders in a population with an ASD. Because persons with ASD present with behavioral symptoms that may mimic symptoms of other disorders (e.g., difficulty with change, difficulty in social situations), it is important to consider the person's baseline presentation when determining a diagnosis of a psychiatric disorder for a person with ASD. A change or increase in impairment is important when considering a diagnosis in addition to an ASD.

Persons with ASD and comorbid psychiatric diagnoses often have greater difficulty with behavioral symptoms. To a varying degree, this may impact all core features of the disorder. Common assessment measures (Table 9.3) for assessment of behavioral and emotional concerns in children with an ASD include:

Table 9.3. Assessment Measures for ASD

Instrument	Brief Description	Age Range	Assessment Type	Number of Items	Ordering and Additional Information
Aberrant Behavior Checklist-2 (ABC-2)	Usually completed by an adult who knows the child well. It has five subscales, including irritability, lethargy/social withdrawal, stereotypy, hyperactivity, and inappropriate speech.	6–54 years	Rating scale	58 items	www.stoeltingco.com/aberrant-behavior-checklist-second-ed-abc-2.html
Behavior Assessment System for Children (BASC-3)	To be completed by teachers, parents, and the child. There also is a structured observation and history taking, to help the assessor understand the behaviors and emotions.	2–5, 6–11, 12–21 years	Rating scale	134–160 items	www.pearsonassessments.com/store/usassessments/en/Store/Professional-Assessments/Behavior/Comprehensive/Behavior-Assessment-System-for-Children-%7C-Third-Edition-/p/100001402.html

(*continued*)

Table 9.3. *(continued)*

Instrument	Brief Description	Age Range	Assessment Type	Number of Items	Ordering and Additional Information
Behavior Problem Inventory (BPI-01)	Filled out by a respondent who knows the child well. It measures self-injurious, stereotypic, and aggressive destructive behavior.	14 and older	Rating scale	52 items	www.bpi.haoliang.me/
Child Behavior Checklist (CBCL)	Completed by a parent or caregiver They rate the child on a variety of areas, including aggressive behavior, anxious or depressed, attention problems, rule-breaking, social problems, somatic complaints, thought problems, and withdrawal.	1.5–5 years, 6–18 years	Rating scale	99 items, 112 items	aseba.org/preschool/#Preschool_CBCL_1%C2%BD5LDS_and_CTRF_Scales
Developmental Behavior Checklist-2 (DBC-2)	A questionnaire completed by parents or other primary caregivers or teachers, to assess behavior or emotional problems.	4–18 years	Rating scale	96 items	www.wpspublish.com/dbc2-developmental-behavior-checklist-2
Repetitive Behavior Scale for Early Childhood (RBS-EC) adapted from the Repetitive Behavior Scale – Revised (RBS-R)	Completed by caregiver. Measures restricted and repetitive behaviors to identify individual differences within the repetitive behavior domain.	Infancy – early school age	Rating scale	34 items	www.cehd.umn.edu/edpsych/research/resources/rbs-ec/

ASD, autism spectrum disorder.

Signs of the Most Common Comorbid Disorders (Mazefsky et al., 2011)

Signs of ADHD

ADHD symptoms in individuals with ASD include inattention, hyperactivity, and impulsivity. When considering a diagnosis of ADHD in an individual with ASD it is important to consider.

- The child's mental age as related to the degree to which behavior is atypical.
- The differences between inattention and skill deficits or hearing impairments.

- Distractibility versus over-focus or preoccupation with irrelevant stimuli (e.g., motor movements or lights).

Signs of an Anxiety Disorder

It is not uncommon for individuals with an ASD to be more likely to experience fears due to their difficulty with change, social situations, and other situations related to the core features of ASD. This is the reason why anxiety disorders are not typically diagnosed separate from an ASD diagnosis. When specific treatment is warranted for anxiety, however, it may be appropriate to do so. Specific anxiety symptoms and classifications may include:

- separation anxiety,
- panic disorder,
- generalized anxiety disorder,
- social phobias,
- obsessive-compulsive symptoms.

Depressive and Anxiety Disorders

Depressive and anxiety disorders may be prevalent in individuals with ASD due to a genetic risk and/or due to environmental stressors. As with all comorbid disorders with ASD, consideration of the severity of symptoms as they relate to ASD versus a mood disorder is important. For this reason, historical information is critically important. For example, measures on the Aberrant Behavior Checklist of social withdrawal are often high for individuals with ASD due to impairments in social functioning. For individuals without an ASD, this may indicate a concern about a mood disorder, however this is typical for individuals with ASD. Some key considerations: Are there changes in affect (which may already be impaired), increased isolation, increased emotional disregulation (e.g., frequent crying) that was not present previously?

ASSOCIATED BEHAVIORAL AND COGNITIVE FEATURES

Severe or serious challenging behaviors are often associated with ASD. The most common behaviors observed are aggression, tantrums, property destruction, and self-injury (Horner et al., 2002). Additional behavioral concerns that can have life-threatening implications are elopement (wandering away) and pica (eating inedible objects). All of the behaviors can significantly affect an individual's quality of life and place the person in danger. If children are exhibiting these behaviors it is important that they are referred to a board certified behavior analyst (BCBA) or a licensed behavior analyst (LBA) and a qualified medical professional with expertise in assessing and treating these behaviors.

Additional behavioral challenges that may be encountered include:

a. Feeding challenges,
b. Sleep challenges,
c. Toileting difficulties.

Each of these may impact the progress that an individual with an ASD can make in the typical environment. Feeding challenges also may impact an individual's health as they may not eat a full range of nutritious foods. Sleep challenges may have an impact on the functioning of the individual and of the family. Toileting difficulties may particularly impede an individual from fully participating in their school and community.

TREATMENT

It is critical that treatment and intervention for ASD is initiated as early as possible. Early intervention is particularly critical as it may result in life-changing beneficial outcomes. Referral to a specialist in diagnosis of ASD is the first step. You may be asked to assist in providing information about professionals in your community who provide treatment. This is where it is important to understand the evidence currently available for the treatment of ASD. Best practice would dictate a well-functioning, interprofessional team to evaluate and assess the presence of the disorder, treat and provide psychiatric and mental health needs, provide training and support for the family, and specific, evidence-based treatment of the child with ASD. There are several resources describing the evidence for treatment of ASD. These include the Centers for Disease Control and Prevention (CDC) (www.cdc.gov/ncbddd/autism/treatment.html), the American Academy of Pediatrics (pediatrics.aappublications.org/content/early/2011/04/04/peds.2011-0426.abstract), and the National Clearinghouse on Autism Evidence and Practice (NCAEP) (ncaep.fpg.unc.edu/research-resources). The review of the literature conducted by the Warren et al. (2011) states that interventions based on Applied Behavior Analysis (ABA) and the Denver Early Start Model have the most evidence for efficacy to date. Additional sources, such as the National Standards Project completed by the National Autism Center (www.nationalautismcenter.org/national-standards-project/) categorize treatments as "established," "emerging," and "unestablished." The National Autism Center lists the following interventions, all based on ABA, as established:

a. Behavioral interventions
b. Cognitive behavioral intervention package
c. Comprehensive behavioral treatment for young children
d. Language training (production)
e. Modeling
f. Natural teaching strategies
g. Parent training
h. Peer training package
i. Pivotal response training
j. Schedules
k. Scripting
l. Self-management
m. Social skills package
n. Story-based intervention

Best practice in treatment for ASD is far from a resolved issue. There are a number of schools of thought on the best treatment approach and there are a number of well-circulated myths or unproven treatments widely used and widely available. Sifting through the evidence can often be time consuming, overwhelming, and difficult for the most sophisticated parent and practitioner. Additionally, new treatments are often developed and advertised without much evidence of their efficacy. There are some tools to help the practitioner in evaluating treatment claims. The Association for Science in Autism Treatment (ASAT) recommends reading the article by Sense About Science (www.senseaboutscience.org/pages/peer-review.html) that discusses the peer review process. On their website ASAT provides a description of autism treatments and the research studies supporting those (asatonline.org/for-parents/learn-more-about-specific-treatments/) and some warning signs of pseudoscientific therapies (asatonline.org/research-treatment/making-sense-of-autism-treatments-weighing-the-evidence/pseudoscientific-therapies-some-warning-signs/).

MEDICATION GUIDE FOR AUTISM SPECTRUM DISORDER

Although the evidence is still emerging, psychopharmacological interventions applied to the core symptoms of social reciprocity and language/communication for ASD are still quite preliminary (Mazzone et al., 2017). Antipsychotic medication (e.g., risperidone) has modest evidence for efficacy on restricted and repetitive behaviors (Zhou et al., 2021). Additionally, oxytocin may have some positive implications for social skills (Parker et al., 2017). The overall lack of medication efficacy for treating core symptoms may be because of the heterogeneity of the disorder

(Hollander & Uzunova, 2017). While there remains minimal evidence to support the use of pharmacotherapy to treat the core symptoms of ASD other than repetitive and restrictive behavior, medication has been used widely to treat behaviors associated with the disorder (e.g., irritability, aggression, self-injury [SIB], inattention, hyperactivity, anxiety and depression.

Symptom based approaches to management using psychopharmacological interventions has afforded youth diagnosed with ASD the opportunity to enjoy improved functioning and quality of life. For example, the FDA approved the prescription of risperidone in 2006 and aripiprazole in 2009 to treat irritability (e.g., moderate to severe tantrums, aggression, and SIB) in youth diagnosed with ASD ages 5 to 16 and 6 to 17 years of age, respectively. When prescribed these agents, youth diagnosed with ASD seem to be afforded improved functioning such as reduction in challenging behaviors (DeVane et al., 2019).

Outside of the medication described, there are few randomized controlled trials that have evaluated the effects of psychopharmacological agents in populations diagnosed with ASD. In essence, providers need to rely on evidence conducted in typically developing populations and extrapolate to individuals diagnosed with ASD. Additionally, in some cases, these medications may exacerbate core symptoms of ASD (i.e., use of stimulants to treat inattention may result in excessive focus on a different and socially inappropriate target). This point is made to simply underscore the importance of careful monitoring of youth diagnosed with ASD and the importance of an interprofessional team to produce the optimized outcome for an individual.

Prior to initiating a psychopharmacological intervention, it is important that individuals have a complete clinical assessment and evaluation that identifies strengths and opportunities in adaptive functioning as well as associated target symptoms. A comprehensive evaluation should include assessments of: (a) developmental psychiatric functioning; (b) medical history; (c) medication history with a focus on the child's response to these interventions (positive and adverse), including dosages, length of trial, and reasons for discontinuation. Given the popular use of supplements, vitamins, and complementary and alternative medicine interventions, review of these agents also should be conducted and assessed for: (a) potential drug-drug interactions; (b) history of current and past educational, psychosocial, and behavioral interventions; and finally, (c) inclusion of behavioral observations and results of rating scales (described previously). Additionally, a functional behavior assessment (FBA) to determine environmental variables contributing to any presenting challenging behavior is recommended and is considered best practice.

Additional assessments, such as physical exam, neurological assessment, imaging studies, audiology and vision evaluation, routine laboratory studies (including lead levels), and EKG should also be included in a comprehensive evaluation when appropriate. Further, psychological assessment (IQ testing, adaptive skills), speech-language-communication assessments (vocabulary, language skills, articulation, and oral-motor skills, pragmatic skills), occupational and physical therapy assessments will likely also be included in a comprehensive assessment of youth diagnosed with ASDs (AACAP, 2014). Each of these evaluations may provide vital information for decisions about psychopharmacological interventions. They will also serve as important points of contrast to evaluate response to response to treatment.

As discussed, there are no current psychopharmacological interventions available to treat the core symptoms of ASD. Educational systems are required to provide functional behavioral assessments to develop behavioral treatment plans, and subsequently evaluate their outcome when associated behaviors that impact the learning environment. Psychopharmacological intervention may be considered when the following criteria are met: (a) the behavioral symptoms persist and continue to interfere with the individual's overall functioning after a behavioral plan is implemented; (b) the behavior or symptom continues to occur at a significant frequency, duration, and/or intensity; and (c) the behavioral symptoms are impacting the safety of the individual or others. If these factors are deemed significant, in spite of behavioral interventions, a targeted medication trial should be considered.

According to Beauvois and Kverno (2020), when medication is appropriate in conjunction with behavioral intervention it is important to collect baseline measures of weight, BMI, blood pressure, among other measures associated with weight gain. Particularly when considering an atypical antipsychotic medication (e.g., apriprizole). Additionally, baseline measures associated with the desired behavioral change and side-effect monitoring are recommended (Zarcone et al., 2008, 2018). Finally the use of appropriate assessment measures, such as anxiety rating scales, the *Pervasive Development Disorder Behavior Inventory*, *Aberrant Behavior Checklist*, and the *Autism Treatment Evaluation Checklist* are recommended (Howell et al., 2021).

Target symptoms that have been demonstrated to be responsive to psychopharmacological intervention for some persons with ASD include: aggression, agitation, anxiety, compulsions, depression, distractibility, hyperactivity, impulsivity, inattention, irritability, obsessions, perseverations, self-injury, or repetitive/restrictive, stereotypic behaviors. It should be noted, however, that the evidence continues to be mild, particularly for severe aggression and self-injury (Adler et al., 2015).

Evidence for psychopharmacological interventions for the listed target symptoms include:

1. Psychostimulants (Cortese et al., 2012)
   - **Agent:** methylphenidate.
   - **Target symptom and/or behavior:** hyperactivity, ADHD-like symptoms.
   - **Adverse events:** irritability, anorexia, sleep disturbance, emotional outbursts, appetite reduction.
2. Alpha Adrenergic Agents (Scahill et al., 2015)
   - **Agent:** guanfacine (Tenex, Intuniv) and clonidine (Catapress, Kapvay).
   - **Target symptom and/or behavior:** hyperactivity, impulsivity.
   - **Adverse events:** hypotension, drowsiness, fatigue, irritability.
3. Norepinephrine Reuptake Inhibitors (Handen et al., 2015)
   - **Agent:** atomoxetine (Strattera).
   - **Target symptom and/or behavior:** ADHD symptoms, noncompliance.
   - **Adverse events:** irritability, GI upset, nausea/vomiting, fatigue, tachycardia.
4. Selective Serotonin Reuptake Inhibitors (Hollander et al., 2005; Thorkelson et al., 2019). **Please review literature as results for SSRIs are quite mixed despite frequency of use.
   - **Agent:** sertraline (Zoloft), fluvoxamine (Luvox), fluoxetine (Prozac), citalopram (Celexa)
   - **Target symptom and/or behavior:** repetitive thoughts and/or behaviors, anxiety symptoms
   - **Adverse events:** activation syndrome (increased activity and/or energy, mood changes, insomnia, agitation), aggression, nausea, sedation, impulsiveness. **Carefully consider Black Box Warning: increased suicidal thinking**
5. Atypical Antipsychotics (Politte & McDougle, 2014; RUPP Autism Network, 2005; Zhou et al., 2021). **Please note, other atypical antipsychotics, such as olanzapine and clozapine have insufficient evidence of efficacy. Additionally, side effects of some, such as clozapine, can be significant and should not be considered without appropriate evaluation and management of symptoms and side effects.
   - **Agent:** aripiprazole (Abilify) and risperidone (Risperdal).
   - **Target symptom and/or behavior:** irritability, mood instability, hyperactivity, restricted/repetitive behaviors, stereotypies, social withdrawal, inappropriate speech, severe tantrums, aggression, and self-injury.

- **Adverse events:** weight gain, increased appetite, vomiting, somnolence, drowsiness, drooling, tremor, fatigue, and dizziness.

6. Mood Stabilizers (Hirota et al., 2014)
   - **Agent:** valproic acid (Depakote) and lamotigine (Lamictal).
   - **Target symptom and/or behavior:** irritability, agitation, aggression, compulsivity, mood.
   - **Adverse events:** insomnia, hyperactivity, irritability, aggression, increased appetite, and skin rash.
   - ***May be best used for irritability/aggression in combination with atypical antipsychotics.**
7. Neuropeptides (Bernaerts et al., 2020; Cai et al., 2018; Parker et al., 2017; Yamasue et al., 2020). **Please review literature as results for neuropeptides are quite mixed despite results of small investigations and interest.
   - **Oxytocin.**
   - **Target symptom and/or behavior:** social reciprocity, social gaze, repetitive behavior.
   - **Adverse events:** Nasal discomfort, tiredness, irritability, skin irritation (none are statistically significant).
8. Hormones (Gringras et al., 2017; Rossignol & Frye, 2014).
   - **Melatonin.**
   - **Target symptom and/or behavior:** sleep disturbance (onset, duration).
   - **Adverse events:** somnolence.

CONSIDERATIONS FOR OFFICE VISITS

Being prepared to support an individual with an ASD and their family when they come for office visits is an important part of primary care. Individuals with an ASD may have difficulty with office visits for a variety of reasons. First, the visit is not part of their typical routine, which may make them anxious. Social situations can be hard for some persons with an ASD, making a visit to a crowded office even more difficult. While waiting can be hard for many children, waiting can be highly problematic for an individual with an ASD. All of these may combine to increase the likelihood the visit will not go smoothly. Some suggestions for easing these concerns might be:

a. Provide the family with pictures of the office, the people in the office, and a description (e.g., story) of what the child can expect.
b. Suggest that the caregivers show the individual the pictures and review the "story" before they come to the office to help the individual prepare.
c. Try and schedule the visit for a time when there are likely to be minimal people in the office and for a time when the wait is likely to be short (e.g., the first appointment in the morning).
d. Be sure to have objects that might be dangerous or that can be thrown both in the exam and waiting rooms out of reach if the individual has a history of displaying challenging behavior.
e. Speak with the person with ASD, not just with the caregiver.
f. Use language that matches the individual's level of comprehension (take your cues from the caregiver).
g. Use visuals to describe what you are doing as often as possible. For example, you might show a picture of a person listening to a child's heart, then say "now this is what I am going to do."

h. Make the visit with the individual with ASD as short as possible. You consider having some toys or play objects in the room to engage the individual with ASD while you speak with their caregiver after the exam.

Individuals with ASD often have impairments in their ability to communicate. This can make your ability to identify symptoms and medical concerns very difficult. Some considerations to help in this process are provided by Mazefsky et al. (2011). These include:

a. A child with an ASD may not look ill, but may display challenging behavior as the only outward symptoms.
b. Challenging behavior may reflect pain that they are not able to communicate. Understanding whether the behavior displayed is part of their typical repertoire or whether it has changed will be critical in detecting whether the behavior is communicating a change in pain.
c. The child with ASD may be in need of care for injuries that are self-inflicted or as a result of a lack of understanding of danger (e.g., ran into the woods).
d. Be aware of the child's history and provide adequate space during an exam if the child has a history of displaying challenging behavior.
e. Consider obtaining information for the appointment in advance via phone call with the caregiver (e.g., history, concerns, and changes).
f. Ask the parent for advice on how to make optimal use of the visit (e.g., reinforcements for the child, communication modalities, whether a second adult would be beneficial).
g. For children who cannot tolerate blood draws, consider prescribing an anesthetic cream in advance for the parent to apply.

There are many publicly available resources to help with office visits. Some examples can be found at the Autism Speak website (www.autismspeaks.org/expert-opinion/autism-and-doctor-visit-communication-tips-success), Children's Hospital of Philadelphia (www.chop.edu/news/tips-more-positive-office-visits-patients-asd), and a variety of social narratives, including a coronavirus toolkit at Massachusetts General Hospital (www.massgeneral.org/children/autism/lurie-center/social-narratives).

REFERENCES

Abrahams, B. S., & Geschwind, D. H. (2008). Advances in autism genetics: On the threshold of new neurobiology. *Nature Reviews, Genetics*, *9*, 344. https://doi.org/10.1038/nrg2861

Adler, B. A., Wink, L. K., Early, M., Shaffer, R., Minshawi, N., McDougle, C. J., & Erickson, C. A. (2015). Drug-refractory aggression, self-injurious behavior, and severe tantrums in autism spectrum disorders: A chart review study. *Autism*, *19*(1), 102–106. https://doi.org/10.1177/1362361314524641

American Psychiatric Association. (2000). *Diagnostic and statistical manual of mental disorders: (4th ed. text revision). DSM-IV-TR.* Author.

American Psychiatric Association. (2013). *Diagnostic and statistical manual of mental disorders: (5th ed.) DSM-5*. Author.

Beauvois, L., & Kverno, K. (2020). Challenges in treating children with autism spectrum disorder: Implications for psychiatric–mental health nurse practitioners. *Journal of Psychosocial Nursing and Mental Health Services*, *58*(12), 7–12. https://doi.org/10.3928/02793695-20201112-02

Bernaerts, S., Boets, B., Bosmans, G., Steyaert, J., & Alaerts, K. (2020). Behavioral effects of multiple-dose oxytocin treatment in autism: A randomized, placebo-controlled trial with long-term follow-up. *Molecular Autism*, *11*(1), 1–14. https://doi.org/10.1186/s13229-020-0313-1

Cai, Q., Feng, L., & Yap, K. Z. (2018). Systematic review and meta-analysis of reported adverse events of long-term intranasal oxytocin treatment for autism spectrum disorder. *Psychiatry and Clinical Neurosciences*, *72*(3), 140–151. https://doi.org/10.1111/pcn.12627

Cortese, S., Castelnau, P., Morcillo, C., Roux, S., & Bonnet-Brilhault, F. (2012). Psychostimulants for ADHD-like symptoms in individuals with autism spectrum disorders. *Expert Review of Neurotherapeutics*, *12*(4), 461–473. https://doi.org/10.1586/ern.12.23

DeVane, C. L., Charles, J. M., Abramson, R. K., Williams, J. E., Carpenter, L. A., Raven, S., Gwynette, F., Stuck, C. A., Geesey, M. E., Bradley, C., Donovan, J. L., Hall, A. G., Sherk, S. T., Powers, N. R., Spratt, E., Kinsman, A., Kruesi, M. J., & Bragg, E. J., Jr. (2019). Pharmacotherapy of autism spectrum disorder: Results from the randomized BAART clinical trial. *Pharmacotherapy: The Journal of Human Pharmacology and Drug Therapy, 39*(6), 626–635. https://doi.org/10.1002/phar.2271

Elsea, S. H., & Girirajan, S. (2008). Smith-Magenis syndrome. *European Journal of Human Genetics, 16*, 412–421. https://doi.org/10.1038/sj.ejhg.5202009

Giles, D. C. (2014). "*DSM-5* is taking away our identity": The reaction of the online community to the proposed changes in the diagnosis of Asperger's disorder. *Health, 18*(2), 179–195. https://doi.org/10.1177/1363459313488006

Gringras, P., Nir, T., Breddy, J., Frydman-Marom, A., & Findling, R. L. (2017). Efficacy and safety of pediatric prolonged-release melatonin for insomnia in children with autism spectrum disorder. *Journal of the American Academy of Child & Adolescent Psychiatry, 56*(11), 948–957. https://doi.org/10.1016/j.jaac.2017.09.414

Handen, B. L., Aman, M. G., Arnold, L. E., Hyman, S. L., Tumuluru, R. V., Lecavalier, L., Corbett-Dick, P., Pan, X., Hollway, J. A., Buchan-Page, K. A., Silverman, L. B., Brown, N. V., Rice, R. B., Jr., Hellings, J., Mruzek, D. W., McAuliffe-Bellin, S., Hurt, E. A., Ryan, M. M., Levato, L., & Smith, T. (2015). Atomoxetine, parent training, and their combination in children with autism spectrum disorder and attention-deficit/hyperactivity disorder. *Journal of the American Academy of Child & Adolescent Psychiatry, 54*(11), 905–915. https://doi.org/10.1016/j.jaac.2015.08.013

Hirota, T., Veenstra-VanderWeele, J., Hollander, E., & Kishi, T. (2014). Antiepileptic medications in autism spectrum disorder: A systematic review and meta-analysis. *Journal of Autism and Developmental Disorders, 44*(4), 948–957. https://doi.org/10.1007/s10803-013-1952-2

Hollander, E., & Uzunova, G. (2017). Are there new advances in the pharmacotherapy of autism spectrum disorders? *World Psychiatry, 16*(1), 101. https://doi.org/10.1002/wps.20398

Horner, R. H., Carr, E. G., Strain, P. S., Todd, A. W., & Reed, H. K. (2002). Problem behavior interventions for young children with autism: A research synthesis. *Journal of Autism and Developmental Disorders, 32*, 423–446. https://doi.org/10.1023/A:1020593922901

Howell, M., Bradshaw, J., & Langdon, P. E. (2021). A systematic review of behaviour-related outcome assessments for children on the autism spectrum with intellectual disabilities in education settings. *Review Journal of Autism and Developmental Disorders, 8*, 67–91. https://doi.org/10.1007/s40489-020-00205-y

Livanis, A., & Mouzakitis, A. (2010). Treatment validity of autism screening instruments. *Assessment for Effective Intervention, 35*, 206–217. https://doi.org/10.1177/1534508410381041

Maenner, M. J., Shaw, K. A., Baio, J., Washington, A., Patrick, M., DiRienzo, M., Christensen, D. L., Wiggins, L. D., Pettygrove, S., Andrews, J. G., Lopez, M., Hudson, A., Baroud, T., Schwenk, Y., White, T., Rosenberg, C. R. R., Lee, L.-C., Harrington, R. A., Huston, M., . . . Dietz, P. M. (2020). Prevalence of autism spectrum disorder among children aged 8 years — Autism and developmental disabilities monitoring network, 11 Sites, United States, 2016. *MMWR Surveillance Summaries, 69*(4), 1–12. http://doi.org/10.15585/mmwr.ss6904a1

Manzi, B., Loizzo, A. L., Giana, G., & Curatolo, P. (2008). Autism and metabolic diseases. *Journal of Child Neurology, 23*, 307–314. https://doi.org/10.1177/0883073807308698

Marlow, M., Servili, C., & Tomlinson, M. (2019). A review of screening tools for the identification of autism spectrum disorders and developmental delay in infants and young children: Recommendations for use in low- and middle-income countries. *Autism Research, 12*(2), 176–199. https://doi.org/10.1002/aur.2033

Martin, J., Mazzone, L., Giovagnoli, G., Siracusano, M., Postorino, V., & Curatolo, P. (2017). Drug treatments for core symptoms of autism spectrum disorder: Unmet needs and future directions. *Journal of Child Neurology, 15*(3), 134–142. https://doi.org/10.1055/s-0037-1602823

Mazefsky, C. A., Filipink, R., Lindsey, J., & Lubetsky, M. J. (2011). Medical evaluation and co-morbid psychiatric disorder. In M. J. Lubetsky, B. L. Handen, & J. J. McGonigle (Eds.), *Autism spectrum disorder: Pittsburgh pocket psychiatry*. Oxford University Press.

Parker, K. J., Oztan, O., Libove, R. A., Sumiyoshi, R. D., Jackson, L. P., Karhson, D. S., Summers, J. E., Hinman, K. E., Motonaga, K. S., Phillips, J. M., Carson, D. S., Garner, J. P., & Hardan, A. Y. (2017). Intranasal oxytocin treatment for social deficits and biomarkers of response in children with autism. *Proceedings of the National Academy of Sciences, 114*(30), 8119–8124. https://doi.org/10.1073/pnas.1705521114

Politte, L. C., & McDougle, C. J. (2014). Atypical antipsychotics in the treatment of children and adolescents with pervasive developmental disorders. *Psychopharmacology, 231*(6), 1023–1036. https://doi.org/10.1007/s00213-013-3068-y

Rea, K. E., Armstrong-Brine, M., Ramirez, L., & Stancin, T. (2019). Ethnic disparities in Autism Spectrum Disorder screening and referral: Implications for pediatric practice. *Journal of Developmental & Behavioral Pediatrics, 40*(7), 493–500. https://doi.org/10.1097/DBP.0000000000000691

Rosen, T., Mazefsky, C. A., Vasa, R. A., & Lerner, M. D. (2018). Co-occurring psychiatric conditions in autism spectrum disorder. *International Review of Psychiatry, 30*(1), 40–61. https://doi.org/10.1080/09540261.2018.1450229

Rossignol, A. D., & Frye, E. R. (2014). Melatonin in autism spectrum disorders. *Current Clinical Pharmacology, 9*(4), 326–334. https://doi.org/10.2174/15748847113086660072

Scahill, L., McCracken, J. T., King, B. H., Rockhill, C., Shah, B., Politte, L., Sanders, R., Minjarez, M., Cowen, J., Mullett, J., Page, C., Ward, D., Deng, Y., Loo, S., Dziura, J., McDougle, C. J., & Research Units on Pediatric Psychopharmacology Autism Network. (2015). Extended-release guanfacine for hyperactivity in children with autism spectrum disorder. *American Journal of Psychiatry, 172*(12), 1197–1206. https://doi.org/10.1176/appi.ajp.2015.15010055

Schaefer, G. B., & Mendelsohn, N. J. (2013). Clinical genetics evaluation in identifying the etiology of autism spectrum disorders: 2013 guideline revisions. *Genetics in Medicine, 15*(5), 399–407. https://doi.org/10.1097/GIM.0b013e31816b5cc9

Simonoff, E., Pickles, A., Charman, T., Chandler, S., Loucas, T., & Baird, G. (2008). Psychiatric disorders in children with autism spectrum disorders: Prevalence, comorbidity, and associated factors in a population derived sample. *Journal of the American Academy of Child & Adolescent Psychiatry, 47*, 921–929. https://doi.org/10.1097/CHI.0b013e318179964f

Smith, A., Boyd, K. E., Brennan, C., Charles, J., Elsea, S. H., Finucane, B. M., Foster, R., Gropman, A., Girirajan, S., & Haas-Givler, B. (2001/2019). Smith-Magenis syndrome. In M. P. Adam et al. (Eds.), *GeneReviews®*. University of Washington.

Taylor, M. J., Rosenqvist, M. A., Larsson, H., Gillberg, C., D'Onofrio, B. M., Lichtenstein, P., & Lundström, S. (2020). Etiology of autism spectrum disorders and autistic traits over time. *JAMA Psychiatry, 77*(9), 936–943. https://doi.org/10.1001/jamapsychiatry.2020.0680

Thorkelson, G., Laughlin, S. F., Turner, K. S., Ober, N., & Handen, B. L. (2019). Select serotonin reuptake inhibitor monotherapy for anxiety disorders in children and adolescents with autism spectrum disorder: A chart review. *Journal of Child and Adolescent Psychopharmacology, 29*(9), 705–711. https://doi.org/10.1089/cap.2019.0001

Walther, S., Stegmayer, K., Wilson, J. E., & Heckers, S. (2019). Structure and neural mechanisms of catatonia. *The Lancet Psychiatry, 6*(7), 610–619. https://doi.org/10.1016/S2215-0366(18)30474-7

Warren, Z., McPheeter, M. L., Sathe, N., Foss-Feig, M. A., Glasser, A., & Veenstra-Vanderweele, J. (2011). A systematic review of early intensive intervention for autism spectrum disorder. *Pediatrics, 127*, e1303–e1311. https://doi.org/10.1542/peds.2011-0426

Yamasue, H., Okada, T., Munesue, T., Kuroda, M., Fujioka, T., Uno, Y., Matsumoto, K., Kuwabara, H., Mori, D., Okamoto, Y., Yoshimura, Y., Kawakubo, Y., Arioka, Y., Kojima, M., Yuhi, T., Owada, K., Yassin, W., Kushima, I., Benner, S., . . . Kosaka, H. (2020). Effect of intranasal oxytocin on the core social symptoms of autism spectrum disorder: A randomized clinical trial. *Molecular Psychiatry, 25*(8), 1849–1858. https://doi.org/10.1038/s41380-018-0097-2

Zarcone, J., Griffith, A., & Rieken, C. J. (2018). Measuring the effects of medication for individuals with autism. In C. McNeil, A. Griffith, & C. J. Rieken (Eds.), *Handbook of parent-child interaction therapy for children on the autism spectrum* (pp. 71–86). Springer Publishing Company. https://doi.org/10.1007/978-3-030-03213-5_5

Zarcone, J., Napolitano, D., & Valdovinos, M. (2008). Measurement of problem behaviour during medication evaluations. *Journal of Intellectual Disability Research, 52*(12), 1015–1028. https://doi.org/10.1111/j.1365-2788.2008.01109.x

Zhou, M. S., Nasir, M., Farhat, L. C., Kook, M., Artukoglu, B. B., & Bloch, M. H. (2021). Meta-analysis: Pharmacologic treatment of restricted and repetitive behaviors in autism spectrum disorders. *Journal of the American Academy of Child & Adolescent Psychiatry*, 60(1): 35–45. https://doi.org/10.1016/j.jaac.2020.03.007

Information for Parents About ASD in Children

There are many resources for parents who are either concerned their child might have autism or whose child has been diagnosed with an ASD.

- Autism Speaks (www.autismspeaks.org/), in particular, has a wealth of information and kits to help parents navigate the often overwhelming dearth of information available on the assessment and treatment of children with ASD. Some resources available on their website include tool kits www.autismspeaks.org/family-services/tool-kits) such as the 100 days kit that helps parents navigate the first 100 days after their child's diagnosis and a variety of others to help families (e.g., tips for successful hair cuts).
- The National Institute of Mental Health has a parent's guide to ASDs (www.nimh.nih.gov/health/publications/autism-spectrum-disorder/index.shtml), the National Autism Center had a Parents Guide to Evidence-Based Practice (www.nationalautismcenter.org/resources/for-families/).
- The American Academy of Pediatrics also has a book for purchase, Autism Spectrum Disorders: What Every Parent Needs to Know, edited by Alan I. Rosenblatt, MD, FAAP, and Paul S. Carbone, MD, FAAP (www.healthychildren.org/English/bookstore/Pages/Autism-Spectrum-Disorders-What-Every-Parent-Needs-to-Know.aspx).

ADDITIONAL INTERNET RESOURCES

- American Academy of Pediatrics AAP Autism Tool Kit, Third Edition

  https://shop.aap.org/autism-caring-for-children-with-autism-spectrum-disorders-a-practical-resource-toolkit-for-clini/
- American Academy of Child and Adolescent Psychiatry (AACAP) https://www.jaacap.org/article/S0890-8567(13)00819-8/pdf
- Association for Science in Autism Treatment: https://asatonline.org
- Autism Speaks https://www.autismspeaks.org
- Centers for Disease Control and Prevention (CDC) Autism Case Training
  - https://www.cdc.gov/ncbddd/actearly/act.html CDC Act Early Campaign
  - https://www.cdc.gov/ncbddd/actearly/
- International Rett Syndrome Foundation: http://www.rettsyndrome.org/
- National Institute of Neurological Disorders and Stroke

  https://www.ninds.nih.gov/Disorders/All-Disorders/Autism-Spectrum-Disorder-Information-Page

CHAPTER 10

Bernadette Mazurek Melnyk and Linda J. Alpert-Gillis

Helping Children and Parents Through Marital Separation and Divorce

FAST FACTS

- It is common for U.S. children to experience divorce of their parents, affecting more than 1 million every year. (Cohen & Weizman, 2016).
- Several decades of research indicate that the outcomes for children and adolescents following divorce are determined by numerous factors that can increase risk or foster resilience. (Kelly, 2012).
- The risk of emotional, behavioral, social, and academic problems for children of divorced parents (25%) is more than double than that of children whose parents are continuously married (10%). However, the differences between children of divorced and married families are modest and not universal.
- Externalizing problems (e.g., acting-out behaviors, impulsivity) have been consistently identified as the most common problems identified in children after divorce.
- Between 75% and 80% of children of divorce fall within the average range or better on objective measures of adjustment 2 to 3 years after parental divorce.
- Interparental hostility and lack of cooperation between parents following divorce is the most consistent predictor of poor outcomes among children.
- Risk factors linked to negative outcomes following divorce with robust empirical support include parental conflict, psychological adjustment of the parents, quality and type of parenting, parent–child relationships, loss of important relationships, parental cohabitation and remarriage, family structure transitions, and economic resources.
- Protective factors linked to resilience in children with strong empirical evidence include: reduced or encapsulated parental conflict, good adjustment of the residential parent, competent parenting of both parents and cooperative or parallel co-parenting styles, higher levels of involvement of the non-residential parent, limited number of family transitions, and economic stability (O'Hara et al., 2019).
- The child's age at the time of divorce affects outcomes related to the developmental tasks associated with that age.
- No consistent gender differences are attributable to divorce.

ADDITIONAL FACTS ABOUT CONFLICT

- Parents' post separation conflict levels are not predicted by level of conflict prior to separation.
- 8% to 12% of parents exhibit high levels of conflict 2 to 3 years after divorce.
- Intensity, conflict style, and focus of marital conflict are better predictors of child outcomes than frequency of conflict or legal conflict.

- There are direct and indirect effects of high levels of conflict on children's adjustment. A direct effect is that children often model their parents' aggressive behavior in their own relationships and do not learn age-appropriate social skills for conflict resolution. Indirect effects are mediated through variables such as quality of parenting, which impacts emotional security.
- The most deleterious impact of post-divorce conflict occurs when parents involve their children directly in the conflict including using them as messengers, as well as when parents talk in a hostile and demeaning manner about the other parent. The amount of legal conflict between parents is not associated with child adjustment.
- Protective factors in families that have high conflict include: warm, competent parenting; not exposing children directly to the conflict; not using children to express anger to the other parent; refraining from making negative comments about the other parent; and positive sibling relationships.
- A good relationship with at least one caregiver or adult mentor and supportive sibling relationships are buffers against the effects of high parental conflict.

Additional Facts About Parents and Parenting

- The adjustment of the parent with primary residential custody is one of the most powerful predictors of children's psychological adjustment following divorce. Parental depression, anxiety, and long-term mental health problems, such as personality disorders, are associated with externalizing, internalizing, and academic problems in children. Significant mental health problems interfere with the quality of parenting and the parent–child relationship which is associated with children's adjustment.
- Shortly after separation, some parents experience a "honeymoon" period in which they feel relieved that a stressful marriage has ended, whereas others feel anxiety, anger/guilt, depression, exhaustion, and helplessness.
- Most adults report that their low point is a year after marital separation, with full adjustment taking 2 to 3 years.
- Quality of parenting is a major predictor of adjustment and academic performance at least of equal importance as conflict in determining risk. Positive adjustment is associated with effective parenting, greater father involvement, and close father–child relationships. Children are found to function best when both parents provide adequate and nurturing parenting in each home and have a cooperative or parallel co-parenting relationship.
- Economic difficulties are associated with increased parental conflict and poorer parental functioning, which then predicts poorer child adjustment.

Additional Facts About Remarriage and Family Transitions

- Remarriage is not a protective factor and does not in itself decrease the risk of adverse outcomes for children.
- Cohabitation is associated with more negative outcomes for children compared to children in remarried families.
- Positive stepfather–child relationships and nonresident father–child relationships are associated with lowered risk for both externalizing and internalizing symptoms.
- Each change in family structure increases the risk of behavioral and social problems, drug use, and poorer academic achievement.

Typical Responses to Marital Separation

Young Children

- Regression
- Irritability and restlessness
- Temper tantrums
- Sleeping difficulties
- Separation problems
- Anger
- Increased whining and crying
- Sadness
- Guilt
- Fear of abandonment
- Excessive clinging
- Withdrawal

School-Aged Children

- Sadness
- Depression
- Longing for parent's return from home
- Withdrawal
- Denial
- Somatic complaints
- Parentification
- Deterioration in school performance
- Low self-esteem
- Anger
- Preoccupation with parent's departure
- Decrease in peer relations
- Shame
- Loyalty conflicts
- Reunification fantasies
- Behavioral problems

Adolescents

- Anger
- Blaming one parent
- Attempts to gain control
- Denial
- Somatic complaints
- Low self-esteem and alcohol usage
- Sadness
- Depression
- Loyalty conflicts
- Acting out or immature behaviors
- Parentification
- Increase in sexual activity and drug use
- Withdrawal

Responses to Marital Separation That Require Immediate Assessment and Intervention

- Self-injury, cutting, or eating disorders;
- Frequent angry/violent outbursts;
- Severe depression and/or withdrawal from primary relationships;
- Significant academic or social difficulty at school;
- Drug or alcohol abuse; and
- Hopelessness or suicidal ideation.

Critical History-Taking Questions When a Divorce or Separation Has Occurred

- Have there been any changes in your family since your last visit? (This is an essential question as parents may not disclose a marital transition unless directly asked.)
- What are the parents' and child's perceptions of the divorce?
- How are the parents and child coping with the divorce and what are their responses? Specifically, how have their emotions and behaviors changed?
- What is the parents' knowledge of the impact of divorce on their children and the typical responses that children have when adjusting to the transition?
- What changes have occurred in parenting practices and daily routines (e.g., limit setting, childcare arrangements)?
- What are the family's other major life stressors (e.g., move to a new home, change in job, and financial difficulties)?
- How much and what type of conflict between the parents is occurring, and is the child a witness or involved in that conflict?
- What social supports do the parent and child have in place to assist them in coping with the separation and divorce?
- What is the level of involvement of the nonresidential parent?
- What is the parent's and child's mood state (e.g., anxiety, depression)? Specifically ask, on a scale of 0 to 10, "How stressed/anxious as well as depressed are you (your child) on a daily basis?"
- What are the parent's and child's current level of functioning (e.g., at work and at school)?
- What is worrying the parent and child most at this time?

Screening for Marital Transitions

Because of the major impact that marital transitions (i.e., separation, divorce, and remarriage) have on families, it is very important to ask the following questions at each healthcare encounter.

For Parents and Children/Teens:

Have there been any changes in your family in the past year, such as marital separation/divorce or remarriage?

On a scale of 0 to 10, if 0 means "there is no fighting" and 10 means "there is a lot of fighting," how much arguing/fighting goes on between family members?

On a scale of 0 to 10, if 0 means you "have no stress" and 10 means you "have a lot of stress," how much stress is your family situation causing you?

On a scale of 0 to 10, if 0 means "not at all" and 10 means "a lot," how much is your family situation affecting your ability to work (for parents) or to do well in school (for children/teens)?

Early Interventions

- Educate parents about risk factors that can lead to child adjustment difficulties: parental conflict, psychological adjustment of the parents, quality and type of parenting and parent–child relationships, loss of important relationships, parental cohabitation and remarriage, family structure transitions, and economic resources.

- Educate parents about protective factors linked to resilience in children: low levels of parental conflict or encapsulated parental conflict, good adjustment of the residential parent, competent parenting of both parents and cooperative or parallel co-parenting styles, higher levels of involvement of the non-residential parent, limited number of family transitions, and economic stability.
- When there are high levels of conflict in the family, it is especially important to share with families the factors that can ameliorate its impact: warm, competent parenting; positive sibling relationships; not exposing children directly to the conflict; not using children to express anger to the other parent; and refraining from making negative comments about the other parent.
- Emphasizing the importance of self-care for the parent and discussing with parents that their own functioning is one of the most powerful predictors of children's psychological adjustment following divorce. Advise the parent to obtain counseling if he or she is having difficulty coping and notice that this is affecting their parenting.
- Inform the parent that it is not helpful to set unrealistic expectations for themselves or their children and that the process of adjustment to this transition may take up to 2 to 3 years.
- Educate the parents about typical age-appropriate responses that children have to separation and divorce.
- Counsel parents about age-appropriate strategies to help their children cope with the transition.
- Provide parents with the handouts "A Dozen Ways to Help Your Child Deal With Divorce," available in this guide.
- Advise parents to consistently reinforce to their child that: (a) the divorce is not the child's fault (as children often feel guilty about it); and (b) that they will not abandon him or her (children need this reinforcement). However, it is important to not make promises that you do not have control over such as frequency of contact with the non-residential parent.
- Encourage parents to help their children openly express their feelings about the divorce (younger children often express their feelings by talking about how their stuffed animal or puppet feels).
- Encourage parents to spend special time with their child every day, even if only for 15 minutes, without interruptions, and to maintain routines.
- Assist the parent with discipline; encourage the importance of setting of limits and reinforcing them consistently. (Although he or she cannot control what happens at the other parent's home, the parent can implement limits at his or her own home.)
- Offer parents the Creating Opportunities for Parent Empowerment (COPE) program, an evidence-based user-friendly program designed to assist parents in helping 3- to 7-year-old children cope with divorce. The program can be obtained from Bernadette Melnyk at cope.melnyk@gmail.com.
- Provide local resources to help parents and children deal with the divorce (e.g., Parents without Partners).
- Inform the parents to contact you with any concerns or worries about their child.

INTERNET RESOURCES

American Academy of Child and Adolescent Psychiatry Facts for Families

www.aacap.org

This website is an excellent source of information on the assessment and treatment of child and adolescent mental health disorders. The AACAP developed *Facts for Families* handouts to provide concise and up-to-date information on issues that affect children, teens, and their families. These handouts are available in English and Spanish and can be duplicated and distributed free of charge as long as AACAP is properly credited and no profit is gained from their use.

Everyday Health

www.everydayhealth.com

This website is committed to providing trusted, real-world, evidence-based health information from the nation's leading healthcare providers and patient advocates, alongside personal patient perspectives and health consumer insights from those on the front lines, in real time.

HELPGUIDE.org

www.helpguide.org

HELPGUIDE is a non-profit organization that maintains a web-site to assist individuals and families with accurate information about a variety of mental health disorders and challenging family issues, such as divorce and remarriage.

Kids Health

www.kidshealth.org

This is an outstanding website that contains health information for healthcare providers, parents, teens, and children. Many of the topics relate to emotions and behaviors (e.g., anxiety, fears, depression) as well as family changes and are developmentally sensitive to specific age groups. Physicians and other healthcare providers review all material before it is posted on this website.

REFERENCES

Cohen, G. J., & Weitzman, C. C., & Committee on Psychosocial Aspects of Child and Family Health; Section on Developmental and Behavioral Pediatrics. (2016). Helping children and families deal with divorce and separation. *Pediatrics, 138*(6), e20163020. https://doi.org/10.1542/peds.2016-3020

Kelly, J. B. (2012). Risk and protective factors associated with child and adolescent adjustment following separation and divorce: Social science applications. In K. Kuehnle & L. Drozd (Eds.), *Parenting plan evaluations: Applied research for the family court* (pp. 49–84). Oxford University Press.

O'Hara, K. L., Sandler, I. R., Wolchik, S. A., Tein, J.-Y., & Abrey Rhodes, C. (2019). Parenting time, parenting quality, interparental conflict, and mental health problems of children in high-conflict divorce. *Journal of Family Psychology, 33*(6), 690–703. doi: 10.1037/fam0000556.

A Dozen Ways to Help Your Child Deal With Marital Separation/Divorce

1. Understand the impact of divorce on children	Marital separation involves stressful and difficult transitions for children and parents. It is common for children to show some behavioral changes in response to such transitions. There are parenting strategies that can help you and your children cope effectively with your family situation.
2. Prepare your children for the changes involved in a divorce.	Give children information about family changes in a way they can understand. Tell children in advance about the changes they are about to experience.
3. Accept children's feelings and encourage talking about them.	Help your children learn to talk about their feelings and express feelings in acceptable ways. When children can put their feelings into words they are much less likely to act out inappropriately.
4. Reassure your children.	Make sure that your children know that you love them and that you will take care of them. Inform your children that you are divorcing the other parent, not them. Provide assurance that a parent's love for a child is a special kind that does not stop.
5. Allow your children to be children.	Avoid having your child take on too many adult responsibilities. Discussing family finances with them or telling them that they are now the "little man or woman of the house" can be a burden. Instead, encourage them to become involved in school activities, clubs, or hobbies that develop their own strength and abilities.
6. Give children permission to love both parents. Support your children's relationship with their other parent.	Children benefit from a positive relationship with each parent; a consistent schedule of when children will be with each parent is very important. Also, not talking in a negative way about the other parent can allow your children a healthier relationship with both parents.
7. Problem solve together.	Talk with your children about how to make things better or more comfortable for them.
8. Work on your relationship with your children.	Set aside special time to spend with each child, doing things together such are reading, playing a game, or taking a walk.

This handout may be distributed to families.

From Melnyk, B. M., & Lusk, P. (2022). *A Practical Guide to Child and Adolescent Mental Health Screening, Evidence-Based Assessment, Intervention, and Health Promotion* (3rd ed.).

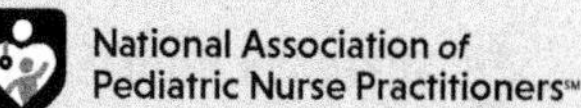

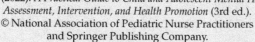

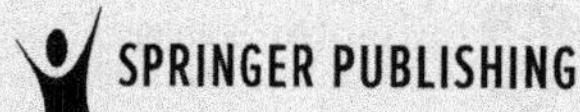

9. Keep conflict away from your children.	Keep arguments with your former spouse as far away from your children as possible, especially if they involve verbal or physical aggression. Intense conflict between parents is likely to lead to adjustment problems in children. Do not use your children as messengers or as weapons to get back at your former spouse.
10. Maintain as much structure and predictability in your everyday routine as possible.	Children thrive on routine, including regular bedtimes, having meals together, and consistent rules. Setting limits on children's inappropriate behavior helps children feel safe and communicates to them that you will provide order and control when they are not able to do so.
11. Listen to children's verbal and non-verbal communication.	Listen to what your children say and watch what they do. Remember children often state things indirectly. For example, "I hate the woman you're dating" may mean "I am worried that you like her more than me."
12. Take care of yourself.	Reach out to resources such as trusted friends, family members, support groups, members of the clergy, and mental health professionals. Research has emphasized the important link between parents' emotional and physical well-being and children's healthy development.

Created by Drs. Bernadette Melnyk and Linda Alpert-Gillis.

CHAPTER 11

Barbara Jones Warren

Evidence-Based Assessment and Management of Substance Abuse and Addiction Spectrum

FAST FACTS

- Children and adolescents make up approximately 27% of the population in the United States (U.S. Census Bureau, 2019).
- While many children and adolescents have normal and healthy developmental processes, approximately 6.1 million children and adolescents between the ages of 12 and 17 years needed treatment for substance-related or addictive disorders between the years of 2015 and 2019 (Substance Abuse and Mental Health Services Administration [SAMHSA], 2011, 2020b), yet only 5 million of these children and adolescents received treatment (SAMHSA, 2020b). Their use of addictive substances intensifies the development of comorbid mental health disorders, developmental delays, and problems with everyday functioning, all of which affect their ability to contribute to society as they emerge into adulthood (Arnett, 2007; SAMHSA, 2011).
- Experimentation may occur for children and teens when they use a substance on a few occasions because they are curious as to "how it feels." This often occurs at parties in response to peer pressure. Failure to identify and intervene with child and adolescent use can evolve into abuse and dependence (Boyd, 2017; SAMHSA, 2020a). The level of use, abuse, and dependence is contingent upon the child's and adolescent's developmental stage, chronological age, and level of protective and risk factors (American Psychiatric Association [APA], 2013; Arnett, 2006, 2007; Boch et al., 2016).
- Appropriate screening and early identification are critical in order to institute evidence-based practice (EBP) approaches for children and adolescents who use addictive substances. This approach includes early detection and treatment of behavioral issues that may affect children and adolescents (Abney et al., 2019). In addition, use of research-based and culturally sensitive strategies are critical to support caregivers, schools, and communities in which the youth live (Warren, 2019).
- Most persons use drugs for the first time when they are children or adolescents.
- The use of many substances has steadily increased for children and adolescents aged 12 to 17 years.
- These drugs include alcohol, cigarettes of any kind, smokeless tobacco, marijuana, inhalants, cocaine, and crack.
- Vaping use is on the increase from 3.5 million to 5 million youth (middle and high school); youth report vaping nicotine, cannabis, and flavorings. Many report daily use.
- Ecstasy and steroid use continues to rise among youth as they view these drugs as safe or less dangerous.

- Marijuana use is on the increase with 7.2% of eighth graders, 17.6% of 10th graders, and 22.6% of 12th graders using marijuana within the past month. This is an increase of 5.7%, 14.2%, and 18.8%, respectively since 2016. Fewer teens smoke cigarettes than marijuana.
- In 2016, 18.5% of 12th graders have used hookah water pipes and another 19.5% report smoking small cigars.
- 6.6% of 12th graders report using marijuana daily.
- The use of synthetic marijuana, known as spice or K2, is a combination of herbal mixtures laced with cannabinoids. K2 is a serious concern in that adolescents perceive it as a safe drug. 11.4% of 12th graders reported using K2 within the past year.
- The non-medical use of prescription drugs is a serious problem for teenagers. In 2016, 15.2 % of 12th graders used a prescription drug non-medically in the past year. The most commonly used abused drugs include Vicodin and Adderall.
- Early marijuana use by children and teens creates a higher risk for the development of depression, anxiety, and attention deficit disorders (Ali et al., 2016; APA, 2013; Barahmand et al., 2016; McCance, 2018; McKnight et al., 2017; SAMHSA, 2020a, 2020b).

TRAJECTORY FOR DEVELOPMENT OF SUBSTANCE USE

The brain continues to develop from birth through childhood and adolescence (into the mid or late 20s) (Boyd, 2017; SAMHSA, 2011). This developmental process creates an increase in behavior that increases learning, expansion of social skills, exploration of society, and testing limits (Arnett, 2006, 2007). It is critical that adults create an environment that fosters these growth patterns but at the same time helps children and teens to avoid destructive behaviors that may lead to substance use and subsequent abuse with cooccurring mental health problems (SAMHSA, 2011). Resilience or the ability of a child's or adolescent's ability to bounce back from difficulties or hardships is one of the most important protective factor that increases their sense of health and well-being (Spher et al., 2019). The level of protective and risk factors is an important determinant of where screening and assessment strategies need to be targeted (Spher et al., 2019). Additional *protective factors* include:

- Presence of a strong bond and involvement between children, adolescents, and their caregivers.
- Provision of financial, emotional, cognitive, and social needs by caregivers for children and adolescents.
- Clear and consistent approaches regarding discipline of children and adolescents.
- Success in academics, extra-curricular activities, and/or religious-based activities.

Risk factors may decrease the level of resilience for children and adolescents. Some include the following:

- Relationship with caregivers or peers who exhibit aggression toward others, use of alcohol or other addictive substances.
- Poverty or homelessness with lack of caregiver or community support.
- Presence of a caregiver, who has an untreated mental illness or engages in criminal behavior.
- Exposure to bullying, physical, sexual abuse, or trauma.
- Incarceration of the child, adolescent, or their caregiver.
- Lack of parenting support and supervision.
- Poor or inadequate coping and stress management skills.
- Poor self-esteem.

- Major transitions in life such as puberty, loss of a parent, and moving.
- Cooccurring mental health disorders (Bougard et al., 2016; Buja et al., 2018; Lopes-Rosa et al., 2017; Mello et al., 2019).

Differences Between Use, Abuse, and Dependence

Use means that a child or teen is regularly using a substance every few weeks or more that affects their functioning. *Abuse* means that a child or teen is using a substance extensively, daily functioning is affected, and negative consequences are occurring within a child's or teen's life; and *dependence* means that the child or teen psychologically and physically needs the substance and that getting the substance becomes the center of their existence (APA, 2013; Curtis et al., 2019; Health Resources and Services Administration [HRSA], 2018).

Findings from studies indicate that approximately one in four children or adolescents may be exposed to abuse by parents before she or he is 18 years of age (Penttinen et al., 2020). The presence of poverty and homelessness coupled with a parent who is a substance abuser increases a child's or adolescent's risk to engage in risky behaviors including substance use and promiscuous sexual exploration (SAMHSA, 2011).

Common Presenting Signs of Abuse

- Changes in peer group,
- Decrease in school performance,
- Drop in school attendance,
- Disciplinary actions at school,
- Changes in sleep patterns,
- Avoidance of family activities,
- Frequent respiratory and stomach complaints,
- Change in overall physical appearance (loss of weight, sloppy appearance, looking fatigued), and
- Stealing money or valuables from others (APA, 2013; SAMHSA, 2011).

The prevention of drug-related problems for children and adolescents is critical to address as it minimizes the damage that can occur once children and adolescents become addicted to substances and develop physiological and psychological problems. Screening within schools, community, and primary care environments can help to identify at-risk children and adolescents or those within the early stages of addictive behaviors.

SCREENING AND ASSESSMENT

The choice of screening, identification, and assessment tools has to be based on the needs of the children, adolescents, caregivers, and the community being served. Public health strategies need to address all three levels of preventive care: primary, secondary, and tertiary (Ewing, 1984; Knight et al., 2002). Primary care involves screening of all available children and adolescents within school and/or community settings. Secondary care entails screening for children and adolescents who have risk factors (e.g., as noted under risk factors) for development of substance and addiction use spectrum disorders (SAMHSA, 2011). Figure 11.1 illustrates the flow for identification and assessment as provided by SAMHSA).

Culturally and linguistically appropriate tools are important to use when screening children and adolescents for possible substance use. Healthcare beliefs, values, and level of literacy are essential components that healthcare providers need to be aware of when developing health and wellness strategies

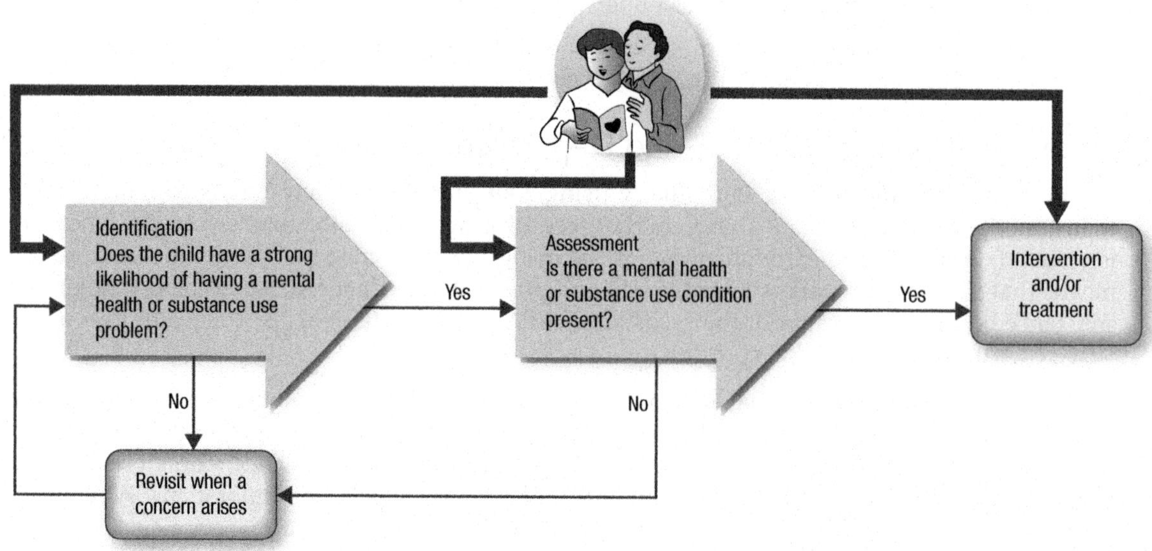

Figure 11.1. Flow for identification and assessment as provided by SAMHSA.

and protocols for children and adolescents who are culturally and ethnically diverse (Warren, 2020, 2013). Failure to incorporate culturally based strategies and protocols often results in poor healthcare outcomes because the recipients of this incompetent approach think that healthcare providers are dismissive regarding the recipients' cultural needs (Carr & Stewart, 2019; HRSA, 2018).

Resources on Cultural and Linguistic Competency (SAMHSA, 2011)

- Care for Diverse Populations
  www.molinamedicare.com/providers/ (see bottom of web page)
- Center for Health and Health Care in Schools: Caring Across Communities:
- Addressing the Mental Health Needs of Refugees and Immigrants (web page)
  www.healthinschools.org/Immigrant-and-Refugee-Children/Caring-AcrossCommunities.aspx
- Culturally and Linguistically Appropriate Services: Review Guidelines (web page)
  www.clas.uiuc.edu/review/index.html
- Indian Health Service (website)
  www.ihs.gov
- National Center for Cultural Competence: Child and Adolescent
- Mental Health Project (web page)
  www11.georgetown.edu/research/gucchd/nccc/projects/camh.html
- National Network to Eliminate Disparities: Resources (web page)
  www.nned.net/index-nned.php/resources/
- Screening and Assessing Immigrant and Refugee Youth in School-Based
- Mental Health Programs (publication)
  www.rwjf.org/files/research/3320.32211.0508issuebriefno.1.pdf
- Technical Assistance Partnership for Child and Family Mental Health:

- Cultural and Linguistic Competence Community of Practice (web page)
  www.tapartnership.org/COP/CLC/default.php

SBIRT: Substance (Use Screening, Brief Intervention), and Referral to Treatment

Both SAMHSA (www.samhsa.gov/sbirt/about) and the American Academy of Pediatrics endorse the SBIRT model of incorporating substance use screening and brief interventions into primary care health settings. From SAMHSA (4/16/2020):

SBIRT is a comprehensive, integrated, public health approach to the delivery of early intervention and treatment services for persons with substance use disorders, as well as those who are at risk of developing these disorders. Primary care centers, hospital emergency departments, trauma centers, and other community settings provide opportunities for early intervention with at-risk substance users before more severe consequences occur.

- Screening quickly assesses the severity of substance use and identifies the appropriate level of treatment.
- Brief intervention focuses on increasing insight and awareness regarding substance use and motivation toward behavioral change.
- Referral to treatment provides those identified as needing more extensive treatment with access to specialty care.

From the American Academy of Pediatrics (AAP, 2016): Committee on Substance Use and Prevention

Because most adolescents (83%) have contact with a physician for an annual physical this time represents a tremendous opportunity for the physician to assess the level of substance use by the adolescent. The Substance Abuse and Mental Health Services Administration recommends universal screening for substance use, brief intervention, and/or referral to treatment (SBIRT) as part of routine health care. Adolescents are the age group at greatest risk of experiencing substance use–related acute and chronic health consequences and, as such, also are most likely to derive the greatest benefit from universal SBIRT.

AAP recommendations for pediatric practices:

- Increase their capacity in substance use detection, assessment, and intervention; and
- Become familiar with adolescent SBIRT practices and their potential to be incorporated into universal screening and comprehensive care of adolescents in the medical home.

The American Academy of Pediatrics advocates for:

- The strong support of continued research to determine the most effective brief intervention strategies applicable to adolescent health care,
- Health insurance providers to:
  - promote and pay for standard screening and brief intervention practices incorporated into medical home health maintenance appointments; and
  - ensure a standard mechanism for payment for confidential follow-up care of adolescents to receive continuity of care for substance use disorders; and
- Parity of access and services for adolescent mental health and substance use disorder treatment compared with general adolescent care and adult health care.

AAP Committee on Substance Use and Prevention. (2016). Substance use screening, brief Intervention, and referral to treatment. *Pediatrics, 138*(1), e20161210. https://doi.org/10.1542/peds.2016-1210 www.pediatrics.aappublications.org/content/138/1/e20161210

What Is a Screening Tool?

A screening tool is a brief list of questions relating to a youth's behavior, thoughts, and feelings. It usually takes only 5 to 15 minutes to answer. A specific method is used to score the answers to the questions, and the score indicates whether the youth is at high likelihood of having a problem or is unlikely to have a problem. As with medical tests, the language used to refer to the results of screening may be confusing. When a score indicates a likely problem, it is called a *positive finding*; when the score indicates that a problem is not likely, it is called a *negative finding*. Like other medical tests, sometimes screening tools might miss problems or are positive when there is not a problem. For examples of a screening tool, see the Pediatric Symptom Checklist forms www2.massgeneral.org/allpsych/psc/psc_forms.htm (SAMHSA, 2011). See Table 11.1 for a matrix of substance use/abuse screening tools.

Materials That Provide Information on the Signs of a Mental Health or Substance Use Problem (SAMHSA, 2011)

For Infants

What Is Infant Mental Health and Why Is It Important? (publication)
www.projectabc-la.org/dl/ABC_InfantMentalHlth_English.pdf

For Children

Mental Illness and the Family: Recognizing Warning Signs and How to Cope (web page)
www.nmha.org/go/information/get-info/mi-and-the-family/recognizingwarning-signs-and-how-to-cope

For Teens—Mental Health

Mental, Emotional, and Behavioral Disorders in Teens (web page)
www.cumminsbhs.com/teens.htm

For Teens—Substance Use

Warning Signs of Teenage Drug Abuse (web page)
www.parentingteens.about.com/cs/drugsofabuse/a/driug_abuse20.htm

General Signs of Alcohol or Drug Use (web page)
www.adolescent-substance-abuse.com/signs-drug-use.html

For Suicide Prevention

Risk Factors for Child and Teen Suicide (web page)
www.healthyplace.com/depression/children/risk-factors-for-child-and-teensuicide/menu-id-68/

Suicide Warning Signs (web page)
www.store.samhsa.gov/shin/content//SVP11-0126/SVP11-0126.pdf (English)
www.store.samhsa.gov/shin/content//SVP11-0126SP/SVP11-0126SP.pdf (Spanish)

Table 11.1. Matrix of Substance Use/Abuse Screening Tools

	Alcohol Use/Abuse Screening Tools			Drug Use/ Abuse Screening Tools	Substance Use/Abuse Screening Tools for Adolescents			
Tool Characteristics	**Adolescent Drinking Index (ADI)**	**Adolescent Obsessive-Compulsive Drinking Scale (A-OCDS)**	**Rutgers Alcohol Problem Index (RAPI)**	**Drug Abuse Screening Test–Adolescents (DAST-A)**	**Adolescent Alcohol and Drug Invol-vement Scale (AADIS)**	**Assessment of Substance Misuse in Adol-escence (ASMA)**	**Crafft**	**Personal Experience Screening Questionnaire (PESQ)**
Target Conditions	Alcohol use problem severity	Craving and problem drinking; differentiates drinkers from experimenters or abusers	Alcohol use problem severity	Drug use problem severity	Alcohol and drug use problem severity	Drug use problem severity	Alcohol and drug use problem severity	Chemical dependency, psychosocial problems, and faking
High-Risk Items[a] Included	Yes	Yes	Yes	Yes—Includes drug-related risks, such as blackouts, withdrawal, and illegal activities	Yes	Yes	Yes—Also includes driving with a driver who has been drinking or is high	Yes—Drug use and certain psychosocial challenges
Informants or Youth Age Range	Youth ages 12–17 years	Youth ages 14–20 years	Adolescents	Adolescents	Youth ages 14–20 years	Adolescents	Adoles-cents	Youth ages 12–18 years
Format (Self-administered unless stated otherwise)	Paper & pencil, (group or individual)	Paper & pencil	Paper & pencil or interview	Paper & pencil	Paper & pencil or structured interview	Paper & pencil	Interview	Paper & pencil

(continued)

Table 11.1. Matrix of Substance Use/Abuse Screening Tools *(continued)*

	Alcohol Use/Abuse Screening Tools			Drug Use/Abuse Screening Tools	Substance Use/Abuse Screening Tools for Adolescents			
Tool Characteristics	**Adolescent Drinking Index (ADI)**	**Adolescent Obsessive-Compulsive Drinking Scale (A-OCDS)**	**Rutgers Alcohol Problem Index (RAPI)**	**Drug Abuse Screening Test–Adolescents (DAST-A)**	**Adolescent Alcohol and Drug Invol-vement Scale (AADIS)**	**Assessment of Substance Misuse in Adol-escence (ASMA)**	**Crafft**	**Personal Experience Screening Questionnaire (PESQ)**
Usual Administration Time	5 minutes	5–10 minutes	10 minutes	5 minutes	5 minutes	5 minutes	5 minutes	10 minutes
Reading Level Required	5th grade	5th grade[b]	6th–7th grade	6th grade	Not specified	Not specified	Appro-priate for youth with poor reading skills	4th grade
Translations				Adult Spanish version could be easily adapted by a bilingual provider			English version could be easily adapted by a bilingual provider	French, Spanish, and Portugese; English version adapted for Alaskans and Native Americans
Settings Where Tool Has Been Studied (*Note:* Tools may have been used successfully in settings where they have not yet been researched.)								
Primary Care						X	X	
Schools	X		X (College)			X		X
Early Care								

(continued)

Table 11.1. Matrix of Substance Use/Abuse Screening Tools *(continued)*

	Alcohol Use/Abuse Screening Tools			Drug Use/ Abuse Screening Tools	Substance Use/Abuse Screening Tools for Adolescents			
Tool Characteristics	**Adolescent Drinking Index (ADI)**	**Adolescent Obsessive-Compulsive Drinking Scale (A-OCDS)**	**Rutgers Alcohol Problem Index (RAPI)**	**Drug Abuse Screening Test–Adolescents (DAST-A)**	**Adolescent Alcohol and Drug Involvement Scale (AADIS)**	**Assessment of Substance Misuse in Adolescence (ASMA)**	**Crafft**	**Personal Experience Screening Questionnaire (PESQ)**
Child Welfare								
Juvenile Justice					X		X	X
Shelters			X	X				
Mental Health Treatment	X							
Substance Abuse Treatment	X	X	X	X	X	X	X	X
Cost	$100 for manual and 25 test booklets	Free	Free	Free or nominal cost	Free	Free	Free	$60 for manual; $43 for 25 forms; $99 for a kit that includes the manual and 25 forms
Appendix B Page #	Page 155	Page 157	Page 176	Page 167	Page 154	Page 160	Page 163	Page 174

[a]High-risk items are those that identify acute mental health or substance use conditions warranting a prompt response. Examples of such conditions are suicidal thoughts, plans for self-harm, or abuse of substances. Specific high-risk items are listed for some tools.

[b]As indicated in Deas et al. (2001).[52]

Source: Substance Abuse and Mental Health Services Administration. (2011). *Identifying mental health and substance use problems of children and adolescents: A guide for child-serving organizations* (HHS Publication No. SMA 12-4670). Author.

Diagnosis of Substance Use and Abuse

DSM Criteria for Spectrum of Substance Use and Addiction

Comprises substance use, abuse, addiction, and dependence for children and adolescents.

Discusses categories associated with the use of alcohol, caffeine, cannabis, hallucinogen, inhalant, opioid, sedative, hypnotic, anxiolytic, stimulant, tobacco.

Additional information is available at: www.dsm5.org/Pages/Default.aspx.

EVIDENCE-BASED MANAGEMENT OF SUBSTANCE USE AND ADDICTION IN CHILDREN AND ADOLESCENTS

Treatment of substance use and addiction spectrum disorders in children and adolescents addresses biobehavioral components. This treatment may involve the use of skills enhancement training in the areas of communication, conflict management, and stress management. Healthcare providers need to help children and adolescents develop health and wellness behaviors that enhance good nutritional, exercise, sleep, and relaxation habits (Alinsky et al., 2020; Boyd, 2012; Lusk & Melnyk, 2011). Medication may be used to target anxiety and attention deficit issues for children and adolescents. However, with the exception of the psychostimulants, other psychiatric medications are off label usage within this population (Boyd, 2012). Moreover, there are three primary principles that guide clinicians, use and choice of any medication within the population of children and adolescents:

- Identification of clear symptoms rationale for use of medication based on screening, assessment, and level of symptoms;
- Remember that children and adolescents are physically different than adults and hence dosage of medications needs to be aimed at their chronological age and size. Prescribing providers need to carefully document why any medication is used and what outcomes occur as a result of the medication; and
- Adherence in taking medications is the responsibility of the parents/caregivers so they must have education regarding the target and side-effect profile for medications their children and/or adolescents are taking.

There also are community guidelines and principles that guide the evidence-based treatment for children and adolescents diagnosed with substance use and addiction spectrum disorders. These include development of the following:

- Age-related assessment of children, adolescents, parent/caregivers and peers;
- Enhancement of parenting skills and training in drug education recognition;
- Preschool, elementary, middle, and high school programs for children's and adolescents' academic and social skills enhancement;
- Child and adolescent peer discussion groups and parent role-playing to enhance education about drug use and abuse;
- Use of research-based prevention and intervention programs within communities and across school settings (Babar et al., 2017; Boyd, 2017)

CRAFFT 2.1

The CRAFFT Screening for youth ages 12 to 21 is most recommended by the American Academy of Pediatrics for SBIRT. It screens youth for "risk" of problematic substance use and provides an opportunity to provide praise and encouragement for healthy habits and also to address with a "brief intervention" such as motivational interviewing, when warning signs, beginning behaviors are identified.

The **CRAFFT 2.1** is the updated version of the CRAFFT, which includes vaping and edibles as methods of administration for marijuana. The CRAFFT 2.1 forms can be obtained online – free of charge and in many languages.

From the CRAFFT website:

www.crafft.org/get-the-crafft/ at www.crafft.org/

There are two versions of the CRAFFT 2.1: a Clinician Interview and a self-Administered Questionnaire. Research has shown that adolescents report greater comfort and likelihood of honesty with self-administered questionnaires (electronic versions or on paper) compared to face-to-face interviews. The self-administered version is also more time-efficient to administer than an interview. Therefore, we recommend the use of the self-Administered Questionnaire whenever possible, under conditions that protect patient privacy and confidentiality. The responses can then be used by the healthcare provider during the appointment to facilitate brief counseling.

The CRAFFT+N versions contain extra questions that are related to tobacco and nicotine use.

These are available as a Clinician Interview and a self-Administered Questionnaire.

Steps for clinicians using the CRAFFT Screening are outlined:

1. ***BEGIN BY ASKING THE OPENING QUESTIONS REGARDING THE FREQUENCY OF THE PATIENT'S SUBSTANCE USE DURING THE PAST 12 MONTHS.***
2. ***ASK THE CRAFFT QUESTIONS.***

   If the patient answered "0" to all the opening "frequency of use" questions, ask the CAR question only. If the patient provided an answer >"0" to the alcohol, marijuana, or "anything else to get high" questions, ask the full set of six CRAFFT questions.

   2.1+N only: If the patient provided an answer >"0" for the nicotine question, ask all 10 Hooked on Nicotine Checklist (HONC) questions.
3. ***ASSESSMENT OF RISK –*** DSM-5 ***CRITERIA FOR A SUBSTANCE USE DISORDER (SUD)***

   Use the bar chart at the top of the second side of the CRAFFT card or the Clinician-Administered CRAFFT Interview to interpret the probability of a patient having a substance use disorder based on their CRAFFT score. The bar chart shows the percentage of adolescents meeting criteria for a *DSM-5* SUD by CRAFFT score. It reflects data from a study testing the CRAFFT screener's validity in identifying adolescents meeting *DSM-5* criteria for a SUD (Mitchell et al., 2014).
4. ***REVISED CLINICIAN TALKING POINTS – THE "5 Rs" OF BRIEF COUNSELING***

   The next step is to have a brief motivational enhancement discussion with the adolescent using the recommended Talking Points for brief counseling. These Talking Points incorporate the latest science on the developing brain and substance use harms, and promote the use of strategies informed by Motivational Enhancement Therapy (MET).

   From this foundation we developed the "5 Rs" of brief counseling:

   i. REVIEW screening results

   ii. RECOMMEND not to use

   iii. RIDING/DRIVING risk counseling

iv. RESPONSE: elicit self-motivational statements

v. REINFORCE self-efficacy

Examples are provided at each step to guide clinicians through the conversation with their patients.

5. *PROVIDE EACH PATIENT WITH THE CONTRACT FOR LIFE.*

For more information on how to use the CRAFFT, please refer to the CRAFFT 2.1 Manual.

Another screening questionnaire that has been around for many years is the CAGE. The CAGE is more helpful for identifying substance dependence.

The CAGE Questionnaire for Alcohol Use (J. A. Ewing)

The CAGE Questionnaire was developed by Ewing (1984) for a clinicians' assessment of an adult's or adolescent's (e.g., over the age of 16 years) use of alcohol. The CAGE may be self- or clinician-administered. An additional use of "or drug use" has been added to the CAGE to assess drug usage. Each question is worth 1 point for a yes response and 0 for a no response. Answering yes indicates a possible problem. Answering yes to two or more questions indicates a possible alcohol or drug abuse problem.

The CAGE involves the following questions:

C – Have you ever felt you should cut down on your drinking or drug use? (Yes or No)

A – Have people annoyed you by criticizing your drinking or drug use? (Yes or No)

G – Do you ever feel bad or guilty about your drinking or drug use? (Yes or No)

E – Have you ever had a drink or used drugs first thing in the morning to steady your nerves or get rid of a hangover? (Yes or No)

Indications for Use: Self-report screening instrument that is well suited for use in busy medical settings where there is limited time for patient interviews. It uses four straightforward yes/no questions that clinicians can easily remember. CAGE can be self-administered or conducted by a clinician. Proven utility for use in routine health screening of adults and adolescents over the age of 16. The screen may identify individuals with alcohol problems that may have been otherwise missed. The CAGE screen may fail to detect low but risky levels of drinking.

Time to Administer: 1 minute

Scoring: Score of **2 or greater** associated with SENSITIVITY of 74% and SPECIFICITY of 91%

Score 1: Evidence of AT RISK. Indicates need for further clinical investigation, including questions on amount and frequency, and so on.

Score 2 or more: Evidence of CURRENT PROBLEM. Indicates need for further clinical investigation and/or referral as indicated by clinician's expertise.

Score 3 or more: Evidence of dependence until ruled out. Evaluate, treat, and/or referral as indicated by clinician's expertise.

Additional information regarding the CAGE may be located at: www.bit.ly/CAGE_inst

SOURCE REFERENCE

Ewing, J. A. (1984). Detecting alcoholism: The CAGE questionnaire. *JAMA: Journal of the American Medical Association, 252*, 1905–1907. https://doi.org/10.1001/jama.252.14.1905

SUPPORTING REFERENCES

Aertgeerts, B., Buntinx, F., Fevery, J., & Ansoms, S. (2000). Is there a difference between CAGE interviews and written CAGE interviews? *Alcoholism: Clinical and Experimental Research, 24*(5), 733–736. https://doi.org/10.1111/j.1530-0277.2000.tb02047.x

Fiellin, D. A., Reid, M. C., & O'Connor, P. G. (2000). Screening for alcohol problems in primary care: Systemic review. *Journal of General Internal Medicine, 15*(Suppl. 1), 65–66. https://doi.org/10.1001/archinte.160.13.1977

Mayfield, D., McLeod, G., & Hall, P. (1974). The CAGE questionnaire: Validation of a new alcoholism instrument. *American Journal of Psychiatry, 131*, 1121–1123.

Reynaud, M., Schwan, R., Loiseaux-Meunier, M. N., Albuisson, E., & Deteix, P. (2001). Patients admitted to emergency services for drunkenness: Moderate alcohol users or harmful drinkers? *American Journal of Psychiatry, 158*(1), 96–99. https://doi.org/10.1176/appi.ajp.158.1.96

REFERENCES

Abney, B. G., Lusk, P., Hovermale, R., & Melnyk, B. M. (2019). Decreasing depression and anxiety in college youth using the Creating Opportunities for Personal Empowerment program (COPE). *Journal of the American Psychiatric Nurses Association, 25*(2), 80–90. https://doi.org/10.1177/1078390318779205

Ali, M., Gray, T. R., Martinez, D. J., Curry, L. E., & Horn, K. A. (2016). Risk profiles of youth, dual, and poly tobacco users. *Nicotine and Tobacco Research, 18*(7), 1614–1621. https://doi.org/10.1093/ntr/ntw028

Alinsky, R. H., Hadland, S. E., Madson, P. A., Cerda, M., & Saloner, B. (2020). Adolescent-serving addiction treatment facilities in the United States and the availability of medications for opioid use disorder. *Journal of Adolescent Health, 67*, 542–549. https://doi.org/10.1016/j.jadohealth.2020.03.005

American Academy of Pediatrics Committee on Substance Use and Prevention. (2016). Substance use screening, brief intervention, and referral to treatment. *Pediatrics, 138*(1), e20161210. https://doi.org/10.1542/peds.2016-1210

American Psychiatric Association. (2013). *Diagnostic and statistical manual of mental disorders-fifth edition (DSM-5)*. Author.

Arnett, J. (2006). *Emerging adults in America: Coming of age in the 21st century*. The American Psychological Association.

Arnett, J. (2007). Suffering, selfish, slacker? Myths and reality about emerging adults. *Journal of Youth Adolescence, 36*, 23–29. https://doi.org/10.1007/s10964-006-9157-z

Babar, T. F., Del Boca, F., & Bray, J. W. (2017). Screening, brief intervention and referral to treatment: Implications of SAMHSA's SBIRT initiative for substance abuse policy and practice. *Society for the Study of Addiction, 112*(Suppl. 2), 110–117. https://doi.org/10.1111/add.13675

Barahmand, I., Khazaee, A., & Hashjin, G. S. (2016). Emotion dysregulation mediates between childhood emotional trauma and motives for substance use. *Archives of Psychiatric Nursing, 30*, 653–659. https://doi.org/10.1016/j.apnu.2016.02.007

Boch, S. J., Warren, B. J., & Ford, J. (2019) Attention, externalizing, and internalizing problems of youth exposed to parental incarceration. *Issues in Mental health Nursing, 40*, 466–475. https://doi.org/10.1080/01612840.2019.1565872

Bougard, B. G., Laupola, T. M., Parker-Dias, J., Creekmore, J., & Stangland, S. (2016). Turning the tides: Coping with trauma and addiction through residential adolescent group therapy. *Journal of Child and Adolescent Psychiatric Nursing, 29*, 196–206. https://doi.org/10.1111/jcap.12164

Boyd, M. A. (2017). Addiction and substance related disorder: Nursing care of persons with alcohol and drug use. In M. A. Boyd (Ed.), *Essentials of psychiatric nursing* (Ch. 25, pp. 448–476). Wolters Kluwer.

Buja, A., Gallimberti, L., Chindamo, S., Terraneo, A., Rivera, M., Marini, E., Gomez-Perez, J., Scafato, E., & Blado, V. (2018). Problemmatic social networking site usage and substance use by young adolescents. *BMC Pediatrics, 18*, 367–378. https://doi.org/10.1186/s12887-018-1316-3

Carr, K. L., & Stewart, M. W. (2019). Effectiveness of school-based health center delivery of a cognitive skills building intervention in young, rural adolescents: Potential applications for addiction and mood. *Journal of Pediatric Nursing, 47*, 23–29. https://doi.org/10.1016/j.pedn.2019.04.013

CRAFFT 2.1. https://crafft.org/

Curtis, B., Ashford, R., Rosenbach, S., Stern, M., & Kirby, K. (2019). Parental identification and response to adolescent substance use and substance use disorders. *Drugs, Education, Prevention and Policy*, *26*(2), 175–183. https://doi.org/10.1080/09687637.2017.1383973

Deas, D., & Thomas, S. E. (2001). An overview of controlled studies of adolescent substance abuse treatment. *American Journal on Addictions*, *10*(2), 178–189. https://doi.org.10.1080/105504901750227822

Ewing, J. A. (1984). Detecting alcoholism: The Cage questionnaire. *Journal of the American Medical Association*, *252*, 1905–1907. https://doi.org/10.1001/jama.1984.03350140051025

Health Resources and Services Administration. (2018). *2018 National Survey of Children's Health (NSCH) data query*. www.childhealthdata.org

Knight, J. R., Sherritt, L., Shrier, L. A., Harris, S. K., & Chang, G. (2002). Validity of the CRAFFT substance abuse screening test among adolescent clinic patients. *Archives of Pediatric and Adolescent Medicine*, *156*(6), 607–614. https://doi.org/10.1001/archpedi.156.6.607

Lopes-Rosa, R., Kessler, F. P., Pianca, T. G., Guimarães, L., Ferronato, P., Pagnussat, P., Moura, H., Pechansk, F., & von Diemen, L. (2017). Predictors of early relapse among adolescent crack users. *Journal of Addictive Diseases*, *36*(2), 130–143. https://doi.org/10.1080/10550887.2017.1295670

Lusk, P., & Melnyk, B. (2011). The brief cognitive-behavioral COPE intervention for depressed adolescents: Outcomes and feasibility of delivery in 30 minute outpatient visits. *Journal of the American Psychiatric Nurses Association*, *17*, 226–236.

McCance-Katz, E. F. (2018). *SAMHSA's 2018 national survey on drug use and health*. SAMHSA.

McKnight, E. R., Bonny, A. E., Lange, H. L. H., Kline, D. M., Abdel-Rasoul, M., Gay, J. R., & Matson, S. C. (2017). Statewide opioid prescriptions and the prevalence of adolescent opioid misuse in Ohio. *The American Journal of Drug and Alcohol Abuse*, *43*(3), 299–305. http://doi.org/10.1080/00952990.2016.1216999

Mello, M. J., Becker, S. J., Bromberg, J., Baird, J., Zonfrillo, M. J., & Spirito, A. (2019). Implementing alcohol misuse SBIRT in a national cohort of pediatric trauma centers - a type III hybrid effectiveness-implementation trial. *Implementation Science*, *13*, 35. https://doi.org/10.1186/s13012-018-0725-x

Mitchell, S. G., Kelly, S. M., Gryczynski, J., Myers, C. P., O'Grady, K. E., Kirk, A. S., & Schwartz, R. P. (2014). The CRAFFT cut-points and DSM-5 criteria for alcohol and other drugs: A reevaluation and reexamination. *Substance Abuse*, *35*(4), 376–380. https://doi.org.10.1080/08897077.2014.936992

Penttinen, R., Hakko, H., Pirkko, R., Isohookana, R., & Riala, K. (2020). Associations of adverse childhood experiences to smoking nicotine dependence among adolescent psychiatric inpatients. *Community Mental Health Journal*, *56*, 333–337. https://doi.org/10.1007/s10597-019-00476-8

Spher, M. K., Zeno, R., Warren, B. J., Lusk, P, & Masciola, R. (2019). Social-emotional screen protocol implementation: A trauma-informed response for children in child welfare. *Journal of Pediatric Health Care*, *33*, 675–683. https://doi.org/10.1016/j.pedhc.2019.05.003

Substance Abuse and Mental Health Services Administration. (2020a). *Reducing vaping among youth and young adults* (SAMHSA Publication No. PEP20-06-01-003). National Mental Health and Substance Use Policy Laboratory, Substance Abuse and Mental Health Services Administration. https://www.samhsa.gov/sbirt/about 04/16/2020

Substance Abuse and Mental Health Services Administration. (2020b). *2019 National Survey of Drug Use and Health (NSDUH) releases*. https://www.samhsa.gov/data/report/2019-nsduh-detailed-tables

Substance Abuse and Mental Health Services Administration. (2011). *Identifying mental health and substance use problems of children and adolescents: A guide for child-serving organizations* (HHS Publication No. SMA 12-4670). Author.

United States Census Bureau. (2019). *National population by characteristics: 2010–2019*. http://www.census.gov/data/tables/time-series/demo/popest/2010s-national-detail.html#par_textimage_1537638156

Warren, B. J. (2013). How culture is assessed in the *DSM-5*. *Journal of Psychosocial Nursing*, *51*(4), 40–45. https://doi.org/10.3928/02793695-20130226-04

Warren, B. J. (2019). Cultural competence in psychiatric nursing. In N. L. Keltner & D. Steele, (Eds.), *Psychiatric nursing* (Ch. 5, 8th ed.). Elsevier.

Warren, B. J. (2020). The synergistic influence of life experiences and cultural nuances on development of depression: A cognitive behavioral perspective. *Issues in Mental Health Nursing*, *41*(1), 3–6. https://doi.org/10.1080/01612840.2019.1675828

The CRAFFT Questionnaire (Version 2.1): To Be Completed by Patient

Please answer all questions honestly; your answers will be kept confidential.

During the past 12 months, on how many days did you:

1.	Drink more than a few sips of beer, wine, or any drink containing **alcohol**? Put "0" if none.	☐ # of days
2.	Use any **marijuana** (cannabis, weed, oil, wax, or hash by smoking, vaping, dabbing, or in edibles) or "**synthetic marijuana**" (like "K2," "Spice")? Put "0" if none.	☐ # of days
3.	Use **anything else to get high** (like other illegal drugs, pills, prescription or over-the-counter medications, and things that you sniff, huff, vape, or inject)? Put "0" if none.	☐ # of days

Read These Instructions Before Continuing:

- **If you put "0" in all of the boxes above, answer question 4, then stop.**
- **If you put "1" or higher in any of the boxes above, answer questions 4 to 9.**

		Circle one	
4.	Have you ever ridden in a CAR driven by someone (including yourself) who was "high" or had been using alcohol or drugs?	**No**	**Yes**
5.	Do you ever use alcohol or drugs to RELAX, feel better about yourself, or fit in?	**No**	**Yes**
6.	Do you ever use alcohol or drugs while you are by yourself, or ALONE?	**No**	**Yes**
7.	Do you ever FORGET things you did while using alcohol or drugs?	**No**	**Yes**
8.	Do your FAMILY or FRIENDS ever tell you that you should cut down on your drinking or drug use?	**No**	**Yes**
9.	Have you ever gotten into TROUBLE while you were using alcohol or drugs?	**No**	**Yes**

NOTICE TO CLINIC STAFF AND MEDICAL RECORDS:

The information on this page is protected by special federal confidentiality rules (42 CFR Part 2), which prohibit disclosure of this information unless authorized by specific written consent.

National Association *of* Pediatric Nurse Practitioners™

SPRINGER PUBLISHING

CHAPTER 12

Pamela Herendeen

Evidence-Based Assessment and Management of Child Maltreatment

FAST FACTS

- Child maltreatment is defined as the causation of a non-accidental injury. It may be physical or sexual abuse. Maltreatment inflicts or allows to be inflicted a physical or sexual offense against a child.
- Child neglect is defined as the omission in care of a child's basic needs that may result in harm or potential harm. It is a significant cause of morbidity and mortality in children.
- Nationally, neglect is the most common form of abuse; nearly 61% of all children are neglected.
- Psychological maltreatment is a repeated pattern of damaging interactions from a parent to a child.
- More than 10% were physically abused only, and 7% were sexually abused only. Statistics indicate a more complex problem where children experience multiple forms of abuse. In 2018, more than 15% of kids were polyvictimized (experiencing two or more forms of abuse).
- About 700,000 children (1% of all children) are maltreated each year; out of these less than 1 million are substantiated. Most of child maltreatment falls under neglect.
- In 2018, an estimated 1,770 children died from child maltreatment; most vulnerable victims are under 6 years of age.
- Annual economic burden of child maltreatment is estimated at $428 billion.
- Most perpetrators are primary caregivers.
- Domestic violence is significantly correlated with child maltreatment. Millions of children witness domestic violence in their lifetime, significantly increasing the risk of child maltreatment.
- Girls who are abused as children may be more likely to become victims of violence as adults. Boys abused as children may be more likely to commit acts of violence as adults.
- Child maltreatment tends to be repetitive and frequently will escalate over time. In many cases the abuser does not intend to hurt the child. Rather, abuse is the result of unrealistic caretaker expectations and poor coping mechanisms of the caregiver.
- Although child maltreatment crosses all socioeconomic, racial, and religious boundaries, high risk socioeconomic factors are associated with an increased risk of abuse and neglect.
- Most children that are victims of sexual abuse will have no sign of genital injury.
- Abusive head trauma (AHT) is the leading cause of fatal head injuries in young children.
- It is essential that every child, regardless of race, religion, or socioeconomic background be screened for child maltreatment in their primary care office.

RISK FACTORS

- Young and/or single caregivers.
- Unrealistic expectations of caregivers.
- Caregivers with a history of being abused.
- Unwanted pregnancy.
- Economic or social stressors.
- Substance abuse/mental illness/developmental delay of the caregiver.
- Domestic violence in the home.
- Children who have fussy/challenging behavior, are less than 3 years old, have chronic medical conditions, developmental disabilities, or special health care needs, and are in foster care

COMMON PRESENTATIONS

Any one indicator is not definitive; it just raises questions. Many primary care providers are resistant to making child protective services (CPS) reports—they feel they "know" the family well and want to spare the "nice" family the aggravation of dealing with CPS, but it is essential to be objective and make referrals to CPS based on the history and indicators.

Triggers of abuse:

- Excessive crying/fussy,
- Acute illness,
- Frequent nighttime awakenings,
- Toilet training,
- Feeding issues, and
- Oppositional behavior.

Behavioral indicators:

- Behavioral extremes and mood swings,
- Mental health disorders/suicidal ideation,
- Anger issues/harming of others or animals,
- Alcohol or substance abuse,
- School problems,
- Poor social interactions with peers,
- Conversion reactions/psychosomatic illnesses,
- Sleep/appetite/behavior changes, and
- Self-injurious behavior.

Behavioral indicators specific for sexual abuse:

- Provocative behavior,
- Aggressive sexual behavior,
- Increased sexual knowledge,
- Regression/new fearfulness,
- New money or gifts, and
- Depression/self-mutilation.

Physical indicators of concern:

- Bruises, burns, fractures not consistent with developmental stage or a delay in care; injuries to mouth (especially in an infant); any bruise/burn/fracture in a non-ambulatory child that lacks a very corroborating history.
- Babies that don't cruise, don't bruise.
- Bruising on the face, neck, wrists, ankles, back, genitals, thighs; bruises in the shape of a hand or object.
- Bites that are too large to be a child's.
- Burns that are patterned, immersion, cigarette shaped.
- Any fracture occurring in a child aged 1 year or younger; fractures of the skull, spine, rib, metaphyseal, spinal, hands/feet, or fractures in multiple stages of healing.
- Head trauma with skull fractures, subdural hematomas, retinal hemorrhages.
- Neglect issues (e.g., inappropriate clothing, poor weight gain, poor medical compliance, lack of appropriate supervision, poor hygiene).
- Itching, discomfort, lesions, bleeding, and discharge in genitals.
- Pain with bowel movements/dysuria.
- New onset encopresis/enuresis.
- Sexually transmitted infections/pregnancy depending on age or situation.
- Any injury that does not fit the history.

Screening Tools

There are very few screening tools that have been methodically tested to assist in the identification of child abuse. Currently, there are a number of studies that are evaluating the feasibility of using a tool for this purpose. However, there is insufficient evidence that these tools will adequately predict child maltreatment, though some have demonstrated promise. Dubowitz has demonstrated that the SEEK Model of focused questions for the caregiver may identify/prevent child maltreatment. The Edinburgh Postnatal Depression Scale or Beck Post-Partum Depression Screening Scale are tools that are currently being utilized in some pediatric practices to screen families. There is evidence to support that a mother who is depressed is at high risk for neglect and abuse of her child. The Guidelines for Adolescent Preventive Services (GAPS) form for adolescents briefly addresses abuse and may provide insight to the provider. PedHITSS is a modification of HITS for adults, and is intended to be completed by parents/guardians of pediatric patients (0–12 years). PedHITSS contains five screening items. A common tool utilized is the ACES Screening Tool; there are many variations of this instrument that medical practices utilize as well. Any of the many tools that are currently being utilized for mood/mental health disorders may be useful in identifying abuse and neglect. Anticipatory guidance regarding child maltreatment and violence should be done at every well child visit. One of the main challenges for healthcare providers is how to add more questions in an already limited time period. Another major concern is how to adequately screen the parent for domestic violence issues with the child in the room, and how to screen the child for abuse issues with the parent in the room. The following brief screening questions may be utilized during a visit to identify abuse and violence in the home.

Questions for Parents

- Because violence is so common, ask about violence in the home.
- Are you in a relationship where you are being hurt physically or emotionally?

- Have you ever been emotionally or physically abused by your partner (e.g., have you ever been hit, kicked, slapped, punched, isolated from your family or someone important to you by your partner?)
- Are you afraid of anyone in your home?
- Do you ever feel so frustrated/overwhelmed that you fear you may hit or hurt your child?
- Have the police come to your home?
- The U.S. Preventive Services Task Force (USPSTF) recommends that clinicians screen women of childbearing age for intimate partner violence (IPV), such as domestic violence, and provide or refer women who screen positive to intervention services. This recommendation applies to women who do not have signs or symptoms of abuse. See www.uspreventiveservicestaskforce.org/uspstf12/ipvelder/ipvelderfinalrs.htm#summary

Screening Tools for Intimate Partner Violence

Several screening instruments can be used to screen women for IPV. Those with the highest levels of sensitivity and specificity for identifying IPV are:

- Hurt, Insult, Threaten, Scream (HITS) (English and Spanish versions available)
- Ongoing Abuse Screen/Ongoing Violence Assessment Tool (OAS/OVAT)
- Slapped, Threatened, and Throw (STaT)
- Humiliation, Afraid, Rape, Kick (HARK)
- Modified Childhood Trauma Questionnaire–Short Form (CTQ-SF)
- Woman Abuse Screen Tool (WAST)

Questions for Children/Teens

- Are you afraid of anyone in your home?
- Whom could you tell if anyone has touched you in your private area? Has this ever happened to you?
- What happens when your parents are angry with you or you get into trouble?
- Do you ever get hit or spanked? What do they hit you with? Are there ever marks left?
- What happens when adults in your home are angry at each other?
- Have the police been to your home?

Assessment

- Thorough psychosocial assessment including current concerns, history of violence in the home, family constellation, day care arrangements, custody issues, economic stressors, child's behavior, and prior involvement with police/child protective services.
- Complete medical history including any presenting physical symptoms, behavior—especially recent changes, psychosocial history, current/past medications, allergies, chronic illnesses.
- Complete physical exam, including the genital area.
  - Carefully examine head-to-toe for any bruises, burns, bites, abrasions, erythema, swelling, old patterned scars (especially in soft tissue areas; extra concern for patterned or shaped injuries), limited mobility of an extremity. Note growth pattern. Genitalia examined for erythema, swelling, bruising, tears, friability, fissures, bleeding, discharge, lesions.

  - Any injury (bruising, burns fractures) in a non-ambulatory child deserves a full child abuse work up unless you have a detailed, corroborating history. For other children it would be dependent on the history provided.
  - Medical photography is advised with any physical injuries for documentation.
  - A full child abuse workup would include a skeletal survey for any child ≤2, head imaging and ophthalmology exam for retinal hemorrhages (especially with any facial bruising, head injury, neurological impairment), labs inclusive of bleeding studies, a trauma panel, abdominal imaging if symptomatic or belly bruising, other labs as indicated such as a urine screen and tox screen.
  - Sexual abuse history/disclosure or symptoms very dependent on timing and community protocols. A disclosure of sexual abuse <96 hours often requires an evidence collection kit. Cultures may need to be obtained; prophylactic medications usually not given to prepubertal children with the exception of possibly HIV meds.
- Many communities now have a child abuse team or child advocacy center staffed with experts to assist you through the process of the assessment and management of child abuse. Please be aware of your community resources and utilize them to help you complete an accurate and safe assessment and plan for your patient.

Diagnosis

The identification of child maltreatment is a very complex diagnosis based on psychosocial factors, social history, medical history, and physical findings. It is advisable to consult a child abuse expert to assist you in your diagnosis. Be extraordinarily careful of your documentation, first presenting the history and your objective findings. It is always recommended to consult with an expert unless you are very sure of your diagnosis as you may find yourself in a legal court of law.

Over 90% of known sexual abuse victims have a normal exam. Please refer to the scale developed by Dr. Joyce Adams for child sexual abuse in the reference section of this chapter.

Management is very specific for the type of child maltreatment that is diagnosed. A child abuse expert should be consulted whenever possible. Foremost, the safe disposition of the child needs to be considered. Use of a child advocacy center is encouraged if there is one located in your region. An interview and/or an exam by a formally trained child abuse specialist is always advised.

Sexual Abuse: A full exam, including genitals with cultures for gonorrhea, chlamydia, with any disclosure is necessary. An evidence collection kit should be considered if the contact was less than 96 hours prior. Blood work for Hep B & C, HIV, and works RPR is recommended. With the exception of HIV (consult Peds ID), no prophylactic treatment of a prepubescent child is recommended. An adolescent needs pregnancy and STD prophylaxis if indicated. Photograph any injuries noted.

Physical Abuse: Very dependent on sustained injuries. Must consider a skeletal survey if ≤2 years old, head imaging, trauma labs, ophthalmology exam, abdominal imaging—this is all very individualized. The history must be correlated with the injuries before you can determine a diagnosis. It is recommended that the skeletal survey be repeated in 2 weeks to ascertain the healing of possible injuries. It is also recommended to consider conducting a skeletal survey on other young children in the home; especially a twin or sibling very close in age.

Neglect: Often CPS and other agencies need to intervene to ensure appropriate resources are implemented. These children all need a full physical, including genitals, and further workups as indicated.

Again, all of these children will benefit from a CAC and/or a child abuse specialist team to guide your care.

EVIDENCE-BASED MANAGEMENT

Prevention Is Key

Child maltreatment is extremely detrimental to children. As healthcare providers, it is important to focus on prevention and to recognize the risk factors early on for our patients. Advocating for children and families is the key to prevention!

Remember: All Healthcare Providers Are Mandated Reporters

You do not have to decide whether or not a child is being maltreated—that is the responsibility of CPS. You are mandated to report if you have a reasonable suspicion of abuse or neglect. There are certain physical or behavioral indicators that should raise a red flag about the possibility. The history must always be integrated together with behavioral and physical indicators. Clearly, some of these indicators may be the result of other stressors in a child's life. Any one indicator is not. Keep in mind that social intuition may play a role in the evaluation process. Often providers will think that a family is too nice to have inflicted injuries, and are quickly discounted as potential abusers. In addition, children who have experienced maltreatment need close follow-up; most children benefit greatly from talking with a therapist that specializes in child maltreatment.

INTERNET RESOURCES FOR FAMILIES

Prevent Child Abuse America

www.preventchildabuse.org

Prevent Child Abuse America has led the way in building awareness, providing education, and inspiring hope for everyone involved in the effort to prevent the abuse and neglect of children. Working with chapters in 39 states and the District of Columbia, this organization provides leadership to promote and implement prevention efforts at both the national and local levels. The organization provides many local programs, prevention initiatives, and events to help to create awareness of this problem and communicate that prevention is possible. It comprises friends, professionals, volunteers, donors, and parents who are preventing child abuse and neglect before it ever starts.

Rape, Abuse, & Incest National Network

www.rainn.org

The Rape, Abuse, & Incest National Network (RAINN) is the nation's largest anti-sexual assault organization. RAINN operates the National Sexual Assault Hotline at 1.800.656.HOPE and carries out programs to prevent sexual assault, help victims, and ensure that rapists are brought to justice.

NATIONAL CHILDREN'S ALLIANCE

Shaken Baby Alliance

www.shakenbaby.com

The mission of the Shaken Baby Alliance is to provide support for families of shaken baby syndrome (SBS) victims (including adoptive and foster parents), advocate for justice for SBS victims, and increase SBS awareness.

SUGGESTED ADDITIONAL READINGS

Adams, J., Farst, K., & Kellogg, N. (2018). Interpretation of medical findings in suspected child sexual abuse: An update for 2018. *North American Society for Pediatric and Adolescent Gynecology, 31*, 225–231. https://doi.org/10.1016/j.jpag.2017.12.011

Brodie, N., McColgan, M., Spector, N., & Turchi, R. (2017). Child abuse in children and youth with special health care needs. *Pediatrics in Review, 38*, 1–13. https://doi.org/10.1542/pir.2016-0098

Choudhary, A., Servaes, S., Slovis, T., Palusci, V., Hedlund, G., Narang, S., Moreno, J., Dias, M., Christian, C., Nelson, M., Silvera, V., Palasis, S., Raissaki, M., Rossi, A., & Offiah, A. (2018). Consensus statement on abusive head trauma in infants and young children. *Pediatric Radiology, 48*(8), 1048–1065. https://doi.org/10.1542/pir.2016-0098

Christian, C., & Committee on Child Abuse and Neglect. (2015). The evaluation of suspected child physical abuse. *Pediatrics, 135*, e1337–e1354. https://doi.org/10.1542/peds.2015-0356

Flaherty, E., Legano, L., & Idzerda, S. (2019). Ongoing pediatric health care for the child who has been maltreated. *Pediatrics, 143*, 59–74. https://doi.org/10.1542/peds.2019-0284

Gillespie, R. (2019). Screening for adverse childhood experiences in pediatric primary care. *Pediatric Annals, 48*, e257–e261. https://doi.org/10.3928/19382359-20190610-02

Hornor, G. (2016). Sexually transmitted infections and children: What the PNP should know. *Journal of Pediatric Care, 31*, 222–228. https://doi.org/10.1016/j.pedhc.2016.04.016

Jenny, C., & Crawford-Jakubiak, J. (2013). The evaluation of children in the primary care setting. When sexual abuse is suspected. *Pediatrics, 132*(2), e558–e567. https://doi.org/10.1542/peds.2013-1741

Keenan, H., Cook, L., Olson, L., Beardsley, T., & Campbell, K. (2017). Social intuition and social information in physical child abuse evaluation and diagnosis. *Pediatrics, 140*(5), e20171188. https://doi.org/10.1542/peds.2017-1188

Miller, E. (2018). Trauma informed approaches to adolescent relationship abuse and sexual violence prevention. *Pediatric Annals, 48*, e274–e279. https://doi.org/10.3928/19382359-20190617-01

Peterson, C., Florence, C., Klevens, J. (2018). The economic burden of child abuse in the United States. *Child Abuse & Neglect, 86*, 178–183. https://doi.org/10.1016/j.chiabu.2018.09.018

Shakil, A., Day, P. G., Chu, J., Woods, S. B., & Bridges K. (2018). PedHITSS: A screening tool to detect childhood abuse in clinical settings. *Family Medicine, 50*(10), 763–769. https://doi.org/10.22454/FamMed.2018.778329.

Simon, J. D., Gandarilla Ocampo, M., Drake, B., & Jonson-Reid, M. (2021). A Review of Screened-Out Families and Child Protective Services Involvement: A Missed Opportunity to Prevent Future Maltreatment With Community-Based Services. Child Maltreatment. https://doi.org/10.1177/10775595211033597

https://www.childwelfare.gov/topics/systemwide/assessment/family-assess/sources/

https://www.nationalchildrensalliance.org

Information for Parents on Child Maltreatment

IMPORTANT FACTS

Child abuse and neglect is defined as causing non-accidental injury or not providing for a child's basic needs. About 3 million reports are filed every year on children that someone suspects may have been abused or neglected. It is unusual for a child that is not walking yet to sustain a lot of bruises, burns, or other physical injuries. You should have a high level of concern if you see these in a child and call the child's healthcare provider.

Child sexual abuse is any use of a child for the sexual gratification of an adult. This includes touching a child's genitals, making a child touch someone else's genitals, pornography, and exposing a person's genitals to a child.

Domestic violence is closely related to child abuse. Millions of children witness domestic violence every day. The risk of these children being abused significantly increases if the mother is being battered. Girls raised in violent homes are at risk for becoming victims of violence as they grow older, while boys are at risk for growing up to be aggressive and violent. Many times the abuser does not intend to hurt the child. Often, they are a loving parent or caregiver who loses control and has unrealistic expectations of the child. Child abuse and violence happens on every level of society. However, it tends to be more frequent in homes that have a lot of stressors.

It also is important to know that the majority of children who are sexually or physically abused are violated by someone they know, often being one of their caretakers.

HOW CAN YOU PROTECT YOUR CHILDREN AND ADOLESCENTS?

- There are some behavioral signs in children that may indicate a child is being abused. However, some of these can be the result of other stressors in a child's life. Any one sign doesn't mean the child is being abused, but the presence of several of these signs should raise concern.
- Appetite changes
- Nightmares/change in sleeping habits
- Mood swings including aggression (especially if child is hurting other people or animals), depression, anxiety, or self-mutilation
- Suicidal ideation
- Provocative behavior
- Extreme fears
- Regression of behavior
- Alcohol/drug abuse
- School problems
- Frequent complaints of headaches, stomachaches, or other illnesses that seem to be excessive and lacks a medical foundation

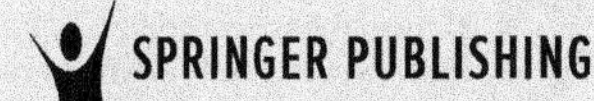

In addition to behavior signs, here are some physical signs to alert you.

- Frequent bruising, especially in a young infant or on the face, chest, back, or genitals
- Pain, extreme redness, discharge, or lesions in the genital region
- Injuries/fractures that are inconsistent with the description of the injury
- Poor weight gain, excessive weight gain, inappropriate clothing, minimal medical care for a child

If you are concerned about any behavioral or physical signs of abuse, please call your primary care provider. They can guide you through the process of how to figure everything out.

It is important to teach children about safety and protecting themselves as they get older. Here are some things that you and your family can do to prevent abuse:

- Adults must watch for signs of abuse as young children cannot protect themselves.
- Be alert to changes in their behavior and discuss it with them.
- Teach your children how and when to say "no." They need to know that they can say no if someone makes them uncomfortable or scared.
- Set privacy boundaries within your family.
- Teach children that special secrets about touching or physical harm are not okay.
- Teach children the correct names of body parts.
- Make sure to keep the lines of communication open. LISTEN AND TALK to your children and adolescents all the time. Make sure they know they can talk to you.
- Do not confuse children with the "stranger danger" concept. This message is not effective, as danger to children is greater from someone they know.
- Screen all caregivers carefully, such as babysitters, day care providers, and coaches.
- Teach your children and adolescents how to get out of a threatening situation. Make a family safety plan!
- Supervise internet use—many sexual predators use this to connect with children.
- Make arrangements ahead of time to be available for your children when they go out with friends. They need to know they can call you for a ride if they find themselves in an uncomfortable position or if they have used substances and feel unsafe to drive home.
- Always report anything suspicious.

Be a parent that is involved in your children's lives. Take the time to listen to your children, which will help them to develop their sense of security. Communication is key. Also, find ways to help yourself if you are feeling stressed. Remember, your stress affects your children.

Information for Adolescents on Child Maltreatment

IMPORTANT FACTS

There are many different forms of child abuse and neglect. It can happen to any child, at any age, including adolescents. Here are some things that could be child abuse:

- An adult is hurting you physically, such as hitting you, especially if it is with an object.
- An adult is touching you in private places such as the breast or genitals, or having any form of genital or oral sex with you.
- One of your friends tries to have sex with you after you have said "NO."
- A boyfriend/girlfriend is physically or emotionally abusive to you.
- You don't have a warm place to stay.
- You don't receive medical care.
- There isn't enough food in the house.
- Your parents keep you out of school.
- Emotional abuse can happen if your caregivers are always mean to you and make you feel bad about yourself.

Adolescents are the group of people most often victimized in the United States. This is especially true for girls. Here are some things that you should be aware of:

- Adolescent girls are the most frequent victims of sexual assault.
- More than 50% of all rape victims are under 18 years old.
- One in 4 college women have been raped or have experienced attempted rape.
- 93% of juvenile sexual assault victims knew their attacker.
- Many sexual assaults are in the victim's home or a friend's home
- Adolescent relationship violence is prevalent; trauma informed care approaches are essential to begin the healing process

The impact of rape includes physical trauma, genital trauma, pregnancy, sexually transmitted infections, psychological symptoms, or economic implications.

Many teenagers experience a lot of problems after being sexually abused or assaulted.

These include:

- Substance abuse,
- Depression and anxiety,
- Difficulty with close relationships,
- Suicide thoughts,

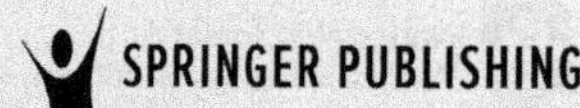

- Violent behavior,
- Nightmares and difficulty sleeping, and
- Frequent headaches, stomachaches, and other medical problems.

HOW CAN YOU PREVENT THIS FROM HAPPENING TO YOU?

- Tell a trusted adult or friend if someone is hurting you emotionally, physically, or sexually at home. Tell a trusted adult or friend if another person in your peer group is forcing you to have sex or hurting you physically.
- Never go out alone! There is always safety in numbers. Don't hitchhike!
- Make sure that an adult knows where you are going and with whom.
- Be careful of the internet. It is NEVER a good idea to meet a stranger with whom you have been communicating online.
- Be very careful about information that you put on Facebook or other social media.
- Never send pictures of yourself partially or fully undressed on your cell phone, even if it is to a friend or boyfriend. This is illegal and you could end up with a federal offense and in lots of legal trouble.
- Don't go to parties or gatherings where there is no adult present. Although it may sound fun and very grown up, there can be lots of activities going on that you aren't ready for, such as alcohol, drug use, and sexual activity.
- Make arrangements with a trusted adult before you go out with friends to be able to call for a ride if you find yourself in an uncomfortable position. This would also work if you have been using drugs or alcohol and feel unsafe to drive home. Remember, **NEVER** get in a car with anyone who has been using drugs or drinking.
- Don't let food or beverages out of your sight! Someone may tamper with it by adding drugs.
- Remember that if someone abuses or assaults you, **IT IS NOT YOUR FAULT!!**

Information for School-Age Children on Child Maltreatment

There are many different ways that a child your age may be abused. Child abuse means that an older child, teenager, or adult is hurting you. It may be one of your parents or someone else that you care about in your family, or even a family friend. It may even be a friend or someone that you know around your age.

HERE ARE SOME THINGS THAT COULD BE CHILD ABUSE OR NEGLECT

- An adult, teenager, or another child is hitting you, biting you, or giving you burns.
- Someone is touching you in your private areas, such as your penis (where boys pee from), rectum (where you poop from), breasts, or urethra/vagina (where girls pee from).
- If they touch you over your clothes or under your clothes, it is not okay.
- It is not okay to touch you in any of your private places with their fingers, any parts of their body, or any kind of object.
- Someone shows you their private parts or asks you to touch them or shows you movies with people that have their clothes off.
- Your parent/guardians do not send you to school.
- There is no heat in your house.
- There is not enough food in your house.
- You do not have enough clothes to keep you warm.
- Your parents/guardians do not bring you to the doctor when you are sick or hurt.

HERE ARE SOME THINGS THAT YOU CAN DO IF SOMEONE IS HURTING YOU OR TOUCHING YOU IN A WAY THAT DOESN'T SEEM RIGHT

- You can say **"NO"** very loudly when that person tries to touch you, and then tell an adult whom you trust.
- Tell someone whom you trust what is happening. Some ideas are teachers, school nurses, police, your doctor or nurse practitioner, other family members, or the other parent that isn't hurting you.
- If someone tells you to keep a secret about hurting or touching, that would be important to tell an adult whom you trust.
- Never get into anyone's car that you don't know very well. If someone tries to force you, yell very loudly and try to run away.
- If you get lost when you are out in public, go to a salesperson or checkout counter or security person and tell them you are lost—don't tell just anyone that you see.

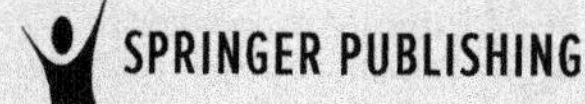

- Never go out alone, and make sure a trusted adult knows where you are at all times.
- Learn your address and phone number.

Remember that if someone is doing something to hurt you or make you feel bad in any way, you need to TELL!!!

It is NEVER your fault.

Your body is your private area; NOBODY has the right to touch it.

CHAPTER 13

Jessica L. Kozlowski and Pamela Lusk

Evidence-Based Assessment and Management of Trauma, Stressor-Related Disorders, Other Adverse Childhood Events, Bullying, and Violence

FAST FACTS

- 50% of children in the United States have at minimum one adverse childhood experience (ACE) (Marsicek et al., 2019).
- ACE terminology began after a study was performed on 17,000 adults in the mid-1990s by the Centers for Disease Control and Prevention and Kaiser Permanente in San Diego, California (Felitti et al., 1998) entitled "Relationship of Childhood Abuse and Household Dysfunction to many of the Leading Causes of Death in Adults: The Adverse Childhood Experiences Study." This study is still seen as a landmark work on this topic (Bachmann & Bachmann, 2018; Bethell et al., 2017; Gilgoff et al., 2020).
- In the Felitti et al. study, the 10 adverse childhood experiences (before age 18 years) were:

  (a) emotional abuse (recurrent), (b) physical abuse (recurrent), (c) sexual abuse (contact), (d) physical neglect, (e) emotional neglect, (f) substance abuse in the household (e.g., living with an alcoholic or a person with a substance-abuse problem), (g) mental illness in the household (e.g., living with someone who suffered from depression or mental illness or who had attempted suicide), (h) mother treated violently, (i) divorce or parental separation, (j) criminal behavior in household (e.g., a household member going to prison).
- There is a dose-response relationship between ACEs and poor health outcome; that is, the higher a person's ACE score, the greater the risk to the person's health. A person with four or more ACEs is twice as likely to develop significant disease (cardiac, cancer, pulmonary problems).
- A pediatrician, Nadine Burke Harris, followed up on this study with children and adolescents and their families in her San Francisco Clinic where she was seeing children exhibiting symptoms that seemed to be related to "toxic stress."
- Dr. Nadine Burke Harris is identified by most as a pioneer in putting a spotlight on childhood ACEs, the importance of universal screening, and treatment. She was recently made Surgeon General in California to improve health disparities and adversity experiences. She has resources and screening questionnaires (English and Spanish) available at the website: Center for Youth Wellness. See centerforyouthwellness.org/translating-aces-science/
- In 2018, Nadine Burke Harris, MD, published "The Deepest Well: Healing the Long-Term Effects of Childhood Adversity," an evidence-based guide to screening, assessment, and management of children and adolescents who have experienced trauma/ACEs.
- From Dr. Burke Harris's pediatric team's work other factors were identified as increasing the risk for toxic stress: (a) community violence, (b) homelessness, (c) discrimination, (d) foster care, (e) bullying, (f) repeated medical procedures or life-threatening illness,

(g) death of caregiver, (h) loss of caregiver due to deportation or migration; and for teens: (i) verbal or physical violence from romantic partner, and (j) youth incarceration.

- Stressors at the household level (the traditional ACEs) seem to have a greater effect on health than stressors at the community level, but this is still being studied. (Burke Harris, 2018, p. 149).
- ACE exposure can limit the development of important healthy coping skills in the child and adult who experience them (Merrick et al., 2019).
- With ACE exposure, the core issue is a dysregulated stress response. Behavioral and learning problems are often indications that ACEs have had a large effect on the child's developing brain.
- According to Burke Harris's work, in response to toxic stress, the child's brain (amygdala) alarm is always on high, the cortisol thermometer is always overheating. The natural antidote to toxic stress is having a well-regulated caregiver who can buffer the stress response (Burke Harris, 2018).
- Less than 47.7% of school-aged children in the United States meet the basic norms for thriving in their day-to-day life (www.childhealthdata.org).
- Healing from toxic stress recommendations for persons of all ages includes promotion of sleep, exercise, nutrition, mindfulness, mental health, and healthy relationships (p. 168).
- ACEs are common events that have been identified as a public health crisis. A 10% reduction in ACEs incidence could equal a savings of $105 billion (Bellis et al., 2019; Gilgoff et al., 2020).
- The impact of ACEs makes prevention, identification, and building resilience a vital part of the primary care provider's clinic day (American Academy of Pediatrics, n.d.; Bethell et al., 2017).
- The importance of a positive adult relationship as a safeguard is vital in preventing toxic stress responses to the child (Gilgoff et al., 2020).
- 1 billion children ages 2 to 17 were victims of violence globally in 2019 (Bellis et al., 2019).
- 1 in 5 high school students were bullied on school property, and 1 in 7 were cyberbullied (CDC).
- Peer victimization when seen along with other ACEs shows a marked increase in substance abuse later in life (Afifi, Taillieu, et al., 2020).
- Conduct disorders occur at lifetime prevalence rates of 12% in males and 7.1% in females (Lillig, 2018).
- Conduct disorders have a higher societal and economic burden than ADHD or autism (Fairchild et al., 2019).

ADVERSE CHILDHOOD EXPERIENCES

Types of Adverse Childhood Experiences

Child maltreatment (see Chapter 12 on Child Maltreatment) and peer victimization:

- Physical abuse
- Sexual abuse
- Emotional abuse
- Physical neglect
- Exposure to intimate partner violence (IPV)

- Spanking
- Peer victimization/bullying

Household challenges (Box 13.1):

- Substance abuse by someone in the home
- Mental health problems of a parent or guardian
- Household gambling
- Parental separation or divorce
- Parental problems with the law
- Foster care placement or Department of Children and Families (DCF) involvement with the family
- Poverty
- Neighborhood Safety (Afifi, Salmon, et al., 2020)

Risk With Adverse Childhood Experience Exposure

Health outcomes:

- Depression
- Substance abuse
- Early introduction of alcohol and alcoholism
- Obesity
- Increased risk of suicide
- Coronary heart disease
- Stroke
- Asthma
- Chronic obstruction pulmonary disease (COPD)
- Kidney disease
- Diabetes

Box 13.1. Social Determinants of Health

Social Determinants of Health are "the conditions in which people are born, grow, live, work, and age as well as the complex, interrelated social structures and economic systems that shape these conditions. Social determinants of health include aspects of the social environment (e.g., discrimination, income, education level, marital status), the physical environment (e.g., place of residence, crowding conditions, built environment [i.e., buildings, spaces, transportation systems, and products that are created or modified by people]), and health services (e.g., access to and quality of care, insurance status)."

"Social determinants of health are linked to a lack of opportunity and to a lack of resources to protect, improve, and maintain health, and taken together, these factors are mostly responsible for health inequities—the unfair and avoidable differences in health status seen within and between populations."

https://www.cdc.gov/nchhstp/socialdeterminants/index.html

- Earlier use of tobacco and vaping products
- Fetal risks (AAP, n.d.; Bellis et al., 2019; Gilgoff et al., 2020; Merrick et al., 2019)

Socioeconomic outcomes:

- Low educational level (not completing high school)
- Unemployment
- No health insurance (Gilgoff et al., 2020; Merrick et al., 2019)
- Teenage pregnancy
- Household poverty

COMMON PRESENTATIONS

Adversity and Toxic Stress

Stress and adversity are not always a negative situation for the child or adolescent. Some stress and adversity can promote strength of character and resiliency, especially, if handled in the correct way (Bachmann & Bachmann, 2018; Dutcher & Creswell, 2018; joiningforcesforchildren.org). Repetitive and prolonged exposures to ACEs, especially four or more, tend to lead to the development of toxic stress (Bachmann & Bachmann, 2018; Dutcher & Creswell, 2018). When that toxic stress persists is when the changes are seen both physiologically and behaviorally (Bachmann & Bachmann, 2018; joiningforcesforchildren.org).

In Nadine Burke Harris's book, "The Deepest Well," she shares stories from her pediatric practice where she would follow children with "failure to thrive," but without response to usual treatment, and learned that the root cause of the child's failure to thrive was not inadequate calories, rather, it was in response to the many ACE's. The child's body was making so many stress hormones that were interfering with their growth. Dr. Burke Harris's work has shown that it is never too late to begin healing. Caregivers have the capacity to calm children's stress response. High-quality, nurturing caregiving improves outcomes. Early identification (screening children for ACEs) in primary care and providing intervention with the parent–child relationship can be an important way to promote the development of the antidote: a warm caring relationship. Integration of behavioral health services into primary care/pediatric practices is a recommended model of care. Child–parent psychotherapy can be provided by clinic therapists.

Screening in primary care settings can contribute significantly to earlier identification of children at risk. Early detection is ideal, but healing can begin with trauma informed care at any time. Children who have high doses of adversity, activate biological pathways and release stress hormones that can affect brain development, the immune system, and the development of hormonal systems. Science shows us that high quality, nurturing caregiving improves outcomes: It improves brain development, immune functioning, and epigenetic regulation. Early home visiting is one of the nationally recognized, evidence-based programs that improves outcomes and leads to better health down the line.

Changes Seen in Response to Toxic Stress

Physiological changes

- Toxic stress causes disruptions in the brain's normal structure during crucial early stages of development.
- Decreased hippocampal volume and dysregulation of the HPA axis, which is significant for dealing with stress.

- Prefrontal cortex inhibition which is important for impulse control, executive function, and overall learning and leads to emotional and cognitive deficits (DiGangi & Negriff, 2020; Dutcher & Creswell, 2018).
- Changes in organ symptoms can be affected due to neuroendocrine–immune feedback loops and the ultimate release of cytokines (DiGangi & Negriff, 2020).

Behavioral changes

- Somatic complaints such as headaches, nausea, chest pain, and abdominal pain.
- Sleep disturbances.
- Learning difficulties.

Box 13.2. Health Equity

Health is influenced by:

- Jobs that pay a living wage
- Safe housing
- Reliable transportation
- Walkable neighborhoods
- Good schools
- Fresh food
- Adequate green spaces

Source: Data from AAP Toolkit to Screen for Food Insecurity link. Retrieved from *https://frac.org›FRAC_AAP_Toolkit_2021*

SCREENING FOR ADVERSE CHILDHOOD EXPERIENCES

In the pediatric primary care setting, screening for ACEs is an important first step in preventing the chronic conditions which are an outcome of exposure (Gilgoff et al., 2020). There are 15 opportunities at well child checkups alone to screen and then provide needed anticipatory guidance before the age of 5. Due to the rate of exposure to trauma and stressors by children and adolescents in the United States, it should be considered at every visit (Gilgoff et al., 2020). There are not any current standardized methods or schedules for the screening of ACEs. Many organizations, such as the American Academy of Pediatrics (AAP), have made recommendations on a suggested timeline and overall importance of screening (Gilgoff et al., 2020):

- Annually after age 2 at their well-child checkup; however, some studies recommend starting at 9 months of age (Marsicek et al., 2019).
- When the child is currently living in poverty.
- Present with any somatic, learning, or behavioral concerns.
- Have previously been identified as having an ACE (Cohen et al., 2008).

How to Screen for Adverse Childhood Experiences

Direct Interview Approach (Taken from the AAP Toolkit for Trauma)

"Has anything bad, sad, or scary happened to you recently?"

"Has anything changed at home for you or your family?

"How do you usually deal with things you find as stressful?"

"You have shared with me some of your concerns about your child's symptoms he/she is presenting with today. Do you have any concerns this may be related to something that maybe stressing or scaring your child?"

Screening Instruments for Adverse Childhood Experiences and Trauma

- Revised Child Impact of Event Scale (CRIES-8).
- Survey of Well-being of Young Children (SWYC) 2 months to 5 years of age.
- Center for Youth and Wellness Adverse Childhood Experience Questionnaire (ACE-Q) Child, Teen (Center for Youth and Wellness is the clinic Nadine Burke Harris was instrumental in founding). Screenings in Spanish/English for Child, Teen (both parent report) and Teen self-report (posted at end of this Section).

When a child has developed a toxic stress response and behavioral concerns arise that are severe in nature and affect their ability to function in their day-to-day life then further diagnoses is necessary.

ASSESSMENT/DIAGNOSIS BASED ON *THE DIAGNOSTIC AND STATISTICAL MANUAL OF MENTAL DISORDERS, FIFTH EDITION*

Adjustment Disorder

- Severe emotional or behavioral symptoms which have developed as a reaction to an identified stressor in the last 3 months.
- The symptoms seen are more severe than the level of the specific stressor or they cause significant difficulty in the day-to-day functioning of the child or adolescent.
- These symptoms should not be a part of a normal grief process and do not continue 6 months after the stressor has completed (O'Donnell et al., 2019).

Acute Stress Disorder

- Severe distress caused acutely after a severe trauma, usually within 1 month, with the symptoms lasting for at least 3 days.
- The child or adolescent should have nine or more symptoms that can include irritability, intrusive thoughts, avoiding anything associated with the trauma, low mood, nightmares, negative thoughts, and guilt (Meiser-Steidman et al., 2017).

Post-Traumatic Stress Disorder

- Symptoms clustered—based categories in which the child or adolescent will see negative changes in awareness and mood (Meiser-Stedman et al., 2017).
- The patient must meet all three categories to achieve the diagnosis along with the symptoms being present for 1 month. The patient also must have significant stress in their level of functioning in day-to-day life.
    - Intrusive recollections
    - Avoidance/numbing symptoms
    - Hyperarousal

Protective Factors in Preventing Development of Toxic Stress

- Strong parent–child relationship from an early age (Bethell et al., 2017).
- Having safe, stable, and nurturing relationships are important (Bethell et al., 2017; Merrick et al., 2019).
- Encouraging resiliency.
- Effective health promotion education (Marie-Mitchell & Kostolansky, 2019).

VIOLENT BEHAVIORS IN CHILDREN AND ADOLESCENTS

Risk Factors

Prenatal

- Maternal smoking
- Maternal alcohol use
- Maternal drug use
- Maternal stress

Perinatal

- Birth complications
- Maternal or paternal mental health disorders
- Malnutrition

Environmental

- Exposure to physical or sexual abuse in childhood.
- Exposure to domestic violence between parents.
- Community violence.
- Poor friend groups that is, those who have truancy issues or abuse substances.
- Harsh discipline.
- Poverty (Fairchild et al., 2019; Lillig, 2018).

Red Flags for Impending Violence in a Child or Adolescent

The Centers for Disease Control and Prevention (CDC) Violence Prevention Program provides key examination findings which could indicate the child or teen requires immediate action to prevent violence (CDC, n.d.). In most cases reaching out to a quick response mental health team or police is the safest option for the child and their family.

- Serious physical fighting with a peer or family member.
- Severe destruction of property.
- Severe anger and rage for what most would think is a minor reason.
- Possession or use of firearms or other weapons.
- Threatened violent act detailed in a written or verbal plan.
- Thoughts or actions of self-harm or suicide.
- Fire setting.
- Animal cruelty.

Screening for Violent Behaviors

- Pediatric Symptoms Checklist (PSC).
- Strengths and Difficulties Questionnaire (SDQ).
- National Institute for Children's Health Quality Vanderbilt Assessment Scales (Lillig, 2018).

Peer Victimization

Bullying has been defined as the planned, violent, and persistent behaviors done by an individual or group over a long period of time. There is normally a perceived social difference in status between the bully and the victim. Globally, one in three students are bullied at least once a month (Mendez et al., 2019). Bullying previously has normally occurred in school, however, now with adolescents spending approximately 9 hours per day utilizing some form of media, cyberbullying has rapidly expanded (Anderson et al., 2017). Cyberbullies typically have incredibly low levels of empathy towards others. Today, ethical–cultural bullying has also become an issue which more people are aware of; education is needed to prevent xenophobia and racism (Mendez et al., 2019). Lesbian, gay, bisexual, transgender, and queer/questioning (LGBTQ+) youth are coming of age in the setting of increased LGBTQ+ rights and visibility, yet they remain vulnerable to higher rates of negative mental health outcomes, including depression, anxiety, eating disorders, self-harm, and suicide (American Academy of Pediatrics, 2021).

Prevention of Peer Victimization

- Empower teachers.
- Teach responsible use of the internet.
- Partnership between the family and school.
- Increase societal awareness.

Diagnosis Based on the *DSM-5*

Conduct Disorder (see Chapter 7 on Disruptive Behaviors in Children and Adolescents)

- Patterns of behaviors in which the rights of others and understood rules of society are persistently ignored or violated by the child or teen. As a provider, identifying when the onset of the behaviors was noted is particularly important (childhood-onset, adolescent-onset, or unspecified-onset).
- Three of the following behaviors seen in the past 12 months with at least one of them occurring in the last 6 months:
    - Aggressive behaviors toward people and animals.
    - Property destruction.
    - Theft or dishonest behaviors.
    - Serious abuses of rules set forth by an adult, school, or workplace (Lillig, 2018).

Treatment

Treatment for conduct disorders can be complex due to the multiple comorbid mental health diagnoses present with the conduct disorder such as ADHD or depression. Most patients will need to be followed much closer by both psychology and psychiatry to maximize level of functioning. These teens are at risk because they have high rates of school dropout, drug use, and criminal behaviors (Lillig, 2018).

Psychosocial Interventions for Children and Adolescents With Adverse Childhood Experiences

High-quality, nurturing caregiving improves outcomes. Early identification (screening children for ACEs) in primary care and providing intervention with the parent–child relationship so that the child receives the antidote: warm caring relationship.

Dr. Burke Harris's research informed her treatment recommendations that child–parent psychotherapy was more effective and more efficient than previous treatments for these children. For ages 0 to 5—young children experiencing adversity—Child Parent Psychotherapy (CPP) is the recommendation. In CPP the parent also receives psychotherapy. Attachment is a main focus of the treatment. Dr. Burke Harris's clinic has integrated behavioral health therapists as part of the treatment team. They provide the child–parent psychotherapy.

In primary care settings, pediatric guidance includes: *Family support*

- Encourage ways to reduce stress levels at home.
- Encourage support through different organizations and community resources.
- Encourage treatment of parental mental health disorders.

Referral to Psychiatric / Behavioral Therapists in the Community

In a recent systematic review of the treatment literature (Dorsey et al., 2017) "Evidence Base Update for Psychosocial Treatments for Children and Adolescents Exposed to Traumatic Events," individual cognitive behavioral therapy (CBT) with parent involvement, individual CBT, and group CBT were deemed "well established"; group CBT with parent involvement and EMDR (eye movement desensitization and reprocessing) were deemed "possibly efficacious" and individual client-centered play therapy, individual mind-body skills, and individual psychoanalysis were deemed "experimental."

Evidence Based Psychotherapies Include

The Young Child

- Parent–Child Interaction Therapy (PCIT).
- Parent Management Training (PMT).
- Triple P-Positive Parenting Program.

Adolescents

- CBT.
- Multisystemic Therapy (MST).
  - Targets antisocial behaviors and is delivered where the patient functions (i.e., school, home) and occurs over a period of 3 to 5 months.
  - Goals: Improving family functioning, parenting skills, improving peer groups, and finally improving the adolescent's emotional regulation, problem-solving, and school performance (Fairchild et al., 2019).

Pharmacologic Interventions

- Currently there are no FDA-approved pharmacologic treatment for pediatric PTSD or ACEs. We will discuss some of the medications we can use for targeting other mental health disorders which can be triggered by this.
- Sleep is a critical need for the growing child. Childhood adversity significantly increases the risk for sleep disturbance/sleep disorders. Nighttime sleep plays a powerful role in

enhancing brain function, hormones, and the immune system. During sleep, levels of cortisol, adrenaline, and noradrenaline drop. Lack of sleep is associated with increased levels of stress hormones and increased stress reactivity.

- Melatonin is a hormone produced in the pineal gland and is available over the counter but not by prescription. Melatonin is effective in reducing time to sleep onset in adults and children with initial insomnia (though there is fewer data with children). Half-life only 40 minutes with peak level of 1 hour. There are studies supporting use in ADHD and autism spectrum disorders. Long-term use side effects are not well understood. Not FDA regulated. Typical dosage 0.5 to 10 mg. Most do not recommend use before 2 years of age.
- Many other medications utilized for sleep (normally based on their side effects) but none are FDA approved for pediatric insomnia. Trazodone is a sleep enhancing antidepressant approved for adults but is sometimes used in low doses for off-label treatment of insomnia in adolescents (Riddle, 2019). The major effect is thought to be on the serotonergic system. The adverse effect profile is like the SSRIs, but is also associated with priapism, which may limit its use in male adolescents.
- Treat comorbid diagnoses such as ADHD. High level of evidence studies have suggested improvement in conduct disorder symptoms with treatment with psychostimulants in aggression improvement (Fairchild et al., 2019; Lillig, 2018).
- Guanfacine for impulsivity/ inattentiveness: For youth with impaired impulse control and inattentiveness due to toxic stress, instead of stimulants there has been reported success with non-stimulants.

  Guanfacine is a nonstimulant that was originally developed to treat high blood pressure but also is used for ADHD. Guanfacine targets specific circuits in the prefrontal cortex where adrenaline and noradrenaline exert their action, improving impulsiveness and concentration, even in situations of high stress. Guanfacine can be helpful for poor impulse and frustration control (Burke Harris, 2018, p. 65) (Riddle, 2019, p. 94–100).

  Guanfacine is not FDA approved for use in youth younger than 6 years.

  Extended release (ER) guanfacine (generic and Intuniv) is FDA approved for ADHD in children and adolescents ages 6 years and older. Initial dose is 1 mg. Max daily dose is 4 mg. Duration of ER guanfacine is up to 24 hours once daily dosing. It should not be taken with a high fat meal Regular checks of blood pressure and heart rate are recommended. Can be used alone or in combination with a stimulant.

  Antidepressants (SSRIs) with increased ACE exposure cause an increased risk of depression and anxiety. With four or more ACEs there is a 460% risk of depression and can lead to adverse effects. The SSRI's approved for pediatric use are covered in the Anxiety and Depression sections (GLAD PC, 2018)
- Medications such as the second-generation antipsychotics approved for use in children and teens (e.g., aripiprazole for disruptive behavior disorders in children and adolescents) are covered in Chapter 7.

PSYCHOSOCIAL INTERVENTIONS

Brief Interventions for Pediatric Primary Care Practices

- Sleep interventions are a first line intervention in primary care. Encourage sleep hygiene.
- Behavioral interventions for sleep can be initiated in the primary care setting at an early age. These interventions begin with sleep hygiene outlined in the Sweet Dreamzzz Early Childhood Sleep Education Program. This is a by-donation program with learning programs

for both healthcare providers and teachers as well. There are free programs with materials for all Title 1 schools which we all know are your lower income schools. The first step is setting up the child's bedroom making sure they have a comfortable bed to sleep in with adequate lighting for comfort but free from excessive stimuli (McDowall et al., 2017). The next step is mapping out the routine at bedtime; this way the child knows the schedule of events before finally laying down to sleep (McDowall et al., 2017). These activities can include shower, bedtime story, or soft music and should always avoid electronics. School-aged children need 9 to 11 hours of sleep and the sleep schedule should not vary on weekends. Reward nights when they stay asleep. Check for anemia (ferritin levels).

Brief Interventions: Skills-Building Worksheets for Primary Care

Brief interventions are discussed in detail in Chapter 17 and some of the worksheets that are evidence-based for children and adolescents who have experienced Trauma/Adverse Childhood Experiences are included. For the child/adolescent experiencing adversity, we borrow from the trauma focused psychotherapies in psychiatry/mental health specialty services and provide psychoeducation and teach/reinforce self-soothing skills.

Psychoeducation

In primary care we can educate about trauma, adverse childhood experiences—there is nothing "wrong with the child/ teen"; rather, they are experiencing the usual, human symptoms that occur when one has experienced something extraordinarily sad or frightening (Weisz, 2017).

Skills Building in Self-Soothing

We can borrow from EMDR and Trauma Focused CBT—teaching and reinforcing individual skills in self-soothing, grounding, and development and strengthening personal resources for times of increased stress/triggering situations.

There is evidence to support brief interventions that address:

1. Attachment to a caring adult.
2. Management of stress.
3. Emotional regulation.

Educational/intervention worksheets provide a way to address the child's symptoms and struggles even in a busy, fast pace practice.

- The worksheets provide an opportunity to instill hope as the team member provides an intervention during that visit and arranges for follow-up to review what the child/teen or parent has learned/practiced and their response. There is active, timely intervention.
- The pediatric team members can use these worksheets to teach the child and parent, "It is not What is wrong with you; rather, What has happened to you?"
- For trauma there is an emphasis on providing worksheets/skill building exercises that increase the young person's ability to develop strategies for self-soothing, grounding, developing personal resources (childtrauma.com)

Worksheets that are helpful in the authors' practice are included at the end of this section.

- Improving the parent/caring adult relationship/attachment (my team of helpers worksheet. guided imagery—peaceful pleasant place)
- Stress management: Healthy coping for stress and worry. Butterfly Hug, Container for strong feelings.
- Emotional Regulation: Strong feelings, anger, hurt, fear, sadness. Positive things about me. Catching, Checking, and Changing self-critical/negative thoughts.

Telehealth

All of these resources can be introduced in the telehealth visit. The provider/team member may need to mail the packet of resources to the child. It increases a connection with that child/teen if, when you mail the worksheets, you include a personal note of encouragement. Also sending some Post-Its or note cards is well received. At the next telehealth visit, the child or teen can show you the skill-building exercise they have worked on and when it was helpful during their week.

An excellent resource for providing telehealth Interventions:

"Telehealth in an Increasing Virtual World," a 2020 Children's Mental Health Report published by The Child Mind Institute (childmind.org/our-impact/childrens-mental-health-report/2020-childrens-mental-health-report/).

Resources for Families

- Child Mind Institute: For Families https://childmind.org/audience/for-families/.
- Ted Talk, Dr. Nadine Burke Harris https://youtu.be/95ovIJ3dsNk.
- Talking about trauma and COVID-19 https://www.pbs.org/parents/thrive/how-to-talk-to-your-kids-about-coronavirus.

Children's Book for Ages 5 to 9

A Terrible Thing Happened

Written by Margaret M. Holmes, illustrated by Cary Pillo

When Sherman, a raccoon, saw something that upset him, he became nervous, did not sleep well, and felt sad. "Through Sherman, the book explains the symptoms of post-traumatic stress disorder in simple terms that young children can understand," says an expert at the Child Mind Institute. Another plus: The story does not specify exactly what happened to Sherman, so the book could be useful in many situations. Ages 5 to 9. Published by Magination Press.

Resources for Providers

- **Book: Worksheets and Skill-Building Exercises to Support Safety, Connection & Empowerment**
- Phifer, L., & Sibbald, L. (2020). Trauma-Informed Social-Emotional Toolbox for Children & Adolescents. PESI Publishing & Media.
- The Resilience Project, American Academy of Pediatrics: https://www.aap.org/en-us/advocacy-and-policy/aap-health-initiatives/resilience/Pages/Clinical-Assessment-Tools.aspx
- The Center for Youth Wellness: https://centerforyouthwellness.org/translating-aces-science/
- Child Mind Institute: https://childmind.org/our-care/clinical-care/
- American Academy of Pediatrics Trauma Toolbox for Primary Care: https://www.aap.org/en-us/advocacy-and-policy/aap-health-initiatives/healthy-foster-care-america/Pages/Trauma-Guide.aspx
- American Academy of Pediatrics Mental Health in LGBTQ+ Youth Pediatric/ Primary care guide to an LGBTQ+ Friendly Practice: https://www.aap.org/en/patient-care/mental-health-minute/mental-health-in-lgbtq-youth/
- Centers for Disease Control's Violence Prevention: https://www.cdc.gov/violenceprevention/index.html

- Ted Talk, Dr. Nadine Burke Harris: https://youtu.be/95ovIJ3dsNk
- Childhealthdata.org
- Joining Forces for Children. *What are ACEs?* http://joiningforcesforchildren.org/what-are-aces/.

REFERENCES

Adler-Tapia, R., & Settle, C. (2017). *EMDR and the art of psychotherapy with children: infants to adolescents* (2nd ed.). Springer Publishing Company.

Afifi, T. O., Salmon, S., Garces, I., Struck, S., Fortier, J., Taillieu, T., Stewart-Tufescu, A., Asmundson, G. J. G., Sareen, J., . . . MacMillan, H. L. (2020). Confirmatory factor analysis of adverse childhood experiences (ACEs) among a community-based sample of parents and adolescents. *BMC Pediatrics, 20*(178), 1–14. https://doi.org/10.1186/s12887-020-02063-3.

Afifi, T. O., Taillieu, T., Salmon, S., Davila, I. G., Stewart-Tufescu, A., Fortier, J., Struck, S., Asmundson, G. J. G., Sareen, J., & MacMillan, H. L. (2020). Adverse childhood experiences (ACEs), peer victimization, and substance use among adolescents. *Child Abuse and Neglect, 106*, 104504. https://doi.org/10.1016/j.chiabu.2020.104504.

American Academy of Pediatrics. (n.d.). *Trauma toolbox for primary care.* https://www.aap.org/en-us/advocacy-and-policy/aap-health-initiatives/healthy-foster-care-america/Pages/Trauma-Guide.aspx.

American Academy of Pediatrics. (2021). *Mental health in LGBTQ+ youth: Pediatric mental health minute series.* https://www.aap.org/en/patient-care/mental-health-minute/mental-health-in-lgbtq-youth/

Anderson, C. A., Bushman, B. J., Bartholow, B. D., Cantor, J., Christakis, D., Coyne, S. M., Donnerstein, E., Brockmyer, J. F., Gentile, D. A., Shawn Green, C., Huesmann, R., Hummer, T., Krahé, B., Strasburger, V. C., Warburton, W., Wilson, B. J., & Ybarra, M. (2017). Screen violence and youth behavior. *Pediatrics, 140*(s2), s142–s147. https://doi.org/10.1542/peds.2016-1758T.

Bachmann, M., & Bachmann, B. A. (2018). The case for including adverse childhood experiences in child maltreatment education: A path analysis. *The Permanente Journal, 22*, 117–122. https://doi.org/10.7812/TPP/17-122.

Bellis, M. A., Hughes, K., Ford, K., Rodriguez, G. R., Sethi, D., & Passmore, J. (2019). Life course health consequences and associated annual costs of adverse childhood experiences across Europe and North America: A systematic review and meta-analysis. *Lancet Public Health, 4*(10), e517–e528. https://doi.org/10.1016/S2468-2667(19)30145-8.

Bethell, C. D., Solloway, M. R., Guinosso, S., Hassink, S., Srivastav, A., Ford, D., & Simpson, L. A. (2017). Prioritizing possibilities for child and family health: An agenda to address adverse childhood experiences and foster the social and emotional roots of well-being in pediatrics. *Academic Pediatrics, 17*(7S), S36–S50. https://doi.org/10.1016/j.acap.2017.04.161

Burke Harris, N. (2018). *The deepest well: Healing the long-term effects of childhood adversity.* Mariner Books, Houghton Mifflin Harcourt.

Centers for Disease Control and Prevention. (n.d.). *Violence prevention.* https://www.cdc.gov/violenceprevention/aces/about.html.

Cohen, J. A., Kelleher, K. J., & Mannarino, A. P. (2008). Identifying, treating, and referring traumatized children: The role of pediatric providers. *Archives of Pediatric Adolescent Medicine, 162*(5), 447–452. https://doi.org/10.1001/archpedi.162.5.447.

DiGangi, M. J., & Negriff, S. (2020). The implementation of screening for adverse childhood experiences in pediatric primary care. *The Journal of Pediatrics, 222*, 174–179. https://doi.org/10.1016/j.jpeds.2020.03.057.

Dorsey, S., McLaughlin, K., Kerns, S., Harrison, J., Lambert, H., Briggs, E., Cox, J., & 7 Amaya-Jackson. (2017). Evidence-based update for psychosocial treatments for children and adolescents exposed to traumatic events. *Journal of Clinical Child and Adolescent Psychology, 46*(3), 303–330. https://doi.org/10.10815374416.2016.1220309

Dutcher, J. M., & Creswell, J. D. (2018). The role of the brain reward pathways in stress resilience and health. *Neuroscience and Biobehavioral Review, 95*, 559–567. https://doi.org/10.1016/j.neubiorev.2018.10.014.

Fairchild, G., Hawes, D. J., Frick, P. J., Copeland, W. E., Odgers, C. L., Franke, B., Freitag, C. M., & De Brito, S. A. (2019). Conduct disorder. *Nature Reviews: Disease Primers, 5*, 1–25. https://doi.org/10.1038/s41572-019-0095-y.

Felitti, V. J., Anda, R. F., Nordenberg, D., Williamson, D. F., Spitz, A. M., Edwards, V., Koss, M. P., & Marks, J. S. (1998). Relationship of childhood abuse and household dysfunction to many of the leading causes of death in adults. *American Journal of Preventive Medicine, 14*(4), 245–258. https://doi.org.10.1016/s0749-3797(98)00017-8

Gilgoff, R., Singh, L., Koita, K., Gentile, B., Marques, S. S. (2020). Adverse childhood experiences, outcomes, and interventions. *Pediatric Clinics of North America, 67*, 259–273. https://doi.org/10.1016/j.pcl.2019.12.001.

Lillig, M. (2018). Conduct disorder: Recognition and management. *American Academy of Family Physicians, 98*(10), 584–592.

Marie-Mitchell, A., & Kostolansky, R. (2019). A systematic review of trials to improve child outcomes associated with adverse childhood experiences. *American Journal of Preventative Medicine, 56*(5), 756–764. https://doi.org/10.1016/j.amepre.2018.11.030

Marsicek, S. M., Morrison, J. M., Manikonda, N., O'Halleran, M. O., Spoehr-Labutta, Z., Brinn, M. (2019). Implementing standardized screening for adverse childhood experiences in a pediatric resident continuity clinic. *Pediatric Quality and Safety, 2*, e154. https://doi.org/10.1097/pq9.0000000000000154.

McDowall, P. S., Galland, B. C., Campbell, A. J., Elder, D. E. (2017). Parent knowledge of children's sleep: A systematic review, *Sleep Medicine Reviews, 31*, 39–47. https://doi.org/10.1016/j.smrv.2016.01.002

Meiser-Stedman, R., McKinnon, A., Dixon, C., Boyle, A., Smith, P., & Dalgliesh, T. (2017). Acute stress disorder and the transition to posttraumatic stress disorder in children and adolescents: Prevalence, course, prognosis, diagnostic suitability, and risk markers. *Depression and Anxiety, 34*(4), 348–355. https://doi.org/10.1002/da.22602.

Mendez, I., Jorquera, A. B., Ruiz-Esteban, C., Martinez-Ramon, J. P., & Fernandez-Sogorb, A. (2019). Emotional intelligence, bullying, and cyberbullying in adolescents. *International Journal of Environmental Research and Public Health, 16*, 4836–4837. https://doi.org/10.3390/ijerph16234837.

Merrick, M. T., Ford, D. C., Ports, K. A., Guinn, A. S., Chen, J., Klevens, J., Metzler, M., Jones, C. M., Simon, T. R., Daniel, V. D., Ottley, P., & Mercy, J. A. (2019). Vital signs: Estimated proportion of adult health problems attributable to adverse childhood experiences and implications for prevention-25 states, 2015-2017. *MMWR, 68*(44), 1000–1005. http://doi.org/10.15585/mmwr.mm6844e1.

O'Donnell, M. L., Agathos, J. A., Metcalf, O., Gibson, K., & Lau, W. (2019). Adjustment disorder: Current developments and future directions. *International Journal of Environmental Research and Public Health, 16*, 2537. http://doi.org/10.3390/ijerph16142537.

Riddle, M. (2019). *Pediatric psychopharmacology for primary care* (2nd ed.). American Academy of Pediatrics.

Weisz, J., Kuppens, S., Ng, M., Eckshtain, D., Ugueto, A., Vaughn-Coaxum, R., Jensen Doss, A., Hawley, K., Marchette, L., Chu, B., Weersing, R., & Fordwood, S. (2017). What five years of research tells us about the effects of youth psychological therapy: A multilevel meta-analysis and implications for science and practice. *American Psychologist, 72*(2), 79–117.

Center for Youth Wellness (CYW) Adverse Childhood Experiences Questionnaire (ACE-Q)—Child

ACE-Q - Center for Youth Wellness

https://centerforyouthwellness.org› uploads › 2018/06

Screening Questionnaires: **Child** (0–12), **Teen** (13–19), and **Teen Self-Report** (13–19)

Today's Date: ______________________________

Child's Name: ______________________ *Date of birth:* ______________________________

Your Name: ______________________ *Relationship to Child:* ______________________

Many children experience stressful life events that can affect their health and well-being. The results from this questionnaire will assist your child's doctor in assessing their health and determining guidance. *Please read the statements below. Count the number of statements that apply to your child and write the total number in the box provided.*

Please DO NOT mark or indicate which specific statements apply to your child.

1) ***Of the statements in Section 1, HOW MANY apply to your child? Write the total number in the box.***
2) ***Of the statements in Section 2, HOW MANY apply to your child? Write the total number in the box.***

Section 1. *At any point since your child was born…*

- ❒ Your child's parents or guardians were separated or divorced.
- ❒ Your child lived with a household member who served time in jail or prison.
- ❒ Your child lived with a household member who was depressed, mentally ill or attempted suicide.
- ❒ Your child saw or heard household members hurt or threaten to hurt each other.
- ❒ A household member swore at, insulted, humiliated, or put down your child in a way that scared your child OR a household member acted in a way that made your child afraid that s/he might be physically hurt.
- ❒ Someone touched your child's private parts or asked your child to touch their private parts in a sexual way.
- ❒ More than once, your child went without food, clothing, a place to live, or had no one to protect her/him.
- ❒ Someone pushed, grabbed, slapped, or threw something at your child OR your child was hit so hard that your child was injured or had marks.
- ❒ Your child lived with someone who had a problem with drinking or using drugs.
- ❒ Your child often felt unsupported, unloved and/or unprotected.

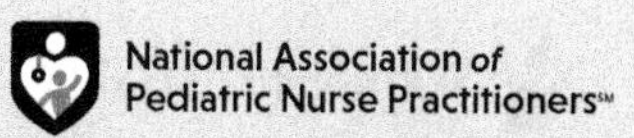

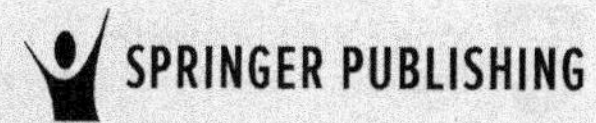

Section 2. *At any point since your child was born…*

- ❒ Your child was in foster care.
- ❒ Your child experienced harassment or bullying at school.
- ❒ Your child lived with a parent or guardian who died.
- ❒ Your child was separated from her/his primary caregiver through deportation or immigration.
- ❒ Your child had a serious medical procedure or life-threatening illness.
- ❒ Your child often saw or heard violence in the neighborhood or in her/his school neighborhood.
- ❒ Your child was often treated badly because of race, sexual orientation, place of birth, disability, or religion.

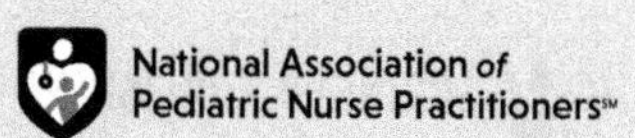

CYW ACE-Q Child (0–12 yo)

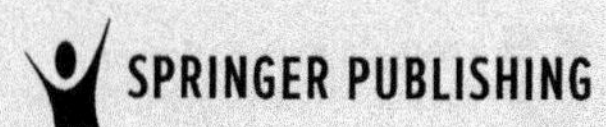

Center for Youth Wellness Adverse Childhood Experiences Questionnaire (ACE-Q)—Teen

Today's Date: ______________________

Child's Name: ______________________ *Date of birth:* ______________________

Your Name: ______________________ *Relationship to Child:* ______________________

Many children experience stressful life events that can affect their health and well-being. The results from this questionnaire will assist your child's doctor in assessing their health and determining guidance. *Please read the statements below. Count the number of statements that apply to your child and write the total number in the box provided.*

Please DO NOT mark or indicate which specific statements apply to your child.

1) ***Of the statements in Section 1, HOW MANY apply to your child? Write the total number in the box.***

2) ***Of the statements in Section 2, HOW MANY apply to your child? Write the total number in the box.***

Section 1. *At any point since your child was born…*

- ❒ Your child's parents or guardians were separated or divorced.
- ❒ Your child lived with a household member who served time in jail or prison.
- ❒ Your child lived with a household member who was depressed, mentally ill or attempted suicide.
- ❒ Your child saw or heard household members hurt or threaten to hurt each other.
- ❒ A household member swore at, insulted, humiliated, or put down your child in a way that scared your child OR a household member acted in a way that made your child afraid that s/he might be physically hurt.
- ❒ Someone touched your child's private parts or asked them to touch that person's private parts in a sexual way that was unwanted, against your child's will, or made your child feel uncomfortable.
- ❒ More than once, your child went without food, clothing, a place to live, or had no one to protect her/him.
- ❒ Someone pushed, grabbed, slapped, or threw something at your child OR your child was hit so hard that your child was injured or had marks.
- ❒ Your child lived with someone who had a problem with drinking or using drugs
- ❒ Your child often felt unsupported, unloved and/or unprotected.

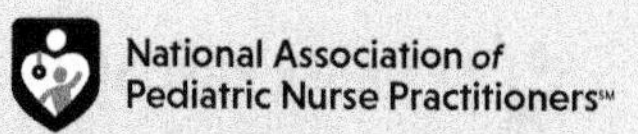

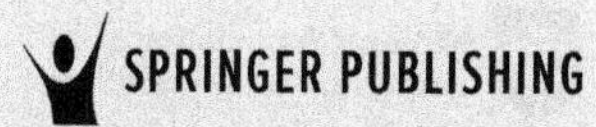

Section 2. *At any point since your child was born…*

- ❒ Your child was in foster care.
- ❒ Your child experienced harassment or bullying at school.
- ❒ Your child lived with a parent or guardian who died.
- ❒ Your child was separated from her/his primary caregiver through deportation or immigration.
- ❒ Your child had a serious medical procedure or life-threatening illness.
- ❒ Your child often saw or heard violence in the neighborhood or in her/his school neighborhood.
- ❒ Your child was detained, arrested, or incarcerated.
- ❒ Your child was often treated badly because of race, sexual orientation, place of birth, disability, or religion.
- ❒ Your child experienced verbal or physical abuse or threats from a romantic partner (i.e., boyfriend or girlfriend).

To be completed by Parent/Caregiver

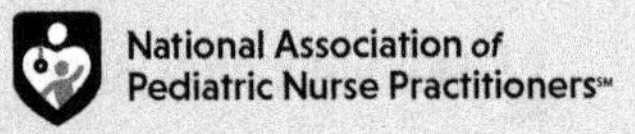

CYW ACE-Q Teen (13-19 yo)

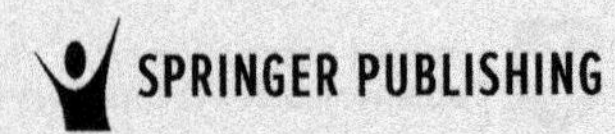

Center for Youth Wellness Adverse Childhood Experiences Questionnaire (ACE-Q)—Teen Self-Report

Today's Date: ______________________________

Your Name: ______________________ *Date of Birth:* ______________________________

Many children experience stressful life events that can affect their health and development. The results from this questionnaire will assist your doctor in assessing your health and determining guidance. Please read the statements below. Count the number of statements that apply to you and write the total number in the box provided.

Please DO NOT mark or indicate which specific statements apply to you.

1) **Of the statements in section 1, HOW MANY apply to you? Write the total number in the box.**
2) **Of the statements in section 2, HOW MANY apply to you? Write the total number in the box.**

Section 1. *At any point since you were born…*

- ❒ Your parents or guardians were separated or divorced.
- ❒ You lived with a household member who served time in jail or prison.
- ❒ You lived with a household member who was depressed, mentally ill or attempted suicide.
- ❒ You saw or heard household members hurt or threaten to hurt each other.
- ❒ A household member swore at, insulted, humiliated, or put you down in a way that scared you OR a household member acted in a way that made you afraid that you might be physically hurt.
- ❒ Someone touched your private parts or asked you to touch their private parts in a sexual way, that was unwanted, against your will, or made you feel uncomfortable.
- ❒ More than once, you went without food, clothing, a place to live, or had no one to protect you.
- ❒ Someone pushed, grabbed, slapped, or threw something at you OR you were hit so hard that you were injured or had marks.
- ❒ You lived with someone who had a problem with drinking or using drugs.
- ❒ You often felt unsupported, unloved and/or unprotected.

Section 2. *At any point since you were born…*

- ❒ You have been in foster care.
- ❒ You have experienced harassment or bullying at school.
- ❒ You have lived with a parent or guardian who died.

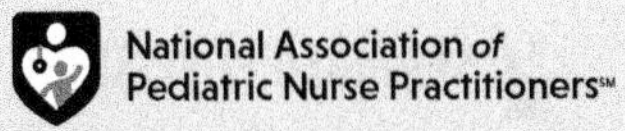

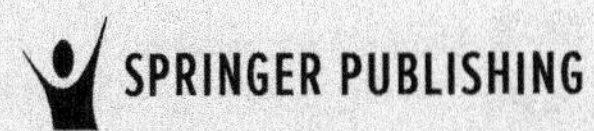

- ❒ You have been separated from your primary caregiver through deportation or immigration.
- ❒ You have had a serious medical procedure or life-threatening illness.
- ❒ You have often seen or heard violence in the neighborhood or in your school neighborhood.
- ❒ You have been detained, arrested, or incarcerated.
- ❒ You have often been treated badly because of race, sexual orientation, place of birth, disability, or religion.
- ❒ You have experienced verbal or physical abuse or threats from a romantic partner (i.e., boyfriend or girlfriend).

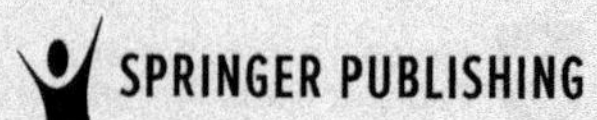

Trauma-Informed Interventions From Evidence-Based Psychotherapies

Grounding and self-soothing interventions from EMDR that you can put together with the child/teen and send with them to assist them in dealing with strong emotions include:

- Deep Breathing for relaxation using the 4-7-8 method: Breathe in for a count of 4; hold for a count of 7; and breathe out for a count of 8;
- Guided imagery—visualizing a safe/calm place; and
- Identifying a "team" of helpers.

From **EMDR** Dr. Robbie Adler Tapia adds:

- Aroma for self-soothing, resourcing.
- Create a container.
- Butterfly Hug breathing (crossing the arms and tapping while hugging yourself).

Container Script

I want you to be able to put all of those thoughts or feelings, or things we talked about into a container. Picture the container and make sure it is strong enough to hold everything you need it to hold. Let us imagine that everything you talked about or worried about today is put in the container and we lock it away, seal it until you come back. If you start thinking about things that bother you that are too hard to handle, you can just imagine putting it into the container and sealing it in there until we meet again. Be sure and use a strong container that can be locked.

Now, imagine putting 100% of the thoughts, feelings, emotions, body and sensations, and disturbance into the container. Seal it tightly, and let me know when you are finished (Adler-Tapia & Settle, 2017).

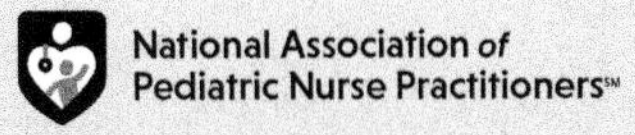

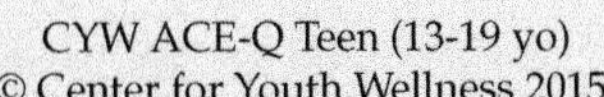

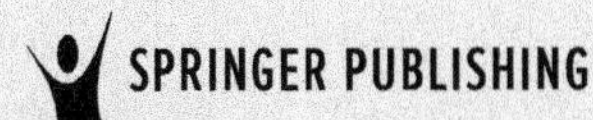

CHAPTER 14

Dianne Morrison-Beedy

Sexuality

FAST FACTS

Growth in stature and appearance of secondary sex characteristics are the most visual changes noted in puberty. The Tanner Stages is the most commonly recognized staging system for this sequence of changes (Emmanuel & Bokor, 2020).

GIRLS

- Puberty is considered early if it is before 8 years of age. Delayed puberty in girls means the absence of breast development by age 13, time lapse of more than 3 years from onset of breast growth to first menses, or no menses by age 16.
- Pubic hair, as well as armpit and leg hair, growth begins at age 9 or 10 years and reaches adult patterns usually by 13 to 14 years.
- The average age of menarche is 12.5 years. Menarche typically occurs 2 years following the development of breasts and pubic hair.
- Although breast budding occurs earlier in African American girls than Whites, there is no difference in onset of menarche.

BOYS

- Delayed puberty in boys is evidenced by no testicular enlargement by age 14 or a lapse of 5 years from the start to completion of genital growth.
- Testicular enlargement is usually the first sign of puberty in boys and occurs on average at age 9 years. Soon after the penis will lengthen. By the age of 16 to 17 years, the genitals are usually adult size and shape.
- Pubic hair, as well as armpit, leg, chest, and facial hair, growth begins around 12 years of age and reaches adult patterns at about 15 to 16 years.
- The onset of sperm emission (spermarche or wet dreams) occurs, on average, at age 14.5 years, but typically starts anywhere from 13 to 17 years.
- African American boys appear to enter puberty sooner than their White counterparts.

SEXUAL RISK BEHAVIOR: THE GOOD, THE BAD, AND THE UNRECOGNIZED

Good News:

- Over the past decade, we have seen a reduction in some sexual risk behaviors in high school students. Those who have ever had sex decreased from 46% to 38%, those with four or more sexual partner contacts decreased from 14% to 9%, and those who have had sex prior to 13 years of age decreased from 6% to 3% (Centers for Disease Control and Prevention [CDC], 2020).
- Teen birth rates have declined significantly largely due to reduced sexual activity and the increase in long-acting reversible contraceptive (LARC) options.

Bad News:

- Condom use among students having sex decreased from 61% to 54% in 2019 (CDC, 2020). This decline follows a period of increased condom use throughout the 1990s and early 2000s.
- Although teens account for only one-quarter of sexually active persons, persons aged 15 to 24 account for half of all new sexually transmitted infections (STIs; CDC, 2019).
- Since 2014, STI rates have been steadily increasing: chlamydia up 19%, gonorrhea up 63%, and syphilis up 71% (CDC, 2019).
- Three out of four teens did not use a method of contraception at their last intercourse.
- The U.S. teen pregnancy rate is substantially higher than in other Western industrialized nations and racial/ethnic and geographic disparities in teen birth rates persist (Romero et al., 2016; Sedgh et al., 2015).
- The majority of teenage girls have intercourse for 18 months before seeking contraception (Romero et al., 2016).
- Teens and emerging adults still face a very real risk of HIV with the highest rates in the United States among young Black men who have sex with men; worldwide heterosexually acquired HIV still predominantly (>90%) occurs in young females.
- Alarmingly, HIV-infected teens are least likely to be connected with appropriate care and, thus, unlikely to effectively suppress their viral load which increases transmission risk to others.

Unrecognized or Connected Risk Factors:

- *Mental health issues* such as depression and anxiety are becoming an epidemic in children and teens. These issues can lead to, or compound, sexual risk behaviors in adolescents (Morrison-Beedy & Mazurek Melnyk, 2019).
- With the numbers of *refugee* adolescents entering the United States, many of whom have had limited to no prior sexual health education, acculturation into U.S. society poses a unique, complicated and often overwhelming challenge, particularly in regard to sexual risk reduction choices.
- *LGBTQ* adolescents are more likely to experience verbal and physical violence as a result of isolation, peer ridicule, abuse, assault, rejection by others, and lack of self-acceptance.
- One out of four LGBTQ youth have experienced sexual dating violence in the prior year and 18% have been forced to have sexual intercourse at some point in their lives (Kann et al., 2016).
- By the time adolescents reach young adulthood, nearly 23% of women and 15% of men have experienced some form of *IPV* (*intimate partner violence*) (Kann et al., 2016).

Evidence-Based Interventions and Legal Issues:

The CDC Compendium lists evidence-based interventions recognized to reduce HIV/STI risk and the Department of Health and Human Services (DHHS) lists recognized Teen Pregnancy Prevention (TPP) programs (DHHS, 2020). Recognized evidence-based interventions (EBIs) have strong evidence for impact and there are a few that address both HIV/STIs and pregnancy risk in teens (e.g., The Health Improvement Project for Teens: *HIPTeens) CDC Synthesis Project (2020)*. EBIs should be considered first for implementation versus "evidence-informed" interventions that have limited weaker evidence of impact. Abstinence education alone is ineffective in reducing sexual risk behaviors and HIV/STIs.

- Most states entitle minors (younger than 18) to receive reproductive health care without parental consent or notification. Check the laws in your state.
- Currently, only 28 states and the District of Columbia mandate sex education. Fifteen states do not require sex education to be any of the following: age-appropriate, medically accurate, culturally responsive, or evidence-based/evidence-informed (Robert Garofalo, 2020).

SEXUAL HEALTH PROTECTIVE/PREVENTIVE OPTIONS

Contraception:

Although many contraceptive options exist, the primary recommendation for teens is the use of LARCs. LARCs are the most effective forms of reversible birth control, are safe and can be removed at any time if pregnancy is desired. Options include:

- **Intrauterine contraceptives (IUCs)**: small, T-shaped devices that are put into the uterus to prevent pregnancy, or;
- **Implants**: a thin, matchstick-sized plastic rod imbedded with hormones that are inserted under the skin of the upper arm.

Emergency Contraception (EC): Two ways to prevent pregnancy after you have unprotected sex:

Option 1: Get a Paragard IUD within 120 hours (5 days) after having unprotected sex. This is the most effective type of emergency contraception.

Option 2: Take an emergency contraceptive pill (AKA the "morning-after pill") within 120 hours (5 days) after having unprotected sex. There are two types of morning-after pills:

- No prescription needed: Brand names are Plan B One Step, Take Action, My Way, After Pill, and others. You can buy these morning-after pills over the counter in most drugstores and pharmacies.
- Prescription needed: You need a prescription from a nurse or doctor to get Brand Name "Ella" emergency contraception, but you can get a fast medical consultation and prescription with next-day delivery. You can take it up to 5 days after unprotected sex, and it works just as well on day 5 as it does on day 1.

Human Papillomavirus Vaccine Recommendations:

- For 9- to 14-year-olds: A two-dose schedule recommended for people who get the first dose before their 15th birthday. In a two-dose series, the second dose should be given 6 to 12 months after the first dose (0, 6–12 month schedule).
- The minimum interval is 5 months between the first and second dose. If the second dose is administered after a shorter interval, a third dose should be administered a minimum of 5 months after the first dose and a minimum of 12 weeks after the second dose.
- For 15- to 26-year-olds: A three-dose schedule recommended for people who get the first dose on or after their 15th birthday, and for people with certain immunocompromising conditions.
- In a three-dose series, the second dose should be given 1 to 2 months after the first dose, and the third dose should be given 6 months after the first dose (0, 1–2, 6 month schedule).
- The minimum intervals are 4 weeks between the first and second dose, 12 weeks between the second and third doses, and 5 months between the first and third doses. If a vaccine dose is administered after a shorter interval, it should be re-administered after another minimum interval has elapsed since the most recent dose.
- For all ages: If the vaccination schedule is interrupted, the vaccine doses do not need to be repeated (no maximum interval).

Provider Impact on Vaccine Uptake:

- If no recommendation or presented as just an option, 20% to 30% elect vaccine.
- If low-quality recommendation, 50%.
- If high-quality recommendation (same way, same day), 70% to 90%. Use the "same way, same day" approach.

PREVENTING NEW HIV INFECTIONS IN TEENS: PRE-EXPOSURE PROPHYLAXIS (PrEP) AND POST-EXPOSURE PROPHYLAXIS (PEP)

PrEP is used by people who are HIV-negative and at high risk for being exposed to HIV through sexual contact or injection drug use. When someone is exposed to HIV through sex or injection drug use, these medicines can work to prevent becoming infected with HIV by keeping the virus from establishing an infection. **PEP** is the use of antiretroviral drugs to stop HIV infection used by people who are HIV-negative after a single high-risk exposure (e.g., sexual assault, needle stick injury). PEP must be started within 72 hours of a possible exposure (the sooner the better) and continued for 4 weeks.

LET'S TALK ABOUT SEX: PARENT, PROVIDER, AND ADOLESCENT COMMUNICATION

- Adolescent sexuality comprises factors over and above the physical changes of sexual maturation and includes developing intimate partnerships, gender identity, and sexual orientation.
- Sexuality is a normal part of childhood and adolescence, with middle adolescence typically the time when teens begin to be interested in more intimate relationships and experimentation.
- Parents can, and should be, the key in helping children and teens develop a healthy sense of their own sexuality; however, addressing these topics can be uncomfortable for both parent and child.
- Primary care providers must talk to their adolescent patients about sexuality at every health maintenance visit and at other appropriate times. The more often providers and parents discuss these issues, the more comfortable they will become in addressing these important needs for children and teens.
- **Talking to teens about sexuality does not promote sexual activity.** Yet, fewer than half of primary care providers asked adolescents about sexual activity and even fewer asked questions about STIs, condom use, sexual orientation, number of partners, or sexual abuse (Robert Garofalo, 2002).
- Healthcare providers should begin discussions with children and parents about the changes of puberty before the onset (approximately age 7 for girls and 9 for boys). By opening up the discussion in your office, parents will be more likely to continue the discussion with their children.
- Young people want to get information about sexuality from their parents and when parents speak to young people about sexuality early, before they become sexually active, adolescents are more likely to delay sexual debut and to be protected when they become sexually active.

CARE SETTINGS

- Discuss sexual health and sexual development (prior to adolescence).
- Discuss healthy behaviors and consent.
- Facilitate communication between parents and children/teens.
- Cervical cancer screening (Pap smear) begins at age 25. Contraception education, with a focus on LARCs, and STI screening should be conducted on all sexually active teens.
- Discuss emergency contraception and HIV testing; familiarize teens with PrEP/PEP.
- Start the HPV vaccine series in girls and boys aged 9–14 years.

- Use a developmental approach to the first pelvic exam. Remember, how the first pelvic exam is conducted will have an influence on further compliance with future pelvic exams.
- Guidelines and up-to-date specific treatments of sexually transmitted diseases (STDs) are available at https://www.cdc.gov/mmwr/volumes/68/rr/rr6805a1.htm

STARTING THE CONVERSATION AND SCREENING

- Explain to a parent or caregiver that you spend a portion of each visit alone with the adolescent.
- Put your patient at ease. Ensure confidentiality except if the adolescent intends to inflict harm or reports being abused. Know your state's laws that affect minor consent and patient confidentiality. The #1 reason that adolescents do not confide in their healthcare providers about their sexuality and sexual risk-taking behaviors is that they have not been assured about confidentiality.
- It is important to inform the adolescent that you will be asking personal questions and that you are asking these questions so you can provide the best possible care. It also is important to let the teen know that you ask these questions of all adolescents. Start with less sensitive topics and use open-ended questions. Clearly explain definitions of sexual terms to ensure understanding.
- It is of great importance that the discussion is open and nonjudgmental. The provider's role is to provide information on healthy behaviors, not to judge the behaviors of the teen. Teens are very sensitive and will likely not return if they feel they are being judged.
- The HEADSS assessment is a good instrument for taking a psychological history from adolescents. Refer to Chapter 1 for additional information about the HEADSS Assessment.

Questions about sexual behaviors Include:

- Some of my patients feel as though they're more of a boy or a girl, or even something else, while their body is going through so many changes. How has this been for you?
- Some patients your age are exploring new relationships. Some people are attracted to guys, some to girls, and some to both. What about you?
- Have you ever had sex with someone? By "sex," I mean vaginal, oral, or anal sex (define).
- Are your sexual activities enjoyable?
- Assess number and gender of lifetime partners, number of partners in the past year. Ask about types of sex (vaginal, oral, anal) and use of protection (condoms and contraception). Satisfaction with methods.
- Have you ever been forced to have sex?
- Have you ever been pregnant (or gotten a girl pregnant)?
- Have you ever been told you have a STI?
- Your body changes a lot during adolescence, and although this is normal, it can also be confusing. What questions do you have about your body and/or sex?

The Guidelines for Adolescent Preventive Services (GAPS) Questionnaire also contain questions about sexuality. These are similar to the HEADSS questions. The GAPS Questionnaire can be completed by the teen while waiting to see the provider, which can save time in a hurried clinical setting. (The GAPS forms are contained in this guide under the Screening and Assessment Section.) A URL for the questionnaire is listed under Resources for Providers.

WHAT SHOULD THE HEALTHCARE PROVIDER DO WHEN A TEEN DISCLOSES THAT HE/SHE IS LESBIAN, GAY, BISEXUAL, TRANSGENDER, OR QUESTIONING?

- Ask whether the teen has disclosed this to his/her family. If yes, what was their reaction? Do they have a trusted adult they can talk to?
- Question carefully about depression and suicidality, as these teens are at higher risk. Refer for mental health services as needed.
- Assess safety at home, school, and work. Ask about bullying or harassment.
- Provide anticipatory guidance around risks that LGBTQ youth may face and discuss concerns about disclosure with teens who have not disclosed to their families. Refer for support and mental health services as needed.
- Counsel about using condoms, contraception, and PrEP/PEP. Adolescents who identify as lesbian or gay may also have sex with members of the opposite sex, which increases the risk for unintended pregnancy.
- Be familiar with resources in the community for teens and parents, such as Parents, Families, and Friends of Lesbians and Gays (www.pflag.org), Healthy Initiatives for Youth (www.hify.org), and The Human Rights Campaign (www.hrc.org), among others.

WHAT TO DO WHEN A TEEN DISCLOSES CURRENT OR FORMER SEXUAL ABUSE OR SEXUAL ASSAULT?

- If the abuse is current, the provider must take the steps required legally for reporting abuse. The teen should be examined by someone certified as a sexual assault nurse/forensic examiner.
- If the abuse or rape was in the past, in addition to providing appropriate physical examination and testing, the provider must ascertain whether the teen has disclosed this before and whether or not he/she received counseling.
- The provider should reassure the teen that what happened was not his/her fault. This reassurance is a key step in providing care to the teen. Discuss the option of counseling.

SUGGESTED RESOURCES FOR PARENTS ABOUT ADOLESCENT SEXUALITY

https://www.cdc.gov/healthyyouth/protective/factsheets/talking_teens.htm

https://www.talkwithyourkids.org/resources-parents/resources-parents.html

https://parentandteen.com/help-parents-talk-comfortably-about-sex/

INTERNET RESOURCES ABOUT SEXUALITY

Amaze

Amaze.org

AMAZE takes the awkward out of sex education with fun, animated videos that provide answers on a wide array of topics including your body, healthy relationships, sex, and personal safety.

The Family Project

www.familiesaretalking.org

The Family Project, which includes the Families Are Talking website and newsletter, is a project of the Sexuality Information and Education Council of the United States (SIECUS, 2020). This project began in 2000 to empower parents and caregivers to communicate with their children about sexuality-related issues, to provide tools to help families communicate about these issues, and to encourage parents, caregivers, and young people to become advocates on the local, state, and national levels for sexuality-related issues including comprehensive sexuality education programs in the schools.

Go Ask Alice!

www.goaskalice.columbia.edu

This is a health question-and-answer internet service produced by Alice! Columbia University's Health Education Program—a division of Health Services at Columbia.

The Teen Health Initiative (THI)

http://www.nyclu.org/thi/frames/thi_frameset.html

The THI was created in 1997 under the auspices of the New York Civil Liberty Union's Reproductive Rights Project (RRP) to work to remove the barriers that prevent young people from accessing critical reproductive health services and information. The THI staff increases awareness of minors' rights to receive confidential reproductive and other healthcare.

INTERNET RESOURCES FOR HEALTHCARE PROVIDERS

The Alan Guttmacher Institute (AGI)

www.agi-usa.org/

This institute is a nonprofit organization focused on sexual and reproductive health research, policy analysis, and public education.

Centers for Disease Control and Prevention (CDC, 2019) Sexual Health

http://www.cdc.gov/sexualhealth/

The CDC provides a wealth of information, including outstanding educational handouts on multiple topics related to sexual health. It also has the current guidelines for STDs.

Guidelines for Adolescent Preventive Services (GAPS) Implementation Materials

www.ama-assn.org/ama/pub/category/1981.html

This site contains multiple resources for how to implement the GAPS tools into clinical practice.

The National Campaign to Prevent Teen Pregnancy

www.teenpregnancy.org/

Founded in February 1996, this is a nonprofit, nonpartisan initiative supported almost entirely by private donations. Its mission is to improve the well-being of children, youth, and families by reducing teen pregnancy.

SIECUS: The Sexuality Information and Education Council of the United States

http://www.siecus.org/

This council has served as the national voice for sexuality education, sexual health, and sexual rights for almost 40 years.

Talking with Kids about Tough Issues

www.talkwithkids.org

This is a national campaign by Children Now and the Kaiser Family Foundation. This website offers practical, concrete tips and techniques for talking easily and openly with young children ages 8 to 12 about some very tough issues, such as sex, HIV/AIDS, violence, drugs, and alcohol. Outstanding educational handouts for dissemination are available.

REFERENCES

Centers for Disease Control and Prevention. (2019). *Sexually transmitted disease surveillance, 2018*. U.S. Department of Health and Human Services. https://www.cdc.gov/std/stats18/STDSurveillance2018-full-report.pdf.

Emmanuel, M., & Bokor, B. (2020). *Tanner stages*. https://www.ncbi.nlm.nih.gov/books/NBK470280/

HIV/AIDS Prevention Research Synthesis Project. (2020). *Compendium of evidence-based interventions and best practices for HIV prevention*. Centers for Disease Control and Prevention.

Kann, L., Olsen, E. O., McManus, T., Harris, W. A., Shanklin, S. L., Flint, K. H., Queen, B., Lowry, R., Chyen, D., Whittle, L., Thornton, J., Lim, C., Yamakawa, Y., Brener, N., & Zaza, S. (2016). Sexual identity, sex of sexual contacts, and health-related behaviors among students in grades 9–12—United states and selected sites, 2015. *Morbidity and Mortality Weekly Report: Surveillance Summaries, 65*(9), 1–202.

Morrison-Beedy, D., & Mazurek Melnyk, B. (2019). Making a case for integrating evidence-based sexual risk reduction and mental health interventions for adolescent girls. *Issues in Mental Health Nursing, 40*(11), 932–941. https://doi.org/10.1080/01612840.2019.1639087. https://pubmed.ncbi.nlm.nih.gov/31403363

National Center for HIV/AIDS, Viral Hepatitis, STD, and TB Prevention. (2020). *Youth risk behavior survey: Data summary & trends report 2009–2019*. Centers for Disease Control and Prevention.

Robert Garofalo, M. D. (2002). Talking to teens about sex, sexuality, and sexually transmitted infections. *Pediatric Annals, 31*(9), 566.

Romero, L., Pazol, K., Warner, L., Cox, S., Kroelinger, C., Besera, G., Brittain, A., Fuller, T. R., Koumans, E., & Barfield, W. (2016). Reduced disparities in birth rates among teens aged 15–19 years—United states, 2006–2007 and 2013–2014. *Morbidity and Mortality Weekly Report, 65*(16), 409–414.

Sedgh, G., Finer, L. B., Bankole, A., Eilers, M. A., & Singh, S. (2015). Adolescent pregnancy, birth, and abortion rates across countries: Levels and recent trends. *Journal of Adolescent Health, 56*(2), 223–230.

SIECUS. (2020). *The SIECUS state profiles 2019/2020*. SIECUS Sex Ed for Social Change. https://siecus.org/state-profiles-2019-2020/

U.S. Department of Health & Human Services. (2021). *Teen pregnancy prevention program*. OASH Office of Population Affairs. https://opa.hhs.gov/grant-programs/teen-pregnancy-prevention-program-tpp

CHAPTER 15

Diana Jacobson, Leigh Small, and Bernadette Mazurek Melnyk

Evidence-Based Assessment and Management of Overweight and Obesity

FAST FACTS

- Although obesity is a chronic medical condition, not a psychological disorder, many researchers and clinicians agree that the psychological and social impact of living with obesity is a risk factor in the development and persistence of mental health problems.
- In adults with mental health disorders, the prevalence of obesity is nearly twice as high as compared to adults without mental health disorders (Allison et al., 2009).
- The research evidence supports the predictive relationship of child emotional and behavioral problems (e.g., high levels of internalizing and externalizing behaviors) and the later life development of obesity or overweight (Duarte et al., 2010; Smith et al., 2020; van Vuuren et al., 2019).
- Psychological and social comorbidities associated with excess body weight in childhood and adolescence include anxiety, depression, poor body image and self-esteem, and decreased social competence and academic achievement (Chao et al., 2020; Harrist et al., 2017; Martin et al., 2018; Small & Aplasca, 2016).
- Routine calculation of body mass index (BMI) of all children 2 years of age and older is essential to identify all children who are overweight or obese. Although not a perfect indicator of body fatness, BMI is a useful tool as an initial screen to classify health risks. Children less than 2 years of age should be routinely assessed for excess body weight through use of weight-for-height calculations that are age and gender adjusted (O'Connor et al., 2017).
- National estimates indicate that over a third of children and adolescents, 2 to 19 years of age, are overweight or obese (Ogden et al., 2016; Hales et al., 2017). In addition, increasing numbers of children and adolescents are now classified as having severe obesity (Skinner et al., 2018).
- Overweight is defined by a BMI greater than the 85th percentile for age and gender. Child and adolescent obesity is defined as having a BMI ≥95th percentile for age and gender. Severe obesity is defined as having a BMI ≥99th percentile.
- The Centers for Disease Control and Prevention (CDC) recommends classifying a BMI of ≥95th percentile as class I obesity; a BMI ≥120% of the 95th percentile as class II obesity; and a BMI ≥140% of the 95th percentile as class III obesity. Using NHANES data from 1999 to 2016, Skinner et al. (2018) determined the following prevalence of pediatric obesity:
  - 26% of preschool children, 2 to 5 years, are overweight or obese; 0.2% class III obesity.
  - 32.8% of school-aged children, 6 to 8 years, are overweight or obese; 1.4% class III obesity.

    - 35.6% of school-aged children, 9 to 11 years, are overweight or obese; 1.0% class III obesity.
    - 38.7% of teens, 12 to 15 years, are overweight or obese; 2.2% class III obesity.
    - 41.5% of teens, 16 to 19 years, are overweight or obese; 4.5% class III obesity.
- About 80% of adolescents with obesity will continue to be obese as adults (Simmonds et al., 2016).
- Waist circumference and waist-by-height ratio is yet another measure of obesity that is an independent predictor of associated severe and chronic comorbid health problems (Lichtenauer et al., 2018).
- The cardiovascular and metabolic consequences of childhood obesity are well known and include insulin resistance, type 2 diabetes, hypertension, dyslipidemia, and atherosclerosis (Expert Panel on Integrated Guidelines for Cardiovascular Health and Risk Reduction In Children and Adolescents, National Heart, Lung, and Blood Institute, 2011).
- Other known health comorbities of excess body weight include polycystic ovary disease, musculoskeletal pain and injury, gastroesophageal reflux, non-alcoholic steatohepatitis, sleep apnea, and increased asthma symptoms (Anderson, 2018; Smith et al., 2020).

Risk Factors (Barlow & Expert Committee, 2007; Smith et al., 2020; Su et al., 2016; Williams et al., 2018)

- Ethnic and minority status (e.g., Hispanic/Latinx, African American, Native American).
- Parental education level.
- Family socioeconomic status.
- Neighborhoods and communities that lack parks, sidewalks, adequate night lighting, and grocery stores that sell fresh produce.
- Neighborhoods and communities with a high crime rate and gun-related violence that prevent children and adolescents from playing or exercising outdoors.
- Adverse childhood experiences.
- Children exhibiting maladaptive internalizing (e.g., withdrawal, depression, and somatization) or externalizing (e.g., hyperactivity and aggression) behaviors.
- Parental or first generation relative who is overweight or obese.
- Family history of first generation or second generation diabetes mellitus (e.g., gestational or type 2 diabetes), metabolic syndrome, hypertension, dyslipidemia, or cardiovascular disease.
- History of low birth weight, large birth, weight, and formula feeding in infancy.
- Rapid weight gain in the first 4 to 12 months of life.
- Adiposity rebound, normally occurring in children who are 5 to 7 years of age, is a critical time during which risk factors can be easily identified and they include:
    - Children with a high BMI during adiposity rebound,
    - Children who experience early adiposity rebound, and
    - Children with rapidly accelerating BMI during adiposity rebound.
- History of psychotropic medications used to treat mental health disorders (see Tables 15.1 and 15.2).
- History of sleep disturbances (e.g., difficulties initiating sleep and/or staying asleep).

Table 15.1 Psychotropic Medications With Increased Risk of Weight Gain

Antidepressants	Mood Stabilizers	Antipsychotics	Anticonvulsant
Paxil (paroxetine)	Lithium (i.e., Eskalith; Lithobid; Lithostat)	Risperdal (risperidone)	Trileptal (oxcarbazepine)
Tricyclic antidepressants (i.e., Elavil (amitriptyline); Norpramin (desipramine) ; Tofranil (imipramine); Vivactil (protriptyline); Sumontil (trimipramine); Anafranil (clomipramine)	Valproate (i.e., Depakote; Depakote ER)	Zyprexa (olanzapine)	
Remeron (mirtazapine)		Clozaril (clozapine)	

Table 15.2 Psychotropic Medications Which Cause Less Weight Gain for Most Children and Adolescents

Antidepressants	Mood Stabilizers	Antipsychotics	Anticonvulsant
Prozac (fluoxetine)	Neurotin (gabapentin)	Abilify (aripiprazole)	Lamictal (lamotrigine)
Luvox (fluvoxamine)	Topamax (topiramate)	Geodon (ziprasidone)	
Lexapro (escitalopram)		Solian (amisulpride)	
Zoloft (sertraline)		Sycrest (asenapine)	
Celexa (citalopram)		Latuda (lurasidone)	
Wellbutrin (buproprion)		Haldol (haloperidol)	
Cymbalta (duloxetine)		Seroquel (quetiapine)	
Effexor (venlafaxine)			

Common Presenting Complaints (Kohut et al., 2019)

- Sleep disturbances;
- Increased asthma symptomology;
- Shortness of breath with activity;
- Depression and/or anxiety, low self-esteem;

- Acanthosis nigricans, striae, or fungal infections of the skin;
- Dysmenorrhea, irregular periods, and hirsutism;
- Gastrointestinal reflux symptoms;
- Hip, knee, and/or foot pain or injury;
- Elevated blood pressure; and
- Somatic complaints (e.g., frequent abdominal pain or headache).

SCREENING FOR OVERWEIGHT AND OBESITY

- Children <2 years of age: Determination of age and gender adjusted height for recumbent weight percentile. Overweight = height for length >95th percentile for age and gender.
- Children 4 to 8 years: Waist circumference ≥ 90th percentile and/or waist-by-height ratio greater than .5.
- Children ≥ 2 years of age: Determination of child/adolescent height and weight with calculation of age and gender absolute BMI and adjusted BMI percentile.
- The U.S. Preventive Services Task Force (USPSTF) (O'Connor et al., 2017), the 2007 Expert Committee (Barlow & Expert Committee, 2007) and the 2011 National Heart, Lung, and Blood Institute Expert Panel (Expert Panel on Integrated Guidelines for Cardiovascular Health and Risk Reduction in Children and Adolescents, National Heart, Lung, and Blood Institute, 2011) recommend that primary care clinicians screen children aged 2 years and older for obesity. The USPSTF found adequate evidence that BMI was an acceptable measure for identifying children and adolescents with excess weight.

Assessment

- Historical information to determine modifiable lifestyle factors (Barlow & Expert Committee, 2007; Cardel et al., 2020; Small et al., 2017; Spear et al., 2007; Taylor, 2020):
    - Overall dietary quality and quantity (e.g., portion sizes, balance of macronutrients (e.g., carbohydrates, fats, saturated fats, and protein) and micronutrients (e.g., vitamins and minerals), meal frequency, and snacking.
    - High intake patterns of energy dense foods and sweetened beverages including fruit juice and sodas.
    - High frequency of fast food and fast/frozen meal consumption.
    - Limited home cooked family meals.
    - Low dietary intake of fruits and vegetables, calcium, and fiber.
    - Limited frequency of breakfast consumption.
    - High frequency of meals and/or snacks consumed while involved in screen time activities.
    - Presence of binge eating, bulimia, boredom eating, emotional eating, and night eating.
    - Assessment of average screen time (e.g., television, computer, gaming, and cell phone texting) use per day.
    - Assessment of the average quality and quantity of physical activity per day
    - Average number of hours of sleep each night and usual bedtime routine. Include distractions from adequate sleep (e.g., TV in bedroom, access to cell phones or technology at night).

- Historical information to identify risk for physical comorbid health problems:
    - Snoring, daily fatigue, sleep difficulties, or daytime sleepiness.
    - Respiratory complaints of shortness of breath, exercise intolerance, frequent coughing, or wheezing.
    - Abdominal pain (recurrent or non-specific), heartburn or chest pain, constipation, and/or encopresis and/or right upper quadrant abdominal pain.
    - Polyuria, polyphagia, and polydipsia.
    - Nocturia, enuresis, and incontinence.
    - Menstrual irregularities and dysmenorrhea.
    - Frequent headache.
    - Lower limb pain or frequent injuries.
    - Acne, striae, hirsutism, skin rash, and/or skin problems.
- Historical information to identify risk for comorbid psychosocial/mental health problems (Hamburger et al., 2011; Herzong & Schmahl, 2018; Miller & Lumeng, 2018):
    - Recipient of weight-related victimization (i.e., bullying or teasing) at home, school, or childcare.
    - Avoidance of social situations appropriate for age, social exclusion, peer rejection, or difficulties with social interactions.
    - Reluctance or avoidance to participate in physical activities (i.e., home, family-associated, or group).
    - Decreased confidence in ability to be physically active.
    - Poor academic achievement or underachievement.
    - School avoidance and school absences for illness or truancy.
    - Sleep problems (e.g., delayed sleep onset, frequent awakenings, early rising, nightmares, insomnia, or hypersomnia).
    - History of sexual, physical, or emotional abuse.
    - Binge eating with or without self-induced vomiting.
    - Fatigue, listlessness, withdrawn, flat affect, depressive symptoms, or apathy.
    - Increased worries relative to other children and/or generalized anxiety.
    - Body dissatisfaction.
    - Low self-esteem or self-neglect.
    - Anger, aggression, irritability, or hyperactivity.
- Historical information to identify risk for socioeconomic factors related to childhood obesity (Adams, 2020; Johnson & Johnson, 2015; Martin et al., 2018; Singh et al., 2010; Williams et al., 2018):
    - Negative family dynamics.
    - Parenting style and food-parenting practices.
    - Low family socioeconomic status.
    - Low parental education.
    - Parental smoking.
    - Limited access or ability to purchase healthy foods.
    - Limited safe play areas (e.g., no sidewalks, parks, or recreation centers).

- Poor housing.
- High stress environments.
- Food insecurity
- School policies related to healthy eating and physical activity opportunities

- Assessment of child and/or parent/caregiver's readiness to change and increase healthy lifestyle behaviors (Miller & Rollnick, 2013; Rosengren, 2018; Taylor, 2020):
  - Consistent with the principles of motivational interviewing, assess the felt importance of the problem, desire to change behaviors, and confidence in ability to change behaviors.
  - Identify personal, familial, social, contextual, and environmental barriers to making behavioral change (i.e., potential and actual family perceptions).
  - Identify personal and familial attributes and strengths, as well as social, contextual, and environmental facilitators of behavior change.
  - Determine the degree of supportiveness in the relationship between the parent and child (parent–child "fit") and potential need for alternative support systems.
  - Identify the child's temperament and/or personality style that may influence the type and methods of environmental and behavioral change strategies.
- Targeted physical examination focus and findings to assess for obesity comorbidities:
  - Blood pressure using the correct cuff size to evaluate for hypertension
    - Diagnostic parameters: ≥95th percentile for age, gender and height on ≥3 separate occasions.
  - Acanthosis nigricans
  - Tonsillar hypertrophy
  - Goiter
  - Genu varum, genu valgum, pes planus
  - Abnormal gait: Limited hip range of motion or pain elicited during exam
  - Fundoscopic examination to rule out papilledema
  - Liver span assessment
  - Tanner stage to examine for precocious or delayed puberty onset, micropenis, and/or undescended testes
  - Acne, striae, and/or hirsutism
  - Assessment of waist circumference at the umbilicus and superior spine of the iliac crests. Determine waist circumference percentile: Intervention initiation indicated if calculated waist-by-height ratio is greater than 0.5 regardless of BMI.
  - Serum blood analyses are evaluated depending upon family history, age, and risk.
    - All overweight or obese children over 2 years of age should have a fasting lipid panel.
    - Children ≥10 years of age with a BMI of 85th to 94th percentile with risk factors for type 2 diabetes should have a lipid panel ordered and if other risk factors are present (e.g., positive family history of hyperlipidemia) should, additionally, have a fasting glucose, ALT and AST levels ordered. These test(s) are repeated every 2 years.
      - Type 2 diabetes risks factors include: family history of diabetes, high-risk racial/ethnic background (e.g., Black, Latinx, or Native American), polycystic

ovarian syndrome, acanthosis nigricans and/or cardiovascular disease risk factors.

- Children ≥10 years of age with a BMI of 95th or greater percentile should have a fasting lipid panel, fasting glucose, ALT and AST levels ordered and repeated every 2 years. If the AST and/or AST levels are above 60 U/L on two occasions, then referral to a gastroenterologist is recommended.

Diagnosis

- Age and gender adjusted weight for recumbent length ≥95th percentile = overweight for children ≤2 years of age.
- BMI percentile ≥85th–94th BMI percentile = overweight for children and adolescents 2 to 19 years of age = overweight.
- BMI percentile ≥95th percentile or absolute BMI ≥30 = obese for children and adolescents 2 to 19 years of age = obesity.
- BMI percentile >99th percentile for children and adolescents 2 to 19 years of age = morbid obesity.

Management of Weight Goals by Age

- 2 to 5 years of age for those with 85 to 94th BMI percentile: Weight maintenance until BMI is <85th percentile or demonstration of slowing of weight gain (e.g., decreasing BMI trajectory).
- 2 to 5 years of age for those with ≥95th BMI percentile: Weight maintenance until BMI is <85th BMI percentile or gradual weight loss of no more than 1 lb. per month if the BMI is >21.
- 6 to 11 years of age for those with 85 to 94th BMI percentile: Weight maintenance until BMI <85th BMI percentile, slowing of weight gain, or decrease in absolute BMI.
- 6 to 11 years of age for those with 95 to 99th BMI percentile: Weight maintenance until BMI <85th BMI percentile, slowing of weight gain, or decrease in absolute BMI (e.g., goal of approximately 1 lb. gradual weight loss per month).
- 6 to 11 years of age for those with >99th BMI percentile: Weight loss (e.g., goal of weight loss is no more than 2 lb. per week).
- 12 to 19 years of age for those with 85 to 94th BMI percentile: Weight maintenance until BMI <85th BMI percentile, slowing of weight gain, or decrease in absolute BMI (e.g., goal of no more than 2 lb. gradual weight loss per week).
- 12 to 19 years of age for those with 95 to 98th BMI percentile: Weight loss of no more than 2 lb. per week).
- 12 to 19 years of age for those with >99th BMI percentile: Weight loss not to exceed 2 lb. per week.
- Parent, family, or other engagement and support has been empirically found to be an important element.
- Behavioral and cognitive strategies are a component of effective healthy weight interventions.

Assessment Tools

Formal assessment tools for bullying behavior (aggressor/perpetrator), victims of bullying, and child social assessment tools are available at no cost from:

1. The National Center for Injury Prevention and Control compendium of assessment tools can be found at www.cdc.gov/violenceprevention/pdf/bullycompendium-a.pdf (Hamburger et al., 2011)
2. Revised the Bullying Prevalence Questionnaire and the Revised Pro-Victim Scale (Rigby, 1997) are available with scoring instruction at www.kenrigby.net/01a-Questionnaires
3. Sizing Me Up—Weight Related Quality of Life (Zeller & Modi, 2009). This instrument is available free of charge after permission is granted from the authors. Information can be found at www.cincinnatichildrens.org/research/divisions/b/psychology/labs/zeller/hrqol-pediatric-obesity/sizing/default/

Perpetrator and victim assessment tools, which are available for a cost:

1. Peer Relations Assessment Questionnaires-Revised (PRAQ-R) (Rigby, 1997) is available for schools to assess the presence of bullying behavior at www.kenrigby.net/01a-Questionnaires.
2. Pediatric Quality of Life Inventory Child-Self-Report (5–18 years of age) and Parent-Proxy Report (2–18 years of age) (PedsQL™) (Varni et al., 2003) are instruments measuring health-related quality of life and are available for clinical practice. These instruments can be found at www.pedsql.org/about_pedsql.html.

Household food insecurity:

1. Although there has been exerted effort to improve the quality of food offered at community food banks, children living in homes with food insecurity often receive supplemental packaged and processed foods that have longer shelf life but are lacking in quality and do not include fresh fruits and vegetables. Food insecurity can be assessed using the U.S. Department of Agriculture (USDA) 18-item Household Food Security Survey. It can be accessed at www.ers.usda.gov/topics/food-nutrition-assistance/food-security-in-the-us/survey-tools/.
2. The Hunger Vital Sign™ (Hager et al., 2010) uses just two of these survey items and has been found to have 97% sensitivity and 83% specificity. Answering "Often true" or "Sometimes true" is a positive screen for the following statements: (a) "Within the past 12 months, we worried whether our food would run out before we got money to buy more."; and (b) "Within the past12 months, food we bought just didn't last and we didn't have money to get more." More information can be found at the Children's HealthWatch website childrenshealthwatch.org/public-policy/hunger-vital-sign/

Adverse Childhood Experiences (also see Chapter 10, Helping Children and Parents Through Marital Separation and Divorce):

Adverse childhood experiences (ACEs) are assessed by the use of the ACE assessment questionnaires. Interrelated and accumulating sources of stress that children experience in early life include physical, sexual, or emotional abuse; physical and emotional neglect; household dysfunction (e.g., parental mental health and substance use disorder); domestic violence; incarcerated family members; and acrimonious parental marital divorce or separation (Herzong & Schmahl, 2018; Hughes et al., 2017). For a complete list of questionnaires that screen for exposure to ACEs, see the excellent review by Oh et al. (2018).

The following screening tools are free to download from the internet:

1. Center for Youth Wellness (CYW)—ACE-Q Materials. These questionnaires are available in English and Spanish. The CYW Adverse Childhood Experiences Questionnaire for Children is 17 items and is completed by the parent/caregiver of children ages 0 to 12 years. The CYW Adverse Childhood Experiences Questionnaire for Adolescents is 19 items and is completed by the parent/caregiver for youth ages 13 to 19 years. The Adverse Child Experiences Questionnaire for Adolescents: Self Report is also 19 items and is completed by youth ages 13 to 19 years. All questionnaires can be found at centerforyouthwellness.org/aceq-pdf/
2. Children's Trauma Assessment Center Trauma Screening Checklist Ages 0 to 5 years and ages 6 to 18 years can be downloaded from wmich.edu/traumacenter/resources-0
3. The Pediatric ACEs and Related Life-events Screener (PEARLS) was developed by the Bay Area Research Consortium on Toxic Stress and Health. The screening tool is available in English, Spanish, and 15 other languages, and can be downloaded from www.acesaware.org/screen/screening-tools-additional-languages/

EVIDENCE-BASED OVERWEIGHT AND OBESITY MANAGEMENT BY STAGE OF OVERWEIGHT AND OBESITY (Barlow & Expert Committee, 2007; Kohut et al., 2019; Spear et al., 2007)

Stage 1: Prevention Plus (Barlow & the Expert Committee, 2007)—Youth between the ages of 2 and 19 years with BMI >85th percentile

- Focus on educating families concerning basic healthy lifestyle eating and activity behaviors utilizing motivational interviewing (Miller & Rollnick, 2013) techniques:
    - Consume ≥5 servings of fruits and vegetables every day.
    - Eliminate sugar-sweetened beverages (i.e., juice, soda, and sports drinks).
    - Decrease screen time to ≤2 hours per day. No television for children under 2 years of age.
    - Increase moderate to vigorous physical activity to at least 60 minutes each day.
    - Limit portion sizes.
    - Prepare family meals at least 5 to 6 times a week to decrease fast and restaurant food consumption.
    - Eat a healthy breakfast every day.
    - Allow child to self-regulate his/her meals and avoid over-restrictive feeding practices.
    - Involve the family in all lifestyle changes respecting cultural differences and developmental age of the child/adolescent.
- Motivational interviewing principles include:
    - Express empathy.
    - Avoid argumentation.
    - Support self-efficacy.
    - Roll with resistance.
    - Develop discrepancy.
- Use patient/family-centered problem-solving including:
    - Identify the barriers.
    - Have a patient/family generate potential strategies to work through unhealthy behaviors contributing to the child/adolescent's energy imbalance.

- Patient/family chooses initial goals to target.
- Evaluate the strategy.

- Follow up for 3 to 6 months, meeting with the child/adolescent and the family in the office setting at mutually agreed upon times.
- If there is no improvement in lifestyle behaviors and in the child's health/weight, the provider offers the next level of weight management.

Stage 2: Structured Weight Management—Children 2 to 19 years of age with BMI >85 to 99th percentile.

- Lifestyle habits as in Stage 1.
- Motivational interviewing techniques continue to be utilized for the family to set healthy lifestyle behavior goals for nutrition and physical activity.
- Include the following as family/patient goals:
  - Three structured, balanced daily eating plan and 1 to 2 planned snacks of foods that are low in energy density and high in fiber; no sugar sweetened beverages.
  - Decreased screen time to ≤ 1-hour each day
  - Planned and supervised physical activity of at least 60 minutes each day.
  - Diet and physical activity logs (e.g., diaries).
  - Planned reinforcement for achieving targeted behaviors.
- More formal nutritional plan may require the expertise of a dietician.
- Monthly follow-up office visits or group sessions.
- If there is no improvement in meeting weight, exercise, and nutrition goals, the provider offers the next level of weight management.

Stage 3: Comprehensive Multidisciplinary Intervention—Children 2 to 19 years of age with BMI >95th percentile

- Maximize primary care office and specialist support given to the child/adolescent and family to increase behavior change.
- Eating and activity goals are similar to Stages 1 and 2.
- Goal setting and food and physical activity monitoring are structured with behavior modification techniques (e.g., food monitoring, goal setting, contingency management).
- Parent involvement and training in improving the home environment is imperative especially with children <12 years of age.
- Child or adolescent must be assessed for mental health issues along with assistance of others in a multidisciplinary team (e.g., registered dietician, exercise specialist, counseling, social worker).
- Primary care provider continues to manage all medical problems and provide a supportive alliance with families.
- Weekly multidisciplinary counseling for a minimum of 8 to 12 weeks, then monthly.
- Generally, not possible in the primary care setting.
- Only increase to Stage 4 after discussing the ongoing risks and patient and family motivation to improve physical activity and dietary habits.

Stage 4: Tertiary Care Intervention—Children >11 years of age with BMI >95 – 99th percentile

- Severely obese youth who have attempted the Stages 1 to 3 recommendations from a multidisciplinary team without success.
- Medications such as sibutramine or orlistat may be initiated for children, 12 years or older, in conjunction with a structured diet and exercise program (safety and efficacy in younger children is untested). Other medications such as Belviq (lorcaserin), Qsymia (phentermine-topiramate), Saxenda (liraglutide), and Contrave (naltrexone-bupropion) have been approved in adults but are not recommended for children under 18 years of age.
- Very low-calorie restrictive diets and weight control surgery may be offered by the tertiary team to adolescents who have not responded to intensive Stage 3 treatment modalities.
- Stage 4 treatments should occur in pediatric weight management centers.

USPSTF RECOMMENDATIONS FOR MANAGEMENT

O'Connor et al. (2017), for the USPSTF, found that effective comprehensive weight-management pediatric primary care programs incorporated counseling and other interventions that targeted diet and physical activity. Interventions also included motivational interviewing and behavioral management techniques to assist in behavior change. Interventions that focused on younger children incorporated parental involvement as a component as did the most intensive interventions for older children and adolescents.

Moderate- to high-intensity lifestyle-based weight loss trials involved participation in interventions that ranged from one session to 122 sessions and contact hours ranged from 0.25 to 122 hours over 2.25 to 24 months.

Findings indicated that weight management interventions with more than 26 contact hours were effective in reducing BMI in children and adolescents after 6 or 12 months. The control group children, across studies, gained 8 to 17 pounds. The trials that did not show statistically significant results did show greater reductions in weight as compared to the control groups. Although the most intensive interventions demonstrated decreases in blood pressure, improvements in fasting insulin, glucose, or lipids were not found regardless of intervention length or intensity.

Although the children and parents were identified, screened, and recruited from pediatric primary care settings, the most effective interventions took place outside of the clinic and included group sessions for both children and parents in dietary management and physical activity. These trials used cognitive behavioral interventions including goal setting, stimulus control, contingency rewards, problem solving, and self-monitoring of behaviors and emotions.

PSYCHOTROPIC MEDICATION USE AND OVERWEIGHT/OBESITY

Weight gain is associated with the use of many psychotropic medications, including antidepressants, mood stabilizers, and antipsychotic drugs (see Tables 15.1 and 15.2). There is an increased risk for reduced life expectancy due to cardiometabolic diseases in persons with severe mental illness (Correll et al., 2015; Mazereel et al., 2020). Recognizing the increased risk of metabolic consequences (e.g., obesity, diabetes mellitus, dyslipidemia) of psychotropic medications is essential for healthcare providers (Nicol et al., 2018). In addition, the younger the age of the child at initiation of psychotropic medications, the more adverse side effects occur over the child's lifetime.

Several management options are available if a child or adolescent is gaining weight at an accelerated pace after the initiation of one of these therapeutic agents. When it is assessed that the child or adolescent taking psychotropic medications is gaining weight abnormally, the practitioner may choose to change to another drug (e.g., collaboratively consult with the mental health provider if not the prescribing provider). In addition, the provider should provide nutritional counseling and encourage increased physical activity. The provider may need to initiate a referral to specialty mental health care for behavioral treatment and management. Prevention of weight gain for children and adolescents requiring psychotropic medications is the best approach and begins by routinely choosing medications that have been shown to cause less weight gain, and by educating and counseling parents and children/adolescents about healthy lifestyles and the weight gain risks of these medications. It is noted that the primary reason adolescents stop taking their prescribed psychotropic medication is due to weight gain.

Upon initiation of any psychotropic medication, routine management should include monitoring of weight, BMI, blood pressure, fasting glucose, fasting cholesterol and triglyceride levels, and glycosylated hemoglobin (hemoglobin A1C). Guidelines from the American Psychological Association (2020) recommend monitoring the child or adolescent's weight monthly for the first 3 months and then at least every 3 months thereafter.

THE COPE HEALTHY LIFESTYLES TEEN PROGRAM FOR THE PREVENTION OF AND MANAGEMENT OF OVERWEIGHT/OBESITY AND DEPRESSION

The Creating Opportunities for Personal Empowerment (COPE) and Healthy Lifestyles TEEN (Thinking, Emotions, Exercise and Nutrition) Program is a manualized 15-session cognitive behavioral therapy based program that can be integrated into middle- and high-school educational curriculum or delivered in small groups or individually in primary care practices and community settings to improve both physical and mental health outcomes in children and youth (Melnyk, 2003). The manualized program, which can be delivered by teachers or health professionals, consists of 15 sessions, including seven cognitive behavioral therapy–based skills-building sessions and eight sessions that focus on nutrition and physical activity (see Table 15.3). Each session incorporates 20 minutes of physical activity to increase youth confidence that they can incorporate it into their daily routine. A 4-hour online training session must be completed before permission is provided to deliver the program. Please see www.COPE2Thrive.com.

Findings from a full-scale cluster randomized controlled trial funded by the National Institutes of Health/National Institute of Nursing Research with 779 culturally diverse adolescents in 11 high schools indicated that the youth who received the COPE TEEN program compared to those who received an attention control program had higher levels of physical activity, a lower BMI, and higher academic competence, social skills, and grade performance post-intervention. Teens in the COPE group with extremely elevated depression scores at pre-intervention had significantly lower depression scores than the attention control group. Alcohol use also was lower in the COPE group. COPE teens had higher health course grades than did control teens. At 6 months post-interventions, COPE teens had a lower mean BMI than teens in the attention control group. The proportion of those overweight was significantly different from pre-intervention to 6-month follow-up with COPE decreasing the proportion of overweight teens, versus an increase in overweight in the attention control adolescents (Melnyk, Jacobson, et al., 2013).

Twelve months following the interventions, COPE teens had a significantly lower BMI than attention control teens. There was a significant decrease in the proportion of overweight and obese COPE teens from baseline to 12 months compared to the attention control group. For youth who began the study severely depressed, COPE teens had significantly lower depression compared to the attention control teens (Melnyk et al., 2015). The National Cancer Institute selected the 15-session COPE TEEN program as an obesity control program for its Research Tested Intervention Programs and gave it the highest rating for its dissemination capability (see ebccp.cancercontrol.cancer.gov/programDetails.do?programId=22686590). Research using COPE with college students also has had similar positive outcomes (Melnyk, Kelly, et al., 2013).

RESOURCES FOR PARENTS AND PROVIDERS

American Academy of Pediatrics, Health Issues/Obesity: https://www.healthychildren.org/English/health-issues/conditions/obesity/Pages/default.aspx

Table 15.3. Content in the 15-Session COPE Healthy Lifestyles TEEN Programs

Session #	Session Content	*Key Constructs From the Conceptual Model and COPE Intervention*
1	Introduction of the COPE Healthy Lifestyles Pre-TEEN program and goals.	*Beginning introduction of cognitive behavioral skills building (CBSB)*
2	Healthy lifestyles and the thinking, feeling, behaving triangle.	*CBSB*
3	Self-esteem. Positive thinking/self-talk.	*CBSB*
4	Goal setting. Problem-solving.	*CBSB*
5	Stress and coping.	*CBSB*
6	Emotional and behavioral regulation.	*CBSB*
7	Effective communication. Personality	*CBSB*
8	Barriers to goal progression and overcoming barriers. Energy balance. Ways to increase physical activity and associated benefits.	*CBSB and Physical Activity Information*
9	Heart rate. Stretching. Physical activity and its positive effects on mental and physical health.	*Physical Activity Information*
10	Food groups and a healthy body. Stoplight diet red, yellow and green.	*Nutrition Information*
11	Nutrients to build a healthy body. Reading labels. Effects of media and advertising on food choices.	*Nutrition Information*
12	Portion sizes "super-size." Influence of feelings on eating.	*Nutrition Information*
13	Social eating. Strategies for eating during parties, holidays, and vacations.	*Nutrition Information*
14	Snacks. Eating out.	*Nutrition Information*
15	Integration of skills to develop a healthy lifestyle plan. Putting it all together	*CBSB*

*Twenty minutes of physical activity is included in each session to build beliefs about engaging in regular physical activity.

- Creates awareness for parents and providers of strategies that will improve both the nutritional intake and physical activity level of children and teens

Centers for Disease Control and Prevention, Division of Nutrition, Physical Activity and Obesity: https://www.cdc.gov/nccdphp/dnpao/resources/child-teen-resources.html

- Provides parent and providers information concerning childhood obesity and resources to support best practices

Centers for Disease Control and Prevention; Healthy Weight, Nutrition and Physical Activity: https://www.cdc.gov/healthyweight/children/index.html

Centers for Disease Control and Prevention, Injury Prevention & Control: Violence Prevention

http://www.cdc.gov/violenceprevention/pub/measuring_bullying.html

- Provides a compendium of bullying assessment tools to assess the behavior of perpetrators, victims and bystanders

Institute of Medicine, Accelerating Progress in Obesity Prevention: https://pubmed.ncbi.nlm.nih.gov/24830053/

- Reports on the state of the science in the most efficacious prevention of overweight and obesity interventions

National Academy of Medicine; Obesity: https://nam.edu/tag/obesity/

- Provides up-to-date resources for providers and parents with a multitude of resources and aggregated obesity treatment strategies, as well as outlining the gaps in the research

Dietary Guidelines for Americans: https://www.dietaryguidelines.gov/

- Provides the most up-to-date dietary guidelines for parents and providers

Let's Move: https://letsmove.obamawhitehouse.archives.gov/learn-facts/epidemic-childhood-obesity

- Provides parents, providers, and communities recommendations for food and nutrition and physical activity for children and families

Mental Health Medications, National Institutes of Mental Health: http://www.nimh.nih.gov/health/publications/mental-health-medications/complete-index.shtml

- Provides information for parents and providers concerning the medications that are commonly prescribed for mental health disorders

Robert Wood Johnson Foundation, Childhood Obesity: https://www.rwjf.org/en/our-focus-areas/topics/childhood-obesity.html

- Discusses the state of improvement in nutrition policies for schools meals in the United States

U.S. Department of Agriculture, Choose My Plate: http://www.choosemyplate.gov/

- Nutritional information and handouts for parents and providers focused on improving meal planning and dietary intake of children and teens.

REFERENCES

Adams, J. (2020). Addressing socioeconomic inequalities in obesity: Democratising access to resources for achieving and maintaining a healthy weight. *PLOS Medicine, 17*(7), e1003243. https://doi.org/10.1371/journal.pmed.1003243

Allison, D. B., Newcomer, J. W., Dunn, A. L., Blumenthal, J. A., Fabricatore, A. N., Daumit, G. L., Cope, M. B., Riley, W. T., Vreeland, B., Hibbeln, J. R., & Alpert, J. E. (2009). Obesity among those with mental health disorders: A national institute of mental health meeting report. *American Journal of Preventive Medicine, 36*(4), 341–350. https://doi.org/10.1016/j.amepre.2008.11.020

American Psychological Association (APA). Guideline Development Panel for Treatment of Obesity. (2020). Summary of the clinical practice guideline for the multicomponent behavioral treatment of obesity and overweight in children and adolescents. *APA, 75*(2), 178–188. https://doi.org/10.1037/amp0000530

Anderson, K. L. (2018). A review of the prevention and medical management of childhood obesity. *Child and Adolescent Psychiatric Clinics of North America, 27*, 63–76. https://doi.org/10.1016/j.chc.2017.08.003

Barlow, S. E., & Expert Committee. (2007). Expert committee recommendations regarding the prevention, assessment, and treatment of child and adolescent overweight and obesity: Summary report. *Pediatrics, 120*(Suppl. 4), S164–S192. https://doi.org/10.1542/peds.2007-2329C

Cardel, M. I., Atkinson, M. A., Taveras, E. M., Holm, J.-C., & Kelly, A. S. (2020). Obesity treatment among adolescents: A review of current evidence and future directions. *JAMA Pediatrics, 174*(6), 609–617. https://doi.org/10.1001/jamapediatrics.2020.0085

Chao, A. M., Wadden, T. A., & Berkowitz, R. I. (2020). Obesity in adolescents with psychiatric disorders. *Current Psychiatry Reports*, *21*(1), 3. https://doi.org/10.1007/s11920-019-0990-7

Correll, C. U., Detraux, J., De Lepeleire, J., & De Hert, M. (2015). Effects of antipsychotics, antidepressants and mood stabilizers on risk for physical diseases in people with schizophrenia, depression and bipolar disorder. *World Psychiatry*, *14*(2), 119–136. https://doi.org/10.1002/wps.20204

Duarte, C. S., Sourander, A., Nikolakaros, G., Pihlajamaki, H., Helenius, H., Piha, J., Kumpulainen, K., Moilanen, I., Tamminen, T., Almqvist, F., & Must, A. (2010). Child mental health problems and obesity in early adulthood. *The Journal of Pediatrics*, *156*(1), 93–97. https://doi.org/10.1016/j.jpeds.2009.06.066

Expert Panel on Integrated Guidelines for Cardiovascular Health and Risk Reduction in Children and Adolescents, National Heart, Lung, and Blood Institute (2011). Expert panel on integrated guidelines for cardiovascular health and risk reduction in children and adolescents: Summary report. *Pediatrics*, *128*(S56), S213–S258. https://doi.org/10.1542/peds.2009-2107C

Hager, E. R., Quigg, A. M., Black, M. M., Coleman, S. M., Heeren, T., Rose-Jacobs, R., Cook, J. T., Ettinger de Cuba, S. E., Casey, P. H., Chilton, M., Cutts, D. B., Meyers, A. F., & Frank, D. A. (2010). Development and validity of a 2-item screen to identify families at risk for food insecurity. *Pediatrics*, *126*(1), 26–32. https://doi.org/101542/peds.2009-3146

Hales, C. M., Carroll, M. D., Fryar, C. D., & Ogden, C. L. (2017). Prevalence of obesity among adults and youth: United States, 2015-2016. *NCHS Data Brief*, *288*, 1–8. PMID: 29155689

Hamburger, M. E., Basile, K. C., & Vivolo, A. M. (2011). *Measuring bullying victimization, perpetration, and bystander experiences: A compendium of assessment tools*. CDC, National Center for Injury Prevention and Control. https://www.cdc.gov/violenceprevention/pdf/bullycompendium-a.pdf

Harrist, A. W., Topham, G. L., Hubbs-Tait, L., Shriver, L. H., & Swindle, T. M. (2017). Psychosocial factors in children's obesity: Examples from an innovative line of inquiry. *Child Developmental Perspectives*, *11*(4), 275–281. https://doi.org/10.1111/cdep.12245

Herzong, J. I., & Schmahl, C. (2018). Adverse childhood experiences and the consequences on neurobiological, psychosocial, and somatic conditions across the lifespan. *Frontiers in Psychiatry*, *9*, Article 420. https://doi.org/10.3389/fpsyt.2018.00420

Hughes, K., Bellis, M. A., Hardcastle, K. A., Sethi, D., Butchart, A., Mikton, C., Jones, L., & Dunne, M. P. (2017). The effect of multiple adverse childhood experiences on health: A systematic review and meta-analysis. *The Lancet*, *2*(8), E356–E366. https://doi.org/10.1016/S2468-2667(17)30118-4

Johnson, J. A., & Johnson, A. M. (2015). Urban-rural differences in childhood and adolescent obesity in the United States: A systematic review and meta-analysis. *Childhood Obesity*, *11*(3), 233–241. https://doi.org/10.1089/chi.2014.0085

Kohut, T., Robbins, J., & Panganiban, J. (2019). Update on childhood/adolescent obesity and its sequela. *Current Opinion in Pediatrics*, *31*, 645–653. https://doi.org/10.1097/MOP.0000000000000786

Lichtenauer, M., Wheatley, S. D., Martyn-St. James, M., Duncan, M. J., Cobayashi, F., Berg, G., Berg, G., Musso, C., Graffigna, M., Soutelo, J., Bovet, P., Kollias, A., Stergiou, G. S., Grammatikos, E., Griffiths, C., Ingle, L., & Jung, C. (2018). Efficacy of anthropometric measures for identifying cardiovascular disease risk in adolescents: Review and meta-analysis. *Minerva Pediatrics*, *70*(4), 371–382. https://doi.org/10.23736/S0026-4946

Martin, A., Booth, J. N., Laird, Y., Sproule, J., Reilly, J. J., & Saunders, D. H. (2018). Physical activity, diet and other behavioural interventions for improving cognition and school achievement in children and adolescents with obesity or overweight. *Cochrane Database of Systematic Reviews*, *1*(3), CD009728. https://doi.org/10.1002/14651858.CD0099728.pub4

Mazereel, V., Detraux, J., Vancampfort, D., van Winkel, R., & De Hert, M. (2020). Impact of psychotropic medication effects on obesity and the metabolic syndrome in people with serious mental illness. *Frontiers in Endocrinology*, *11*, Article 573479. https://doi.org/10.3389/fendo.2020.573479

Melnyk, B. M. (2003). *The creating opportunities for personal empowerment (COPE) healthy lifestyles TEEN (Thinking, Emotions, Exercise and Nutrition) program*. COPE2Thrive, LLC.

Melnyk, B. M., Jacobson, D., Kelly, S. A., Belyea, M. J., Shaibi, G. Q., Small, L., O'Haver, J., & Marsiglia, F. F. (2013). Promoting healthy lifestyles in high school adolescents: A randomized controlled trial. *American Journal of Preventive Medicine*, *45*(4), 407–415. September 10, 2013. [Epub ahead of print] https://doi.org/10.1016/j.amepre.2013.05.013

Melnyk, B. M., Jacobson, D., Kelly, S. A., Belyea, M. J., Shaibi, G. Q., Small, L., O'Haver, J. A., & Marsiglia, F. F. (2015). Twelve-month effects of the COPE healthy lifestyles TEEN program on overweight and depression in high school adolescents. *Journal of School Health*, *85*(12), 861–870.

Melnyk, B. M., Kelly, S., Jacobson, D., Arcoleo, K., & Shaibi, G. (2013). Improving physical activity, mental health outcomes and academic retention of college students with freshman 5 to thrive: COPE/healthy lifestyles. *Journal of the American Academy of Nurse Practitioners*, *26*(6), 314–322.

Miller, A. L., & Lumeng, J. C. (2018). Pathways of association from stress to obesity in early childhood. *Obesity*, *26*, 1117–1123. https://doi.org/10.1002/oby.22155

Miller, W. R., & Rollnick, S. (2013). *Motivational interviewing: Helping people change* (3rd ed.). The Guilford Press.

Nicol, G. E., Yingling, M. D., Flynn, K. S., Schweiger, J. A., Patterson, B. W., Schechtman, K. B., & Newcomer, J. W. (2018). Metabolic effects of antipsychotics on adiposity and insulin sensitivity in youths: A randomized controlled trial. *JAMA Psychiatry*, *75*(8), 788–796. https://doi.org/10.1001/jamapsychiatry. 2018.108824

O'Connor, E. A., Evans, C. V., Burda, B. U., Walsh, E. S., Eder, M., & Lozano, P. (2017). Screening for obesity and interventions for weight management in children and adolescents: A systematic evidence review for the U.S. Preventive services task force. Evidence synthesis No. 150. *Agency for Healthcare Research and Quality*, *317*(23), 2427–2444. https://doi.org/10.1001/jama.2017.0332

Ogden, C. L., Carroll, M. D., Lawman, H. G., Fryar, C. D., Kruszon-Moran, D., Kit, B. K., & Flegal, K. M. (2016). Trends in obesity prevalence among children and adolescents in the United States, 1988-1994 through 2013-2014. *Journal of the American Medical Association*, *315*(21), 2292–2299. https://doi.org/10.1001/jama.2016.6361

Oh, D. L., Jerman, P., Boparai, S. K. P., Koita, K., Briner, S., Bucci, M., & Harris, N. B. (2018). Review of tools for measuring exposure to adversity in children and adolescents. *Journal of Pediatric Health Care*, *32*(6), 564–578. https://doi.org/10.1016/j.pedhc.2018.04.021

Simmonds, M., Llewellyn, A., Owen, C. G., & Woolacott, N. (2016). Predicting adult obesity from childhood obesity: A systematic review and meta-analysis. *Obesity Reviews*, *17*(2), 95–107. https://doi.org/101111/obr.12334

Singh, G. K., Siahpush, M., & Kogan, M. D. (2010). Socioeconomic status and other factors associated with childhood obesity. *Health Affairs*, *29*(3), 503–512. https://doi.org/10.1377/hlthaff.2009.0730

Skinner, A. C., Ravanbakht, S. N., Skelton, J. A., Perrin, E. M., & Armstrong, S. C. (2018). Prevalence of obesity and severe obesity in US children, 1999-2016. *Pediatrics*, *141*(3), e20173459. https://doi.org/10.1542/peds.2017-3459

Small, L., & Aplasca, A. (2016). Childhood obesity and mental health: A complex interaction. *Child and Adolescent Psychiatric Clinics of North America*, *25*(2), 269–282. https://doi.org/10.1016/j.chc.2015.11.008

Small, L., Thacker, L., Aldrich, H., Bonds-McClain, D., & Melnyk, B. (2017). A pilot intervention to address behavioral factors that place overweight/obese young children at risk for later-life obesity. *Western Journal of Nursing*, *39*(8), 1192–1212. https://doi.org/10.1177/01939459/7708316

Smith, J. R., Fu, E., & Kobayashi, M. (2020). Prevention and management of childhood obesity and its psychological and health comorbidities. *Annual Review of Clinical Psychology*, *16*, 351–378. https://doi.org/10.1146/annurev-clinpsy-100219-060201

Spear, B. A., Barlow, S. E., Ervin, C., Ludwig, D. S., Saelens, B. E., Schetzina, K. E., & Taveras, E. M. (2007). Recommendations for treatment of child and adolescent overweight and obesity. *Pediatrics*, *120*(Suppl. 4), S254–S288. https://doi.org/10.1542/peds.2007-2329F

Su, S., Jimenez, M. P., Roberts, C. T. F., & Loucks, E. B. (2016). The role of adverse childhood experiences in cardiovascular disease risk: A review with emphasis on plausible mechanisms. *Current Cardiology Reports*, *17*(10), 88. https://doi.org/10.1007/s11886-015-0645-1

Taylor, J. (2020). Looking beyond lifestyle: A comprehensive approach to the treatment of obesity in the primary care setting. *The Journal for Nurse Practitioners*, *16*, 74–78. https://doi.org/10.1016/j.nur.pra.2019.09.021

Rigby, K. (1997). Attitudes and beliefs about bullying among Australian school children. *Irish Journal of Psychology*, *18*(2), 202–220. https://doi.org/10.1080/03033910.1997.10558140

Rosengren, D. B. (2018). *Building motivational interviewing skills: A practitioner workbook*. (2nd ed.). The Guilford Press.

van Vuuren, C. L., Wachter, G. G., Veenstra, R., Rijnhart, J. J. M., van der Wal, M. F., Chinapaw, M. J. M., & Busch, V. (2019). Associations between overweight and mental health problems among adolescents, and the mediating role of victimization. *BMC Public Health*, *19*, 612. https://doi.org/10.1186/s12889-019-6832-z

Varni, J. W., Burwinkle, T. M., Seid, M., & Skarr, D. (2003). The PedsQL™ 4.0 as a pediatric population health measure: Feasibility, reliability and validity. *Ambulatory Pediatrics*, *3*, 329–341. https://doi.org/10.1367/1539-4409(2003)003<0329:tpaapp>2.0.co:2

Williams, A. S., Ge, B., Kruse, R. L., McElroy, J. A., & Koopman, R. J. (2018). Socioeconomic status and other factors associated with childhood obesity. *The Journal of the American Board of Family Medicine*, *31*(4), 514–521. https://doi.org/10.3122/jabfm.2018.04.170261

Zeller, M. H., & Modi, A. C. (2009). Development and initial validation of an obesity-specific quality of life measure for children: Sizing Me Up. *Obesity*, *17*, 1171–1177. https://doi.org/10.1038/oby.2009.47

Information for Parents: Overweight/ Obesity in Children and Teens

WHAT IS CONSIDERED OVERWEIGHT OR OBESE IN CHILDREN AND TEENS?

Body mass index (BMI) percentile is a measurement used to determine if a child or adolescent is overweight or obese. Children found to be greater than the 85th percentile for age and gender are considered overweight. Children found to be greater than the 95th percentile for age and gender are considered obese. These guidelines were established by many professional organizations, including the American Academy of Pediatrics. If you are unsure whether your child or teen is overweight, have your child's healthcare provider calculate their BMI percentile for you or consult one of the many webs that will help you to calculate your child's BMI (www.cdc.gov/healthyweight/bmi/calculator.html). Heavily muscled athletes may be over*weight*, but not over*fat*, and excess body fat is the primary cause of the medical complications associated with a high BMI.

HOW CAN OVERWEIGHT AFFECT SOMEONE'S HEALTH?

Excessive weight can cause a wide variety of health problems, including:

- Type 2 diabetes,
- High blood pressure,
- Worsening of asthma,
- Heart disease,
- Sleep apnea,
- Gastro esophageal reflux, and
- Poor coping and more mental health problems (e.g., depression, anxiety, low self-esteem).

WHAT CAUSES OVERWEIGHT?

An unhealthy environment can increase a person's risk for gaining excess weight. Stress, inability to exercise, and in ability to buy healthy foods add to a person's chance of becoming overweight. Sometimes, the kinds of food and how much is eaten each day can be more than what the person needs for their energy and activity levels. If this energy imbalance continues, the body will store the extra energy as fat and put on extra weight.

WHICH CHILDREN/TEENS ARE AT RISK TO BECOME OVERWEIGHT?

Scientists who study overweight in children and teens have identified things that place certain children and teens at high risk for overweight.

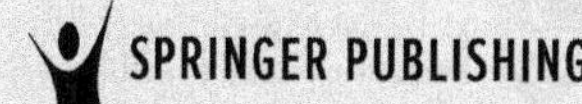

Those risk factors include:

- Overweight in the toddler and preschool years.
- Sitting for most of the day (e.g., too much computer or television viewing time).
- Family members, parents or caretakers who are overweight or obese.
- Food intake that is high in calories from fat and sugar but also low in fiber.
- Decreased servings of fruits and vegetables each day.
- High stress levels.
- Not enough sleep.

WHAT ARE THE TREATMENTS FOR OVERWEIGHT IN CHILDREN AND TEENS?

It is important that overweight in children and teens be treated using a focus on increasing healthy lifestyle habits. Discuss with your healthcare provider how you can increase:

- Healthy dietary intake.
- Regular exercise or activity.
- Manage stress in healthy ways.

WHAT CAN YOU DO TO HELP YOUR CHILD WITH THEIR WEIGHT?

There are a few simple steps that you can begin with your child or teen to help them to make positive, healthy lifestyle changes:

- Decrease the amount of sugared beverages (e.g., soda, fruit punch, sports drinks). Mostly drink water every day. Skim milk provides essential nutrients and may satisfy hunger but drink no more than two glasses each day.
- Decrease the amount of television viewing time and/or game computer time to 2 hours per day.
- Provide a moderately low fat diet by baking and roasting instead of frying foods.
- Provide healthy snacks for your family such as fruit, whole grain crackers, and low-fat cheese.
- Engage in healthy family activities on a regular basis. Reward your child or teen with trips to the park, the mall, a board game, a walk or a bike ride.
- It is best to improve the whole family's diet instead of restricting food for only one child or teen.
- Be a positive and supportive influence on your child or teen and model regular healthy eating and activity habits.
- Build your child's or teen's self-esteem by focusing on their special characteristics and strengths.

- Help your child or teen build their beliefs and confidence in their ability to start and keep healthy behaviors.
- Agree to work on one healthy lifestyle goal at a time instead of tackling too much at one time.

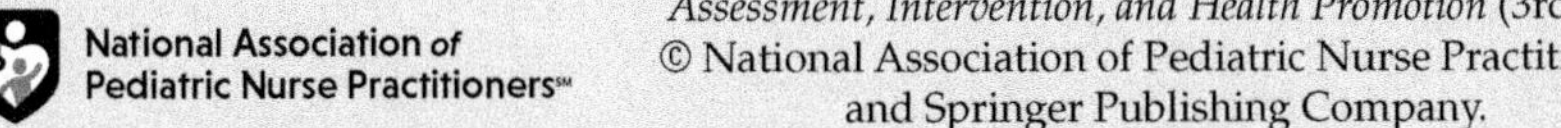

SPRINGER PUBLISHING

CHAPTER 16

Neil Herendeen

Reimbursement for Mental/Behavioral Health Services in Primary Care

FAST FACTS

- Getting reimbursed for the time and effort that you spend caring for children with psychosocial and mental health issues requires a working knowledge of the diagnostic coding system and local practices of your third-party payers.
- There are two parts to your billing submission, the service code and the diagnosis code. The Current Procedural Terminology (CPT) code set is maintained by the American Medical Association and describes medical, surgical, and diagnostic **services**. It is designed to communicate uniform information about medical services and procedures as well as help to establish reimbursement values for each type of service. The CPT code is often referred to as the *level* of billing.
- *The International Classification of Diseases (ICD)* coding book is updated yearly (the current version is *ICD-11*) and has thousands of diagnostic codes from which to choose. Although these are nationally accepted tools, you may risk a rejected claim if your local insurers have restrictions on certain codes. The list in Table 16.1 is meant to save time sorting through the entire coding book, but you may want to ask your local insurance company if they recognize a specific code before you submit your bill.

ROUTINE EVALUATION AND MANAGEMENT CODES FOR OFFICE VISITS

No two offices are the same when it comes to providing for the psychosocial needs of your primary care patients. Many offices are integrating mental/behavioral health therapists in their medical home. However, given limited access to psychology and psychiatry resources for children, many primary care providers also are finding themselves taking over the prescribing duties for psychoactive medications. Certain billing codes are meant for primary care providers or psychiatric nurse practitioners while others are restricted for use by psychologists and master's level therapists.

The year 2021 brought revisions to billing for outpatient visits with less emphasis on specific elements of the review of systems or physical exam and more emphasis on the level of medical decision-making or total length of time spent caring for the patient. Medical decision-making is considered straightforward, low, moderate, or high based on two out of three elements of medical decision-making.

1. Number and complexity of problems addressed.
2. Amount and/or complexity of the data to be reviewed and analyzed.
3. Risk of consequences and/or morbidity or mortality of patient management (Table 16.1).

Documentation of the history and physical exam is essential for medical communication and assumed to be completed by the medical provider with the appropriate level of detail. It will be up to the provider to determine the most appropriate criteria to bill under based on the individual patient

Table 16.1 CPT Codes for Billing of Services in Established Patients

CPT Code Established Patient	Medical Decision-Making	Time Spent	
99212	Straightforward	10–19 min	
99213	Low	20–29 min	
99214	Moderate	30–39 min	
99215	High	40–54 min	
99354 face to face time	Prolonged service >54 min	+15 min increments	99358 (non-face to face)

CPT, Current Procedural Terminology.

circumstances. For patients with a long list of minor complaints or a single concern for which you spend a long time in motivational interviewing and counseling, the time-based billing criteria may be in your best interest. For well-known patients with high levels of medical complexity or high-risk behavior who you can see in less than 30 minutes, you may be best served using medical decision-making criteria. For established patient visits that exceed 55 minutes, you may add a prolonged service code for each additional 15 minutes spent caring for the patient on the day of the encounter (i.e., 99358 ×2 for 16–29 minutes of prolonged service).

Reimbursable activities have been expanded to include:

- Preparing to see the patient (e.g., review of tests).
- Obtaining and/or reviewing separately obtained history.
- Performing a medically appropriate examination and/or evaluation.
- Counseling and educating the patient/family/caregiver.
- Ordering medications, tests, or procedures.
- Referring and communicating with other healthcare professionals.
- Documenting clinical information in the electronic or other health record.
- Independently interpreting results and communicating results to the patient/family/caregiver.
- Care coordination.

As was true before, the time counted is the time personally spent by the billing provider on the calendar date of the encounter (not the time spent by medical students, residents, or nurses who contribute to the overall office experience). Suggested wording to add to your documentation is: "I personally spent __ minutes on the calendar day of the encounter, including pre- and post-visit work."

For Mental/Behavioral Health Integration:

Starting in January of 2017, the Centers for Medicare and Medicaid Services (CMS) approved payment for services provided to patients with mental/behavioral health disorders who are participating in psychiatric collaborative care programs or are receiving mental/behavioral health integration services. The CMS has classified this group of services as "Behavioral Health Integration" (BHI) services and it includes three codes describing Psychiatric Collaborative Care Management services (CoCM) (G0502, G0503, G0504) and General BHI service (G0507). Coverage for these services includes patients with a behavioral health or substance use disorder who receive coverage through a traditional Medicare plan or Medicare advantage plan.

What is Collaborative Care Management (CoCM)?

Psychiatric CoCM typically is provided by a primary care team consisting of a primary care provider and a care manager who work in collaboration with a psychiatric consultant, such as a psychiatrist. Care is directed by the primary care team and includes structured care management with regular assessments of clinical status using validated tools and modification of treatment as appropriate. The psychiatric consultant provides regular consultations to the primary care team to review the clinical status and care of patients and to make recommendations. The treating primary care provider (PCP) submits the claims for these services. The consulting psychiatrist and the care manager are then paid by the PCP through a contract, employment, or other arrangement. Although meant for adults with Medicare, these codes may be available to you in the care of children depending on local insurer policies.

CODING FOR REVIEWING SCREENING TOOLS AND FORMS

Codes 96110 Developmental screening (e.g., developmental milestone survey [ASQ/M-CHAT], speech and language delay screen) and 96127 Brief emotional/behavioral assessment (e.g., depression inventory [PSC 17/SCARED], attention-deficit/hyperactivity disorder [Vanderbilt] scale), with scoring and documentation, per standardized instrument are both practice expense only codes. They are not meant to be reimbursement for provider work but can be added on to well child or follow-up visits.

G8431 and G8510 cover all postpartum depression screenings of mothers provided during the infant's medical checkups or follow-up visits. Each state and commercial insurer stipulates the payment ($2.50 to $30) and how often you can bill for maternal screening.

DOCUMENTING THE FOLLOW-UP PLAN

The follow-up plan is the proposed outline of treatment to be conducted as a result of clinical screening. Follow-up for positive depression screening must include one or more of the following: additional evaluation, suicide risk assessment, referral to a practitioner who is qualified to diagnose and treat depression, pharmacological interventions, other interventions, or follow-up for the diagnosis of depression. The documented follow-up plan must be related to positive depression screening, for example: "Patient referred for psychiatric evaluation **due to** positive depression screening."

CODING FOR THE DELIVERY OF BRIEF COGNITIVE BEHAVIORAL SKILLS BUILDING PROGRAMS FOR DEPRESSION AND ANXIETY

The delivery of brief cognitive behavioral skills building intervention programs, such as the Creating Opportunities for Personal Empowerment (COPE) program for children, teens, and college youth/young adults (Melnyk, 2003, 2020) (see brief interventions section) can be billed as 99214.

99214 is the code assigned to the medical service that meets the following requirements:

1. The patient is an established one; this is not their first visit to the office.
2. It must be an outpatient visit.
3. It must meet the definition of moderate level of medical decision-making OR the time spent by the provider on direct and indirect patient care and coordination equals 30 to 39 minutes.

CODING FOR TELEMEDICINE

The CPT manual lists 79 standard CPT codes for which a "95" modifier can be used to indicate that the service was provided via a real-time, interactive audio and video telecommunications system. A number of these codes are used daily in most pediatric practices. For example, the list includes the commonly used office or other outpatient evaluation and management (E/M) codes for new patient (99201–99205) and established patient visits (99212–99215). A variety of consultation codes are included as well (e.g., 99241–99245). Behavioral health codes also are on the list (e.g., behavioral change intervention codes 99406–99408). Some insurers prefer the use of GQ or GT as modifiers for synchronous video visits or store and forward visits so you will need to check with your local insurers for appropriate billing procedures. During the COVID-19 pandemic, many restrictions have been lifted for the patient originating site, provider location, types of services, telemedicine platform security, and payment parity, however, it is unclear which policies will continue after the emergency status is lifted.

COMMON DIAGNOSES USED IN PRIMARY CARE PEDIATRICS

These are some of the more common diagnoses that you will use when caring for the psychosocial needs of your pediatric patients:

ICD 10 code

F41.9	Anxiety state: unspecified
F41.1	Generalized anxiety disorder
F48.9	Suicide ideation
F34.1	Dysthymic disorder
F43.21	Brief depressive reaction
F33.0	Major depressive disorder, recurrent mild
F31	Bipolar disorder, unspecified
313.81	Oppositional disorder
F43.22	Adjustment disorder *with* anxious mood
F43.25	Adjustment disorder *with* mixed emotions and conduct
F43.24	Adjustment disorder *with* conduct disturbance
F43.21	Adjustment disorder *with* depressed mood
F43.29	Adjustment disorder *with* physical symptoms
F43.10	Post-traumatic stress disorder, unspecified
G47.9	Sleep disturbance, unspecified
Z55.3	Academic underachiever disorder
F90.0	Attention deficit hyperactivity disorder, inattentive
F90.2	Attention deficit hyperactivity disorder, combined type
E66.01	Obesity, morbid
E66.9	Obesity, unspecified
Z71.3	Dietary counseling
R62.0	Delayed developmental milestones
F84.0	Autism
Z62.820	Counseling for parent/child problem
Z71.1	Feared condition, not present
F99	Other unknown and unspecified cause (still trying to figure it out)
T43.95XA	Adverse effects of psychoactive medication
F99	Mental disorder, not otherwise specified

REFERENCES

Melnyk, B. M. (2003). *Creating Opportunities for Personal Empowerment (COPE) programs for children, teens and college youth/young adults*. COPE2Thrive, LLC.

Melnyk, B. M. (2020). Reducing healthcare costs for mental health hospitalizations with the evidence-based COPE Program for child and adolescent depression and anxiety: A cost analysis. *Journal of Pediatric Health Care, 34*(2), 117–121. https://doi.org/10.1016/j.pedhc.2019.08.002

CHAPTER 17

Pamela Lusk and Bernadette Mazurek Melnyk

Brief Evidence-Based Interventions for Child and Adolescent Mental Health

FAST FACTS

- One in five U.S. children and adolescents between the ages of 6 and 17 has a treatable mental health disorder, such as depression and anxiety problems, yet 50% of these children do not receive necessary treatment or counseling from a health professional. Primary care providers (PCPs) have become the main providers of mental health services for their patients (Whitney & Peterson, 2019).
- Building on long-standing relationships with children and their families along with an emphasis on development, early intervention, and prevention, pediatric practices are the ideal setting for the integration of mental health into primary care.
- Federal, organizational, and professional initiatives strongly support integration. The American Academy of Pediatrics and private foundations are supporting initiatives to develop the evidence base and provide tools for primary care providers to implement mental health services in order to improve access and evidence-based treatment.
- The primary care setting is ideal for initiating services to children with emerging developmental and behavioral problems as well as common mental health disorders.
- A paradigm shift is needed in the United States from sick and crisis care to prevention and wellness as a majority of chronic diseases, including mental health conditions, can be prevented with healthy lifestyle behaviors such as physical activity, healthy eating, stress reduction, and not smoking or using drugs and alcohol.
- Childhood is the foundation for the rest of adult life; children and teens must be equipped with coping and problem-solving skills in order to deal with the stressors they will encounter and prevent mental health problems.
- One model for working with families that is being used successfully in many healthcare settings is SBIRT. SBIRT information is located on the SAMHSA–HRSA Integrated Health Solutions website. The SBIRT model grew out of an Institute of Medicine (now called the National Academy of Medicine) recommendation that called for community-based screening for health risk behaviors, including substance use.
- SBIRT stands for:

  Screening

  Brief **I**ntervention

  Referral

  Treatment

- In the SBIRT model, effective strategies for intervention are started in primary care prior to more extensive or specialized treatment.
- As with other approaches that started as models for alcohol/drug prevention and intervention in primary care, the SBIRT approach is being endorsed by mental health organizations to address other mental health concerns, such as depression and anxiety.
- Use of screening tools for children and teens (e.g., the Pediatric Symptom Checklist, Vanderbilt ADHD parent form) is the first step in the SBIRT model and are easily incorporated into pediatric outpatient practices as an evidence-based way to assess patients for mental health problems.
- Referral to and consultation with mental health professionals for specialty psychiatric treatment is always a consideration in primary care, depending on the presentation of the child and family, and availability of psychiatric treatment providers in the community. In many communities, there are long wait lists for child psychiatric evaluation and treatment, which is why equipping pediatric healthcare providers with excellent skills in preventing, screening, assessing, and providing evidence-based treatment for common mental health disorders is so important.
- Continuing education courses, such as the KySS Online Child and Adolescent Mental Health Course housed at The Ohio State University College of Nursing prepares primary care providers to screen, assess, and manage common mental health problems in primary care settings. See nursing.osu.edu/offices-and-initiatives/office-continuing-education/kyss-mental-health-fellowship-child-and
- Ideally, the intensity of the mental health services will match the intensity of the child's needs.

The **brief interventions** presented in this chapter are evidence-based interventions that can be provided by primary care providers in the context of brief office visits or several standard office visits. Brief interventions can be used as a stand-alone treatment for those at risk as well as a vehicle for engaging those in need of more intensive specialized care.

With brief interventions, the clinician can begin to actively address the child/teen and family's mental health concerns within the time constraints of busy outpatient practices even as the child is awaiting psychiatric services.

Some Important Points About Brief Interventions

- Commonly used by clinicians to talk to patients about health issues or medication adherence.
- Designed for use in busy clinical settings.
- Can be started right away with the resources found in outpatient practices.
- Generally 5 to 15 minutes in duration, but no more than 30 minutes.
- Can be used as stand-alone treatment as well as a vehicle for engaging those in need of more intensive specialized care.
- Include behavioral approaches, supportive counseling, parent focused interventions, motivational interviewing and cognitive behavioral therapy (CBT)–based skills-building techniques.

  From: The National Institute on Alcohol Abuse and Alcoholism (NIAAA) and SAMHSA http://www.samhsa.gov/prevention/SBIRT/index.aspx, http://nihcm.org/pdf/PediatricMH-FINAL.pdf

WHEN DELIVERING BRIEF INTERVENTIONS

- Use an empathetic, non-confrontational style.
- Engage the child/teen/family and offer choices.
- Emphasize patient responsibility and accountability.
- Convey confidence in the child, teen, and/or family's ability to change.

MENTAL HEALTH PROMOTION AND EARLY INTERVENTION WITH PARENTS

The one evidence-based change in practice that can provide the greatest impact for children and families is modifying the parent's perception of their child, and how that child compares with other children by emphasizing the child's individual positive strengths.

Parent based interventions are evidence-based for many common child and adolescent mental health disorders (American Academy of Pediatrics—Evidence-Based Psychosocial Interventions).

It has long been recognized that parents' perceptions of their children (i.e., how they see their children compared to other children) may be a powerful determinant in a child's future well-being.

It is often the case that modifying the parent's perception of their child (cognitive reframing) can make a huge difference in the quality of the parent–child relationship and significantly improve that child's life (Yearwood et al., 2021).

Parents value the expertise and opinion of their PCP and generally want to be seen as "good" parents. They are accustomed to anticipatory guidance at their child's visits. Therefore, PCPs are in an ideal position to intentionally modify a parent's healthy perceptions of their children.

Some individuals have struggles with parenting. There are some parents who have harsh and critical parenting styles, while others are too permissive or seem indifferent to the child. No matter what challenging behaviors the parent displays, the best way to help a child is to work hard to develop a provider/parent working relationship and "nurture" the parent into being the best parent they are capable of being. Sometimes, this will seem a very slow process with only tiny glimpses of progress, but it is well worth the effort for the child.

Clinicians can leverage the parent's trust in the healthcare provider and belief in the provider's expertise in all aspects of children's health to "normalize" behaviors that concern parents but are fairly common at certain developmental stages. If there are diagnosable mental disorders, it is important to de-stigmatize those disorders as having a neurodevelopmental base.

A specific strategy for working with parents is modification of their perception of the child (cognitive reframing).

- Starting at the very first visit, the positive traits of that individual child can be identified by the provider and documented. Documentation implies importance for the parent and helps the provider keep the list of the child's strengths in the chart as important clinical data.
- This same approach is followed with the parents. The parents' particular strengths and the contributions the parents have made to the child's development of skills are recognized. Strengths in the parent/child relationship are pointed out by the clinician as they are observed. Even "super challenging" parents will have one or two positives that can be noted and reinforced.
- Not only does this approach serve to engage parents into a working alliance, but it provides an opportunity to role model the positive approach employed with the child. This intervention can be used with all ages and stages of children, even the very young.

Engagement with the child and family is enhanced when the clinician provides positive feedback for behaving in developmentally appropriate ways or when the parent is praised for responding sensitively to their child during the visit.

Clinicians can role model at every visit, focusing on the child's unique strengths (instead of only talking about problem behaviors) with the goal of guiding the parent into changing negative perceptions of the child to a more positive view.

Clinical Example of the Cognitive Reframing Technique for Parents

> The parent says: "Johnny is tearing up everything in the house. He takes apart everything, his toys, his sister's things, the vacuum cleaner, everything. ………".
>
> The provider might say, "Johnny seems to be very curious and that can be an outstanding trait. Probably famous inventors like Edison or the new inventors of smart phones were boys like that. Johnny, what do you learn from taking toys apart, have you discovered the parts inside the toys? Are you good with tools?" Then the parent can be asked, "Who in the family shares Johnny's curiosity? Who else is good with their hands and tools?"
>
> "Is there a way to promote Johnny's curiosity, but not have other family members' things taken apart?" "Let's set a rule today about what is off limits for Johnny's toolkit and then when he comes in for his next appointment, he can tell me about some new discovery he has made."

Pediatric providers can serve as the parents' support and coach and, in the SBIRT model, provide referral information (along with brief intervention), to connect that family with support services and a network of other parents in a similar situation. Providing written materials for home reading also reinforces what the clinician is teaching.

Brief Interventions Provided Routinely by Pediatric Practitioners

Pediatric providers routinely provide brief psychosocial interventions in their practices. The literature increasingly supports the importance of brief psychosocial interventions in increasing families' abilities to problem solve. Psychosocial interventions include:

- **Active Monitoring**: When a symptom or concern first presents, the PCP often uses screening tools and reschedules the family for a return visit, which is sooner than would normally be scheduled so that active monitoring of the child's symptom can occur. The PCP counsels the family about developmental parameters, when to ignore the child's symptoms, and when the presentation requires immediate attention.
- **Behavioral Interventions**: Most pediatric clinicians have an assortment of favorite behavior strategies that they use in counseling parents about behavior management: checklist/monitoring, reward charts, special times, logical consequences, planned ignoring, goal setting/target behaviors, positive and negative reinforcements, and time-outs and time-ins.
- **Supportive Counseling**: Related to developmental changes or significant losses, such as loss by death of a family member or pet or environmental stresses (e.g., moving, changing schools).

As more practices move toward integration of mental health/behavioral health care into primary care, professionals in the practice will be educated in specific brief evidence-based interventions, such as motivational interviewing (MI) and cognitive behavioral approaches.

Motivational Interviewing to Modify Health Behaviors in Primary Care

One approach that has been used successfully to change or modify health behaviors in primary care settings is MI. MI has been used to address many of the basic health concerns we see with young people of all ages (e.g., alcohol use, smoking, exercise, unhealthy eating) (Miller & Rollnick, 2012).

MI is a counseling intervention, based on the Stages of Change Theory and Rogerian client-centered psychotherapy, which has been found to be effective in eliciting behavior change to promote health and reduce risk in adults. Evidence is accumulating to support similar effects of MI with adolescents, especially in the area of substance abuse prevention and early intervention, but also with peer violence and overweight/obesity. Although risky behaviors are a leading cause of preventable morbidity and mortality, behavioral counseling interventions to address them are not commonly used in healthcare settings.

Developmentally, young people are likely to be receptive to self-guided behavior change strategies, a cornerstone of brief interventions.

What is MI?

MI is a "client-centered, directive method for enhancing intrinsic motivation to change by exploring and resolving ambivalence" (Miller & Rollnick, 2012). Originally, it was designed for multiple sessions of 30 minutes or longer, but MI has been adapted for brief (5 to 15 minute) encounters in a variety of settings.

Essential principles of motivational interviewing:

- Express empathy,
- Develop discrepancy,
- Roll with resistance, and
- Support self-efficacy.

Spirit of MI:

- Readiness to change is a state (such as depression), not a trait (such as optimism).
- Change comes from the client.
- Resolving ambivalence is the client's task.
- Helping client explore ambivalence:
  - Avoid direct persuasion,
  - Quiet, eliciting, respectful style.
- Provider–client partnership.

How Do Clinicians Facilitate Change?

Clinicians need to understand why people do change, do not change, and how they change.

Why People Do Not Change

People do not change when the sum of the forces discouraging change is greater than the sum of the forces encouraging change (e.g., when what a person likes about smoking is greater than what they don't like about smoking, or their fear about quitting may be greater than the imagined benefits of quitting).

Why People Change

People change when the sum of the forces encouraging change is greater than the sum of the forces discouraging change (e.g., when the perceived negative consequences of drinking outweigh the benefits of drinking).

How People Change

Stages of Change	Intervention by Healthcare Provider
Pre-contemplation – not considering change	Increase awareness
Contemplation – considering change, but ambivalent	Facilitate resolution of ambivalence
Preparation – willing to accept direction, anxious about change	Help the client develop an action plan
Action – learning the new behavior	Solve problems related to new behavior
Maintenance – stable in the new behavior	Review successes, reinforce healthy behavior
Relapse – reappearance of old behavior – a process, not an event	Move into action once again

TOOLS FOR MOTIVATIONAL INTERVIEWING

- Agenda Setting: Client determines priorities, e.g., "What would you like to talk about today?"
- Getting Permission: e.g., "I'd like to spend a few minutes talking about…Is that okay with you?"
- Open-ended questions to get started, e.g., "Tell me about……" "Help me understand….."
- Reflective Listening: e.g., "It sounds like you are feeling…" "It sounds like that is important to you."
- Summarizing: e.g., "So it sounds like you have two strong reasons why you want to quit, but on the other hand you worry that you will experience stress during the quitting process."
- Eliciting Self-Motivational Statements: Change talk.
- Willing: e.g., "On a scale of 1 to 10 – with 0 being not willing to 10 being very willing, how willing (motivated, interested) are you to walk the dog every day?"
- Importance: e.g., "On a scale of 0 to 10 with 0 being not confident at all to 10 being very confident, assuming you decided to … (begin exercising, quit smoking), how confident are you that you can succeed?"

Eliciting Strengths and Barriers

Example: "You said your confidence to change is a 7. Why did you say 7 instead of 0 or 1"?

Example: "You said your level of interest was 5. Why isn't it a 9 or 10. "

Providing Information without Interpreting for the Client

Example: "Chlamydia can increase a woman's risk of pelvic infections and infertility. What do you think about that?"

Closing the Deal

Example: "Where does that leave you?" "Where do we go from here?"

Markers of a Productive MI Encounter

- Client does most of the work.
- Client accepts the possibility for change.
- Client accepts the responsibility for change.
- Upward slope of commitment language within or between sessions.
- Dancing, not wrestling.

BRIEF COGNITIVE BEHAVIOR–BASED INTERVENTIONS

Following is the American Academy of Pediatrics' (AAP) Evidence-based Child and Adolescent Psychosocial Interventions chart. The interventions in the AAP chart generally represent treatment protocols that involve 60-minute visits over a period of time in specialty practices that have been replicated in university and community settings. The interventions that have the strongest research evidence to support them are listed, and it is clear that there is strong support for cognitive behavioral approaches for a variety of mental health conditions in children and adolescents.

- Cognitive behavioral approaches have the strongest level of evidence to support efficacy for child and adolescent anxiety, depression, substance abuse, and traumatic stress—mental health problems that commonly present at pediatric primary care visits.
- While cognitive behavior therapy (CBT) should be conducted by mental health professionals who have appropriate education and sufficient training to conduct this type of therapy, there are key components of CBT or cognitive behavioral skills that can be learned and incorporated into practice by other healthcare professionals (e.g., PCPs) in targeting symptoms such as stress, anxiety, and mild to moderate depression as well as assisting children and teens in coping with life stressors and learning to problem-solve and goal set.
- Cognitive behavioral concepts combined with skills-building exercises can be delivered in primary care and pediatric settings as a brief intervention.
- CBT-based brief interventions integrated into medication management visits can "jump start" improvement and increase adherence to treatment plans (Sudak & Taormina, 2018).
- Depending on the child's age and developmental level, parents will be involved in the CBT-based intervention in different ways. It is important that the parent understand *how* ***these*** interventions can benefit their child and family.
- Incorporating CBT interventions into medication management visits is effective

EVIDENCE-BASED CHILD AND ADOLESCENT PSYCHOSOCIAL INTERVENTIONS

This report is intended to guide practitioners, educators, youth, and families in developing appropriate plans using psychosocial interventions. It was created for the period October 2018 – April 2019 using the PracticeWise Evidence-Based Services (PWEBS) Database, available at www.practicewise.com. If this is not the most current version, please check the AAP mental health website (www.aap.org/mentalhealth) for updates.

Please note that this chart represents an independent analysis by PracticeWise and should not be construed as endorsement by the AAP. For an explanation of PracticeWise determination of evidence/level, please see below or visit www.practicewise.com/aap.

Problem Area	Level 1-BEST SUPPORT	Level 2-GOOD SUPPORT	Level 3-MODERATE SUPPORT	Level 4-MINIMAL SUPPORT	Level 5-NO SUPPORT
Anxious or Avoidant Behaviors	Attention Training, Cognitive Behavior Therapy (CBT), CBT and Medication, CBT for Child and Parent, CBT With Parents, Education, Exposure, Modeling	Assertiveness Training, Attention, CBT and Expression, CBT and Parent Management Training (PMT), CBT With Parents Only, Cultural Storytelling, Family Psychoeducation, Hypnosis, Mindfulness, Relaxation, Stress Inoculation	Contingency Management, Group Therapy	Behavioral Activation and Exposure, Biofeedback, Play Therapy, PMT, Psychodynamic Therapy, Rational Emotive Therapy, Social Skills	Assessment/Monitoring, Attachment Therapy, Client Centered Therapy, Eye Movement Desensitization and Reprocessing (EMDR), Peer Pairing, Psychoeducation, Relationship Counseling, Teacher Psychoeducation
Autism Spectrum Disorders	CBT, Intensive Behavioral Treatment, Intensive Communication Training, Joint Attention/Engagement, PMT, Social Skills	Family Psychoeducation, Imitation, Peer Pairing, PMT and Medication, Theory of Mind Training	None	Massage, Peer Pairing and Modeling, Play Therapy	Attention Training, Biofeedback, Cognitive Flexibility Training, Communication Skills, Contingent Responding, Eclectic Therapy, Executive Functioning Training, Fine Motor Training, Modeling, Parent Psychoeducation, Physical/Social/Occupational Therapy, Sensory Integration Training, Social Skills and Peer Pairing, Structured Listening, Working Memory Training

Problem Area	Level 1-BEST SUPPORT	Level 2-GOOD SUPPORT	Level 3-MODERATE SUPPORT	Level 4-MINIMAL SUPPORT	Level 5-NO SUPPORT
Delinquency and Disruptive Behavior	Anger Control, Assertiveness Training, CBT, Contingency Management, Multisystemic Therapy, PMT, PMT and Problem Solving, Problem Solving, Social Skills, Therapeutic Foster Care	CBT and PMT, CBT and Teacher Training, Communication Skills, Cooperative Problem Solving, Family Therapy, Functional Family Therapy, Mindfulness, PMT and Classroom Management, PMT and Medication, PMT and Social Skills, Rational Emotive Therapy, Relaxation, Self Control Training, Transactional Analysis	Client Centered Therapy, Moral Reasoning Training, Outreach Counseling, Peer Pairing	CBT and Teacher Psychoedu-cation, Exposure, Physical Exercise, PMT and Classroom Management and CBT, PMT and Self-Verbalization, Stress Inoculation	Behavioral Family Therapy, Catharsis, CBT With Parents, Education, Family Empowerment and Support, Family Systems Therapy, Group Therapy, Imagery Training, Play Therapy, PMT and Peer Support, Psychodynamic Therapy, Self Verbalization, Skill Development, Wraparound
Depressive or Withdrawn Behaviors	CBT, CBT and Medication, CBT With Parents, Client Centered Therapy, Family Therapy	Attention Training, Cognitive Behavioral Psychoeducation, Expression, Interpersonal Therapy, MI/Engagement and CBT, Physical Exercise, Problem Solving, Relaxation	None	Self-Control Training, Self-Modeling, Social Skills	CBT and Anger Control, CBT and Behavioral Sleep Intervention, CBT and PMT, Goal Setting, Life Skills, Mindfulness, Play Therapy, PMT, PMT and Emotion Regulation, Psychodynamic Therapy, Psychoeducation
Eating Disorders	CBT, Family-Focused Therapy, Physical Exercise and Dietary Care and Behavioral Feedback	Family Systems Therapy, Family Therapy With Parents Only	Family Therapy and Usual Care	Physical Exercise and Dietary Care	Behavioral Training and Dietary Care, CBT With Parents, Client Centered Therapy, Dietary Care, Education, Family Therapy, Family Therapy With Parent Consultant, Goal Setting, Psychoeducation, Yoga

(*continued*)

(continued)

Problem Area	Level 1-BEST SUPPORT	Level 2-GOOD SUPPORT	Level 3-MODERATE SUPPORT	Level 4-MINIMAL SUPPORT	Level 5-NO SUPPORT
Elimination Disorders	Behavior Alert, Behavior Alert and Behavioral Training, Behavioral Training, Behavioral Training and Biofeedback and Dietary Care and Medical Care, Behavioral Training and Dietary Care and Medical Care	Behavioral Training and Dietary Care, Behavioral Training and Hypnosis and Dietary Care, CBT	Behavior Alert and Medication	None	Assessment/Monitoring, Assessment/Monitoring and Medication, Behavioral Training and Medical Care, Biofeedback, Contingency Management, Dietary Care, Dietary Care and Medical Care, Hypnosis, Medical Care, Psychoeducation
Mania	None	CBT for Child and Parent, Cognitive Behavioral Psychoeducation	None	None	Cognitive Behavioral Psychoeducation and Dietary Care, Dialectical Behavior Therapy and Medication, Family-Focused Therapy, Psychoeducation

Problem Area	Level 1-BEST SUPPORT	Level 2-GOOD SUPPORT	Level 3-MODERATE SUPPORT	Level 4-MINIMAL SUPPORT	Level 5-NO SUPPORT
Substance Use	CBT, Community Reinforcement, Contingency Management, Family Therapy, MI/Engagement	Assertive Continuing Care, CBT and Contingency Management, CBT and Medication, CBT With Parents, Family Systems Therapy, Functional Family Therapy, Goal Setting, Goal Setting/Monitoring, MI/Engagement and CBT, MI/Engagement and Expression, Multidimensional Family Therapy, Problem Solving, Purdue Brief Family Therapy	CBT and Family Therapy, Drug Court, Drug Court and Multisystemic Therapy and Contingency Management, Eclectic Therapy	Psychoeducation	Advice/Encouragement, Assessment/Monitoring, Behavioral Family Therapy, Case Management, CBT and Community Information Campaign, ClientCentered Therapy, Drug Court and Multisystemic Therapy, Drug Education, Education, Family Court, Feedback, Group Therapy, Mindfulness, MI/Engagement and CBT and Family Therapy, Multisystemic Therapy, Parent Psychoeducation, PMT, Therapeutic Vocational Training
Suicidality	None	Attachment Therapy, CBT With Parents, Counselors Care, Counselors Care and Support Training, Interpersonal Therapy, Multisystemic Therapy, Parent Coping/Stress Management, Psychodynamic Therapy, Social Support	None	None	Accelerated Hospitalization, Case Management, CBT, Communication Skills, Counselors Care and Anger Management

(*continued*)

(continued)

Problem Area	Level 1-BEST SUPPORT	Level 2-GOOD SUPPORT	Level 3-MODERATE SUPPORT	Level 4-MINIMAL SUPPORT	Level 5-NO SUPPORT
Traumatic Stress	CBT, CBT with Parents, EMDR	Exposure	None	CBT and Expression, Play Therapy, Relaxation and Expression	Advice/Encouragement, Client Centered Therapy, CBT and Medication, CBT With Parents Only, Education, Expressive Play, Interpersonal Therapy, Problem Solving, Psychodynamic Therapy, Psychoeducation, Relaxation, Structured Listening

Adapted with permission from PracticeWise.

Note: CBT, cognitive behavior therapy; EMDR, eye movement desensitization and reprocessing; MI, motivational interviewing; PMT, parent management Training; Level 5 refers to treatments whose tests were unsupportive or inconclusive. This report updates and replaces the "Blue Menu" originally distributed by the Hawaii Department of Health, Child and Adolescent Mental Health Division, Evidence-Based Services Committee from 2002–2009.

The recommendations in this publication do not indicate an exclusive course of treatment or serve as a standard of medical care. Variations, taking into account individual circumstances, may be appropriate. Original document included as part of Addressing Mental Health Concerns in Primary Care: A Clinician's Toolkit.

Introduction to Cognitive Behavioral Skills Building

Cognitive Theory (CT): The cognitive theory of depression and psychotherapy as developed by Aaron Beck (2021) focuses on identifying and correcting "cognitive distortions" or automatic negative thoughts, such as catastrophizing (e.g., I got a D on my test, I will flunk this course and drop out of school and never get a job), labeling (e.g., I'm stupid; I can never get anything right), and should statements (e.g., I should be a better daughter or parent).

Beck proposed a negative cognitive triad—A negative view of:

a. Oneself,
b. One's environment,
c. The future.

This pattern of thinking leads to hopelessness, anxiety, and depression.

Seligman's Learned Helplessness Theory proposes that depression results from experiencing uncontrolled negative events with the belief that one cannot influence the outcomes with behavior.

From the cognitive theoretical perspective, a person who has negative thoughts or beliefs is more likely to have negative emotions (e.g., anxiety, depression) and display negative behaviors (e.g., risk taking, poor school performance).

CBT is rooted in the Cognitive Theory of Depression as developed by Beck and also adds behavioral theories as developed by Skinner and Lewinsholn.

- Lewinsohn stressed that the lack of positive reinforcement from pleasurable activities and other people leads to negative thought patterns.
- Behavior theory suggests that individuals are depressed and anxious not only because of a lack of positive reinforcements, but also a lack of skills to elicit positive reinforcement from others or to terminate negative reactions from others.

CBT consists of cognitive restructuring (i.e., understanding the connection between thoughts and feelings as well as behaviors), problem-solving, and behavioral activation and change.

Active components of CBT include:

- reducing negative thoughts (cognitive restructuring),
- increasing pleasurable activities (behavioral activation) even when you do not feel like doing them, and
- Improving assertiveness and problem-solving skills.

Important points about CBT:

- Homework or skills building is an essential component of CBT so that individuals can put into practice the skills that they are learning.
- Important skills in CBT are positive re-appraisal ("Okay, I'm not at my ideal weight, but with healthy eating and exercise, I can get there") and positive self-talk ("I can learn to eat healthy and exercise; I am calm; I am able to deal with stress well. I am too blessed to be stressed.")
- In CBT, individuals are taught to become aware of antecedent events (e.g., a trigger event, such as being called ugly by a friend) as well as physical symptoms being experienced, so that cognitive reappraisal and behaviors to reduce negative symptoms can be instituted early in the process.

- CBT emphasizes collaboration and active participation.
- CBT is goal oriented and problem focused.
- CBT initially emphasizes the present and focuses on present concerns.
- CBT sessions are structured.
- CBT uses a variety of techniques and exercises to change thinking, mood, and behavior.

The Thinking, Feeling, and Behaving Triangle: Individuals are taught that how they think is related to how they feel and how they behave (i.e., the thinking, feeling, and behavior triangle).

- By changing (reframing) the thinking about a situation, emotions and subsequent behaviors can be positively impacted.
- Everyone is prone to negative thoughts and perceptions of ourselves or others. Many of our negative thoughts are automatic, almost reflexive. We develop these automatic negative thoughts through our life experiences, and we practice thinking this way so much that we assume the thoughts are true.
- The good news is that with brief cognitive behavioral–based intervention, thoughts can be changed to be more positive.
- When feeling stressed, angry, anxious, or depressed, individuals are taught to stop and ask themselves "What am I thinking? Is this thought true or helpful? Is there evidence to back the thought up?" The answer is usually no, so by reframing our thoughts from negative to positive, we can respond more positively to situations and feel better.
- **This core concept of Cognitive Theory is used when parents are assisted to reframe negative perceptions of their child to more positive perceptions (like the earlier example of helping the parent see their son as a "curious boy" versus a destructive child).**

The core concept of Cognitive Behavioral Theory is that thinking affects emotions and behaviors, otherwise known as **the thinking, feeling, behavior triangle(Figure 17.1)**

How a person *thinks* is related to how he or she *feels and acts.*

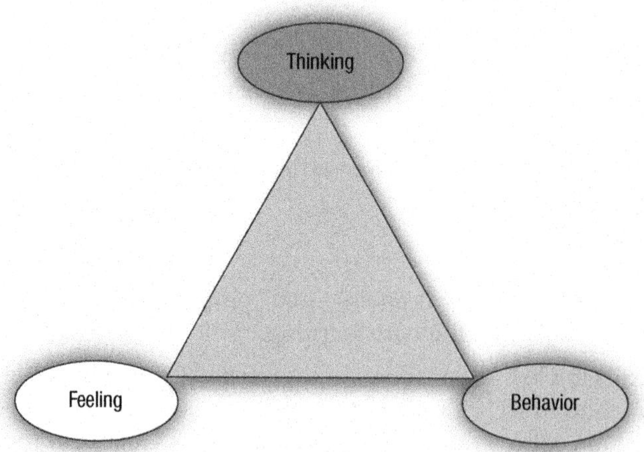

Figure 17.1. Thinking, feeling, behavior triangle

Source: From the COPE for Teens Manual (copyright, Bernadette Melnyk)

The following is an example of a segment from a brief cognitive behavior skills building session by a healthcare provider (HP) with a depressed teen from the COPE/Healthy Lifestyles Program for Teens by Bernadette Melnyk, 2004.

The Clinical Case

Anna is a 15-year-old girl who has been mildly depressed for the past few weeks, according to her mother. She does not want to go to her gymnastics class or hang out with her friends (new behaviors for her). Her appetite also has not been good lately. On interview, you find out that she received a D on a math test she took a couple of weeks ago, which seems to be a major cause of how she is feeling. It also did not help that a couple of her friends laughed at her score on the test.

During her interview, you discover that she believes that she is stupid, which is causing her to feel depressed and to not want to study anymore.

HP: Anna, I understand from your mom that you have been feeling down lately.	Anna: I sure have.
HP: On a scale of 0 to 10, with 0 meaning "not at all" to 10 meaning "a lot," how down or depressed have you been feeling over the past 2 weeks?	Anna: a 9.
HP: Anna, I'm going to continue to ask you some questions that will seem very personal, but all of the questions have to do with your health. What you tell me is confidential between the two of us, unless you tell me that you want to hurt yourself or that someone else has hurt you. Then, I need to tell another professional about it. I also want you to know that I ask all teens who are feeling down this question.	Anna: Okay.
HP: Have you ever wished that you were dead or thought about hurting yourself?	Anna: Yes, one time—last week.
HP: Did you think about how you would hurt yourself, that is, did you make a plan?	No, I really wouldn't ever try to kill myself because my parents would never forgive me.
HP: What do you think is causing you to feel so down lately?	Anna: I just feel I can't do anything right lately. A couple of weeks ago, I got a D on my math test when I studied for it. My close friends laughed at me, saying that I was getting dumber by the year. I don't even want to try anymore because I think "what's the use?"
HP: I can understand how you feel. I have felt the same way at times in my life, but you know what I found? Thinking like that only makes you feel down and depressed, and then you give up and don't try as hard. That only makes things worse.	Anna: I guess that's true, but I don't know what to do. Everything I do lately seems to go wrong.
HP: Anna, I could teach you a few tips on how you can start to feel better—not so down. Do you want to hear about them?	Anna: Sure.

(*continued*)

(*continued*)

HP: There is something called the "thinking, feeling, behavior triangle." What that means is how you think affects how you feel and how you behave. For instance, if something bad happens, like getting a D on your test, you believe that you are stupid, which makes you feel bad and not want to try anymore. Can you think of another example?	Anna: Yeah. When my dad screams at me because I didn't clean my room, and I think "I flubbed up again," then I feel rotten about myself.
HP: That's right. Can you think of how you can turn that negative thought (i.e., "I flubbed up again") into a positive one?	Anna: Well, I guess I could think, "Okay, I put off cleaning my room, but that's okay; I'll get it done now."
HP: That's great, Anna. Now you are getting it. You have to start to monitor the way you are thinking when things happen and change the negative thought around as soon as it starts to happen into a positive thought, which will help you to feel a lot better. I'd like you to keep a log this week of all the things that happen that start making you have negative thoughts. I want you to write those down—the event that happened that triggered you to have a negative thought—and then, I want you write a positive thought that could replace the negative thought you had. Would you be willing to do that?	Anna: Sure, but do you really think this will help me?
HP: Yes, I do. It works for a lot of teens, and adults, too. When you come back, we'll work on more things and before you know it, you'll be feeling much better.	Anna: Okay, I'll try.

The following courses are designed to be used by mental health professionals, however, they provide some useful resources and examples of cognitive behavioral skills-building with teens.

The Adolescent Coping with Stress Course (for teens at high risk for depression) and

The Adolescent Coping with Depression Course (for teens who are depressed) are both available at http://www.kpchr.org/public/acwd/acwd.html

COPE: A Cognitive Behavioral Skills-Building Intervention

Creating Opportunities for Personal Empowerment (COPE) is a seven-session manualized cognitive behavioral skills building (CBSB) intervention developed by Bernadette Melnyk for children, teens, and young adults (child version for 7 to 11 year olds; teen version for 12 to 18 year olds; and young adult version for 18 to 25 year olds) (see www.cope2thrive.com). The program is designed to be feasible for delivery by healthcare providers, health promotion professionals, social workers, psychologists, mental health counselors, and teachers in a variety of settings, including primary care settings, schools, school-based health centers, private practices, and community mental health clinics after a 4-hour on-line training workshop. Findings from numerous studies over the past two decades support that COPE, delivered individually, in group format, or integrated into school/university curricula reduces anxiety, stress, depressive symptoms, anger and suicidal ideation as well as improves self-concept, academic performance, and healthy lifestyle behaviors (Erlich et al., 2018; Hart Abney et al., 2019; Hoying et al., 2016; Hoying & Melnyk, 2016; Kozlowski et al., 2015; Lusk & Melnyk, 2011; Melnyk et al., 2007, 2009, 2013; Melnyk, Amaya, Szalacha et al., 2015 Melnyk, Kelly, & Lusk, 2014). Healthcare providers are being reimbursed to deliver this program in primary care with the 99214 CPT code. Findings from a recent cost analysis indicated a cost savings of $14,262 for every hospitalization prevented by delivering COPE to depressed adolescents, resulting in $146.2 million dollars of cost savings for the U.S. healthcare system (Melnyk, 2020).

A 15-session COPE Healthy Lifestyles TEEN (Thinking, Emotions, Exercise and Nutrition) program also is available that adds eight nutrition and physical activity sessions. This 15-session program was evaluated in a NIH/National Institute of Nursing Research funded clinical trial that found teens in high school classrooms who received COPE from their teachers had decreases in depression, alcohol use, and overweight/obesity, and increases in physical activity, social skills, and academic competence compared to adolescents who received an attention control program (Melnyk et al., 2013; Melnyk, Jacobson, Kelly et al., 2015). These positive findings sustained for 12 months after completion of the program. The COPE TEEN program is designated as a research tested intervention program by the National Institutes of Health (see ebccp.cancercontrol.cancer.gov/programDetails.do?programId=22686590). In addition, a digital on-line interactive teen COPE program is available.

Information About COPE

- The evidence-based COPE program is manualized and delivered weekly for 7 weeks, exactly as written in the manual.
- The COPE sessions fit nicely into 20 to 30-minutes office visits for individual children and teens; 45 minutes if delivered in group format.
- The COPE 7 session manual is developmentally appropriate and covers all the elements of successful CBT-based interventions, and also provides skills-building activities and assignments.
- The COPE program has "**ease of use.**" Once a provider is trained to use COPE through a 4-hour on-line training seminar, when the child or teen arrives, the manual is ready to use and has everything the provider needs to implement the program, including the skills building assignments.
- COPE, as with other CBT interventions, is designed to be time limited.
- COPE is goal oriented and problem-solving focused.
- COPE emphasizes collaboration and active participation by the child or teen.
- COPE can be delivered to children/teens/young adults and their parents.
- In the COPE program, children and adolescents are taught the **ABCs**, including:

  Antecedent or Activating Event: "My friends call me 'chubbo.'"

  Belief that is negative: "I'm fat; I'll always be fat."

  Consequences -Emotional Outcome: Depression

  Behavioral Outcome: "I give up; I won't try eating healthy anymore."

  In the ABCs, the child/teen/young adult is taught to turn the initial negative belief around (e.g., "I may be overweight now, but I will change that with regular exercise and healthy eating ") so that they feel better and engage in healthy behaviors (e.g., eating healthier foods).

- Incorporating skills-building activities and reinforcing the practice of these skills is a critical element in the child/teen's improvement. (Examples of a few concepts taught in the COPE program can be found in handouts at the end of this chapter.)
- Self-regulation of behavior is a key coping strategy reinforced throughout the program.
- COPE is a CBSB program that actively promotes mastery of child/adolescent developmental tasks by each participant. The child/teen is an active participant in the intervention and the provider maintains positive belief in their abilities with statements such as:

  > "You can do it. You can develop skills to COPE with whatever you are facing. By monitoring your thoughts and changing negative thinking to positive thinking, you can change/regulate your feelings and behaviors, and feel better."

The COPE handouts contained at the end of this chapter are designed to facilitate talking to school-age children about their thoughts, feelings, and behaviors as well as helping them to cope with stress and worry. These handouts can be reproduced for use during office visits. However, they do not replace the COPE 7-session program.

Training to deliver the 7- and 15-session COPE programs is available through a workshop at www.COPE2Thrive.org.

Resources for Healthcare Providers and Parents

Evidence-based intervention programs, which offer training for clinicians and resources for parents.

Collaborative Problem-Solving: Clinicians find this approach helpful in addressing the very challenging disruptive behaviors of children. http://www.livesinthebalance.org/

Incredible Years (IY) is a program with several levels. There is some evidence that reading the IY manual can be helpful for parents who cannot engage in the program. Incredible Years also has CDs that cover key concepts and that may be a help. http://www.incredibleyears.com/

Cognitive behavioral skills building: COPE (Creating Opportunities for Personal Empowerment) for children, teens and young adults: See www.cope2thrive.com

Triple P – Parenting Program: See www.triplep.net/

Motivational Interviewing: See www.motivationalinterview.org/

Web Resources

American Academy of Pediatrics – Evidence-based Psychosocial Interventions http://www2.aap.org/commpeds/dochs/mentalhealth/docs/CR%20Psychosocial%20Interventions.F.0503.pdf

SBIRT: http://www.samhsa.gov/prevention/SBIRT/index.aspx

Integration of Mental Health into Pediatric Practices: http://nihcm.org/pdf/PediatricMH-FINAL.pdf

Guidelines for Adolescent Depression in Primary Care (GLAD-PC): http://pediatrics.aappublications.org/content/120/5/e1313.full.html

Strengths and Difficulties Questionnaire: www.sdqinfo.com

The REACH Institute: www.thereachinstitute.org/

2020 Children's Mental Health Report: Telehealth in an Increasingly Virtual World. Child Mind Institute

https://childmind.org/our-impact/childrens-mental-health-report/2020-childrens-mental-health-report/

The National Academy of Sciences, Engineering, and Medicine (NASEM). Five cognitive behavioral skills micro-learning modules for children and teens (i.e., belly breathing; increasing favorite activities; mindfulness; catch it, check it, change it-labeling; and catch it, check it, all or nothing thinking) are freely available in English and Spanish at https://www.nationalacademies.org/our-work/promoting-emotional-well-being-and-resilience#sl-three-columns-a006043a-0181-42fe-8dff-e6ee6557ff34

REFERENCES

Beck, J. (2021). *Cognitive therapy: Basics and beyond* (3rd ed.). Guilford Press.

Erlich, K. J., Li, J., Dillon, E., Li, M., & Becker, D. F. (2018). Outcomes of a brief cognitive skills-based intervention (COPE) for adolescents in the primary care setting. *Journal of Pediatric Health Care, 33*(4), 415–424. https://doi.org/10.1016/j.pedhc.2018.12.001.

Hart Abney, B. G., Lusk, P., Hovermale, R., & Melnyk, B. M. (2019). Decreasing depression and anxiety in college youth using the Creating Opportunities for Personal Empowerment Program (COPE). *Journal of the American Psychiatric Nurses Association, 25*(2), 89–98. https://doi.org/10.1177/1078390318779205.

Hoying, J., & Melnyk, B. M. (2016). COPE: A pilot study with urban-dwelling minority sixth grade youth to improve physical activity and mental health outcomes. *Journal of School Nursing, 32*(5), 347–356. https://doi.org/10.1177/1059840516635713.

Hoying, J., Melnyk, B. M., & Arcoleo, K. (2016). Effects of the COPE cognitive behavioral skills building TEEN program on the healthy lifestyle behaviors and mental health of appalachian early adolescents. *Journal of Pediatric Health Care, 30*(1), 65–72.

Kozlowski, J., Lusk, P., & Melnyk, B. M. (2015). Pediatric nurse practitioner management of child anxiety in the rural primary care clinic with the evidence-based COPE. *Journal of Pediatric Health Care, 29*(3), 274–282.

Lusk, P., & Melnyk, B. M. (2011). The brief cognitive-behavioral COPE intervention for depressed adolescents: Outcomes and feasibility of delivery in 30-minute outpatient visits. *Journal of the American Psychiatric Nurses Association, 17*(3), 226–236.

Melnyk, B. M. (2004). *COPE (Creating Opportunities for Personal Empowerment) for children, teens and young adults: A 7-session cognitive behavioral skills building program*. COPE2thrive.

Melnyk, B. M. (2020). Reducing healthcare costs for mental health hospitalizations with the evidence-based COPE program for child and adolescent depression and anxiety: A cost analysis. *Journal of Pediatric Health Care, 34*(2), 117–121. https://doi.org/10.1016/j.pedhc.2019.08.002.

Melnyk, B. M., Jacobson, D., Kelly, S., Belyea, M., Shaibi, G., Small, L., O'Haver, J., & Marsiglia, F. F. (2013). Promoting healthy lifestyles in high school adolescents: A randomized controlled trial. *American Journal of Preventive Medicine, 45*(4), 407–415. [Epub ahead of print]. https://doi.org/10.1016/j.amepre.2013.05.013.

Melnyk, B. M., Jacobson, D., Kelly, S. A., Belyea, M. J., Shaibi, G. Q., Small, L., O'Haver, J. A., & Marsiglia, F. F. (2015). Twelve-month effects of the COPE healthy lifestyles TEEN program on overweight and depression in high school adolescents. *Journal of School Health, 85*(12), 861–870.

Melnyk, B. M., Jacobson, D., Kelly, S., O'Haver, J., Small, L., & Mays, M. Z. (2009). Improving the mental health, healthy lifestyle choices and physical health of Hispanic adolescents: A randomized controlled pilot study. *Journal of School Health, 79*(12), 575–584.

Melnyk, B. M., Kelly, S., & Lusk, P. (2014). Outcomes and feasibility of a manualized cognitive-behavioral skills building intervention: Group COPE for depressed and anxious adolescents in school settings. *Journal of Child and Adolescent Psychiatric Nursing, 27*(1), 3–13. https://doi:10.1111/jcap.12058

Melnyk, B. M., Small, L., Morrison-Beedy, D., Strasser, A., Spath, L., Kreipe, R., Crean, H., Jacobson, D., Kelly, S., & O'Haver, J. (2007). The COPE healthy lifestyles TEEN program: Feasibility, preliminary, efficacy, & lessons learned from an after school group intervention with overweight adolescents. *Journal of Pediatric Health Care, 21*(5), 315.

Miller, W. R., & Rollnick, S. R. (2012). *Motivational interviewing: Preparing people for change* (3rd ed.). The Guilford Press.

Sudak, D., & Taormina, S. (2018). Integrate brief CBT interventions into medication management visits. *Current Psychiatry, 17*(2), e3–e4.

Whitney, D. G., & Peterson, M. D. (2019). US National and state-level prevalence of mental health disorders and disparities of mental health care use in children. *JAMA Pediatrics, 173*(4), 389–391. https://doi.org/10.1001/jamapediatrics.2018.5399.https://jamanetwork.com/journals/jamapediatrics/fullarticle/2724377?utm_campaign=articlePDF&utm_medium=articlePDFlink&utm_source=articlePDF&utm_content=jamapediatrics.2019.5991

Yearwood, E., Pearson, G., & Newland, J. (2021). *Child and adolescent behavioral health: A resource for advanced practice psychiatric and primary care practitioners in nursing* (2nd ed.). Wiley-Blackwell.

COPE for Children: The Thinking-Feeling-Behaving Triangle

The Thinking-Feeling-Behaving Triangle

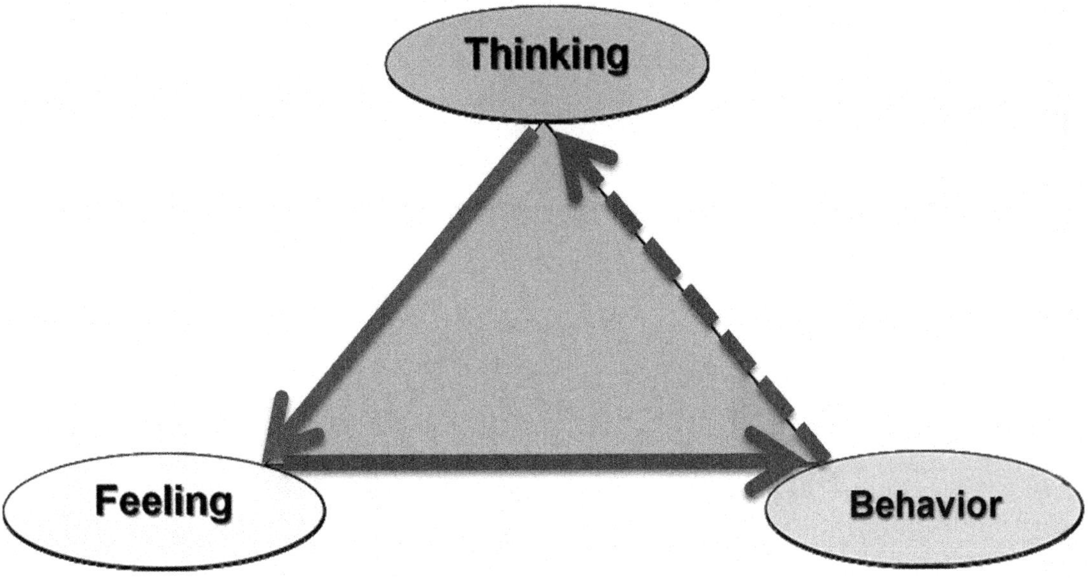

How you think affects how you feel and how you act or behave.

Here's an example:

- Alex is starting his first day of the school year at a new school. He is **thinking** that he doesn't know anybody at his new school and that maybe no one will like him. This makes him **feel** worried and sad. So, he **acts** very scared when he gets to school and doesn't talk to any other kids.

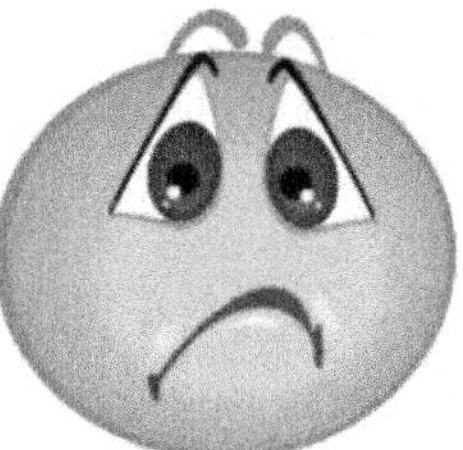

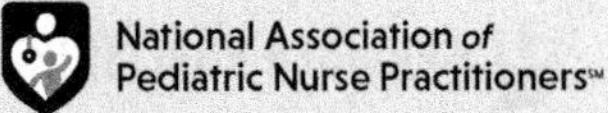

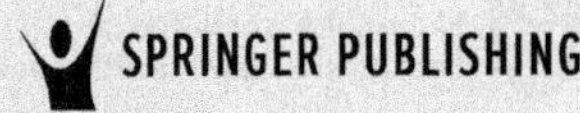

- **How Alex thinks affects how he feels and how he acts.**

Let's think of an example from your school.

We can change our thoughts from negative to positive. When we change to positive thoughts, we will feel better.

How we think affects how we feel (and how we act follows)

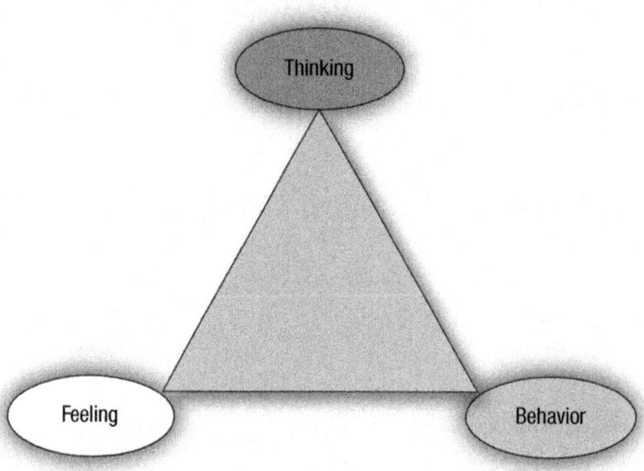

Let's change the thought (negative) to positive on the triangle. How might Alex feel with a different, more positive thought.

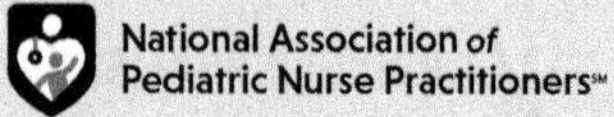

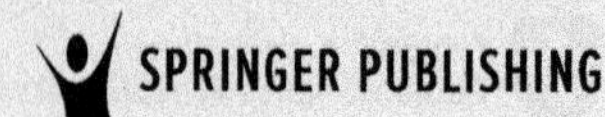

COPE for Children: Healthy Coping for Stress and Worry

Healthy Coping for Stress and Worry

Healthy coping is when you deal with stressful things in positive ways that don't hurt you or other people.

Did you know that your body tells you when you are stressed?

Here are some different ways that our bodies can respond when we are feeling worried or sad:

- Heart beating fast or pounding
- Breathing fast
- Sweating
- Anger
- Restlessness (feeling like you have to keep moving)
- Headaches
- Stomachaches
- Not being hungry
- Tightness in your neck or shoulders
- Problems thinking clearly
- Trouble sleeping or sleeping too much
- Feeling tired all the time

How does *your* body feel when you're stressed?

Here are some ideas for healthy coping:

- Talking about how you feel
- Exercise/playing outside
- Going to family or friends for help
- Writing your thoughts and feelings in a journal/diary
- Changing a negative thought into a positive one
- Using positive self-talk (positive self-statements)
- Doing relaxation exercises (we will do one today)
- Trying something new
- Doing something that you enjoy (like reading or drawing)

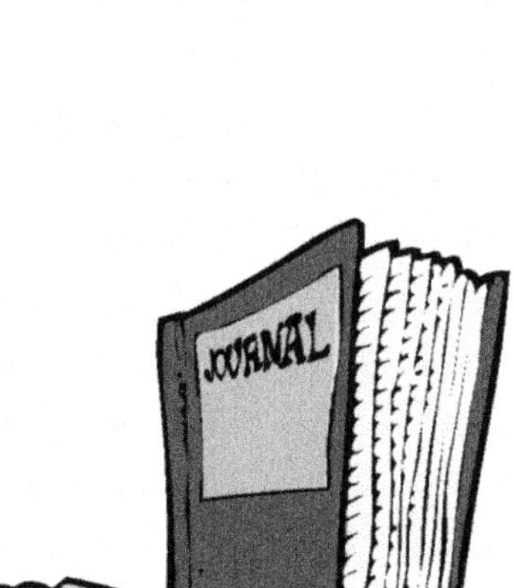

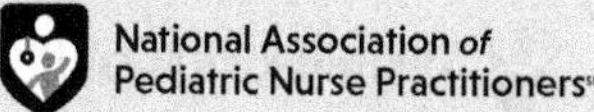

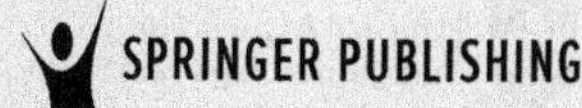

Write down three healthy coping skills/activities that sound fun to you.

1. ________________________________
2. ________________________________
3. ________________________________

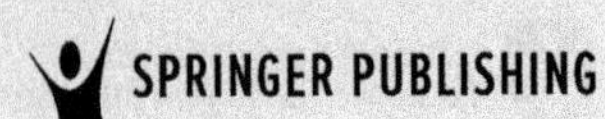

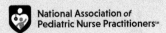

CHAPTER 18

Patrice Rancour and Rosie Zeno

Helping Children and Adolescents to Deal With Grief and Loss

"When we can talk about our feelings, they become less overwhelming, less upsetting, and less scary. The people we trust with that important talk can help us know that we are not alone."

—Mr. Rogers

Fast Facts

- These three things are true: We live in a death-phobic society, children do grieve, and while it can be excruciating, grief is a normal healing response to all loss.
- Each year, an estimated 7.2% (5.2 million) of U.S. children younger than 18 years old experience a parental death (Burns et al., 2020).
- Prolonged grief disorder (PGD), also commonly referred to as "complicated grief" (CG), is estimated to affect 10% of bereaved individuals (Lundorff et al., 2017).
- Normal grief requires facilitation, while CG requires intervention.
- Parentally bereaved children experience an increased incidence of depression, post-traumatic stress disorder (PTSD), and long-term functional impairments that can be ameliorated by the identification and preventive treatment of depression early in the course of grief (Pham et al., 2018).
- Comorbid conditions of CG, like PTSD, also require treatment to attenuate functional impairments that can track across the lifespan.
- While a parental loss is one of the most traumatic childhood experiences children can experience, other significant life changes and loss can result in CG like family relocation, foster placement, and parental divorce/separation or incarceration.
- Nearly 80% of adults who lost a parent before age 20 report that losing a parent was the hardest thing they ever faced; 57% report that support from family and friends tapered off within the first 3 months of the loss; and 53% report struggling to find grief resources following a parental loss (New York Life Foundation, 2017).
- Helping children come to terms with loss and grief becomes a teachable moment in learning to adapt to the cycles of change throughout the lifetime.

FACILITATING NORMAL GRIEF IN CHILDREN

The goal of grief facilitation is to help children to redefine their relationship with their lost loved one or object, to hold onto meaningful memories that continue the relationship, and to maintain an inner connection with the deceased as they continue to grow and develop (Bergman et al., 2017; Griese et al., 2017, 2018; Haine et al., 2008). The Transitional Events Model, a framework to guide interventions with parentally bereaved children, posits that the primary goal of interventions is to decrease children's exposure to stressful changes and strengthen child and family resources for dealing with those stressors following a traumatic loss (Haine et al., 2008).

Young children respond to loss and grief according to their stage of development. Common questions following a parental loss may include:

- "Can I catch this too?" (Fear of contagion)
- "Who will take care of me now?" (Fear of abandonment)
- "I told Mommy I wished she was dead last week. Did I cause this?" (Magical thinking)

These become opportunities to teach children about fundamental concepts that help to make sense of death. By age 5 to 7 years, children can begin to understand four key concepts that help to comprehend and cope with death: irreversibility, finality, causality, and universality. With help, children's understanding of these concepts can be accelerated.

- "Will Mommy still come to my birthday?" Help children understanding that death is not reversible (irreversibility).
- "Won't Daddy be cold when he's buried?" Reassure children that death is final; people no longer feel pain, cold, loneliness, sadness, and so forth (finality).
- "Did Mommy do something bad?" or "Did Mommy die because I did something bad?" Help children understand that death is inevitable for everyone and does not occur as a consequence or punishment for thoughts or actions (universality), and likewise that the child's thoughts and behaviors cannot cause death (causality).

Table 18.1 details responses to loss and grief by age group.

Table 18.1. Age-Related Responses to Loss and Grief

Age Stage	Concept	Presentation	Assistance
Infants and Toddlers (0–2)	No understanding of death. No language. Recognizes changes in family.	Separation anxiety, anxious, crying, problems with appetite or sleep, fearfulness, needy, irritable.	Provide parental warmth and physical closeness, meet needs, maintain routine, include in family rituals as much as possible, provide verbal love and reassurance.
Pre-School (3–5)	Believes death is temporary, magical thinking, fantasies.	Crying, anxious, irritable, regressed behavior, temper tantrums, problems eating or sleeping, separation anxiety, acting out.	Provide parental warmth and physical closeness, maintain routines, include in family rituals as much as possible, be honest in responses to questions, listen to and accept children's need to express themselves, make time for play.

(*continued*)

Table 18.1. Age-Related Responses to Loss and Grief (*continued*)

Age Stage	Concept	Presentation	Assistance
School-Age (6–9)	Now understands that death is permanent. Starts to wonder what happens after death.	Asking questions, problems with sleeping/appetite, withdrawn, anxious, guilty, nightmares, problems in school, acting out, crying, angry.	Provide parental warmth and closeness, be honest, answer questions, accept feelings, encourage use of play and art to express self, maintain routines, work with school, encourage inclusion in family mourning rituals.
Pre-Teen (10–12)	Understanding finality of death, magical thinking, understanding that life will go on without the loved one.	Confusion, denial, shock, lonely, angry, anxious fearful, problems with sleep/appetite, acting out, problems in school, may self-isolate, guilty, physical problems, questioning existential issues.	Provide opportunities to tell his/her story, include in family rituals, provide parental warmth, encourage expressive arts, be honest, work with school, provide information.
Teenagers (13–18)	Understanding of the universality and finality of death, magical thinking, understanding that life will go on without the loved one, spiritual concepts evolving.	Confusion, denial, shock, sadness, lonely, angry, self-conscious, guilty, anxious, fearful, acts out, problems with sleep/appetite, problems in school, self-isolation, other physical problems.	Provide parental warmth, be honest, opportunities for expressive arts, peer group support, anticipate risky behaviors, include in family mourning rituals, work with school, be honest.

Source: Adapted from Lyles, M. (2004). *Navigating children's grief: How to help following a death.* Children's Grief Education Association. https://www.tiporangecounty.org/pdfs/How_to_help_chart.pdf

STRATEGIES FOR FACILITATING GRIEF

Pediatric providers must be equipped to support grieving children and their families. Evidence-based and expert-informed guidance includes:

- To help others come to terms with death and process their grief, it is important to become more comfortable with *facing your own mortality* so that death is a discussible subject.
- The best way to ensure healthy grieving in children is to ensure that the surviving parent remains supported and healthy in their own grief work. CG in the surviving parent is a predictor of CG in the child.
- For caregivers who display symptoms of CG, mood disorders, substance abuse, or PTSD, it is important to ensure mental health screening for the early identification and treatment of conditions that may impact their parenting and their children's mental health. Evidence shows that when parents are supported, they can demonstrate an enhanced capacity to support their children.

- Be alert to signs of child abuse or neglect. Following parental death, some children may remain with the surviving parent, while others may live with another family member or foster parent. Household and family changes following the death of a parent can cause additional stressors (single parent, financial strain, parental grief, etc.) that may predispose a child to maltreatment.
- Counsel parents to be truthful with children. Use developmentally appropriate language to hold brief, truthful conversations in a safe environment and allow the child to ask questions.
- Advise the use of accurate, concrete language. Do not say the person "passed away" or "went to sleep." Use the word "died." Otherwise, children may be afraid that they also might die in their sleep or that perhaps the lost one will "pass back." Helping children to understand that death is *final* and *irreversible* ultimately facilitates the grief process. Talking about the death does not trigger the pain. The pain and loss are already present. Remind parents that they can choose to be sad together or be sad separately.
- Provide informational resources about the grief process to children and their caregivers. Reassure caregivers that misbehaviors and regression are a common way that children express their grief.
- Encourage patients to express their feelings openly and normalize them. For example, "I feel sad today because I miss Daddy." However, parents should not seek emotional support from their children. Encourage parents to seek grief support from other adults.
- Reassure parents that crying is a normal, healthy human emotion. Sharing sadness with children shows them that the parent can handle sadness, and therefore, so can the child.
- Reassure children that they are not responsible for fixing parental distress. Explain that these feelings are normal and will improve over time.
- Counsel parents to include children in the family's process of grief and mourning as much as possible. This means encouraging them to attend funerals and other mourning rites where they see their family members come together for support. Packing a bag of drawing materials, paper, small toys, and books will help occupy young children as they watch adults cry, tell stories, and reduce the sense of isolation. Many adults who were prevented from attending funerals of deceased friends and relatives as children report feeling resentment from being excluded. As a result, they had difficulty developing life skills related to loss and grief. Children tend to fantasize the worst when left to their own devices.
- Parents should let children know the ground rules and what to expect during these mourning rituals to prepare them to participate. Let children know that if they feel overwhelmed by their experiences, they can take breaks and that their adults will talk with them and answer questions when they are ready.
- Become familiar with the family's cultural and spiritual beliefs about what happens when people die, their customs surrounding mourning, any particular rituals, prayers, and devotionals important to them. Ask them to share their beliefs in order to avoid inadvertently offending their sensibilities.
- Referral for family therapy may be in order if the loss exacerbates pre-existing dysfunction.
- Play therapy utilizes therapeutic storytelling, drama, role play, puppets and masks, dance and movement, and sand and clay trays to help children work through feelings for which they often do not have the vocabulary.
- Support groups are particularly effective for teenagers whose need for peer support steadily increases as they work toward self-acceptance and acceptance by their peers. In particular, group work helps normalize their feelings when they feel self-conscious or when they believe that expressing vulnerable emotions makes them look weak.

- Social media networking, online blogs, chat rooms, and other web-based communication portals can be therapeutic and reduce a sense of social isolation. However, teens need to be counseled about internet safety. Ensure that a responsible adult is able to monitor safe internet use, particularly during times of increased vulnerability.
- Animal-assisted therapy is an intervention whereby children can receive support through non-threatening contact with specially trained service animals in helping them cope with loss. Interaction with therapy animals or even a child's family pet often helps to reduce child stress levels.
- Cognitive behavioral therapy may be useful for children whose language skills have developed to a level whereby their myths about death can be challenged, and more healthy thought substitutions can help them transform maladaptive coping with healthier grief work.
- Creative visualization/relaxation training can maximize children's innate tendency to use their imaginations by helping them induce a relaxation response before taking them to a safe space. Remember that children will not have learned to censor unusual sensory experiences that adults have censored. They will report auditory, visual, olfactory, tactile, and other sensory stimulation that adults might feel uncomfortable with and identify as hallucinatory. Unless there are other disturbing symptoms, accept these experiences that children report as normal. Children can also be guided into having conversations with their lost loved one to speak with them, especially if they did not have a chance to say good-bye before the death.
- Bibliotherapy and movies provide a non-threatening introduction of how other children and teenagers respond to loss and grief. Exploring an age-appropriate book or movie provides a natural opportunity for the child to share their feelings. It can also be a prelude to the child or teen writing their personal story to work through their experiences.
- Expressive arts like music, journaling, and painting give children and teenagers a creative outlet that can release emotional material in non-threatening ways. For example, giving sentence-completion exercises such as answering questions like "The day my dog died…." Alternatively, "The thing that I am most afraid of now that my mother has died is…." Asking children to paint pictures of their family before the loss occurred and then afterward can act as a springboard for discussion.
- For children with difficulty accessing emotional vocabulary, "visualizing hurt" can be a useful technique. For example, "If your tears could talk, what would they say?"
- Holidays and anniversary dates present unique challenges for incorporating the lost person into the life of the family. Lighting candles, decorating graves with flowers on select dates of remembrances, and other meaningful rituals can help keep the memories of deceased family members alive so that children and families can feel connected to their loved one.
- Encourage weekly "family fun time" as a way to break from grief.
- Therapeutic letter writing, for example, writing a letter to the parent explaining what it has been like since they died, can be helpful in processing grief and maintaining a connection with the loved one.
- Creating a farewell ceremony such as writing a message and sending it off on a balloon can help the child find ways to create their own rituals.
- Use the death of pets as intentional teachable moments about coping with loss.
- Create memory boxes, collages, or scrapbooks. Use photos, souvenirs, and other related memoirs to build a concrete reminder of positive memories of time spent together.

(Bergman et al., 2017; Centers for Disease Control and Prevention [CDC], 2019; Haine et al., 2008; Revet et al., 2020; Sandler et al., 2013; Schonfeld & Demaria, 2016).

Table 18.2. Differences Among Normal Grief, Complicated Grief (CG), Depression, PTSD, and General Anxiety Disorder

Normal Grief	CG	Depression	PTSD	General Anxiety Disorder
Sadness	Yearning	Sadness	Numbness	Anxiety
Improves over time	Overwhelmed by the loss	Does not improve over time	Disconnection	Does not improve over time
Childhood attachment issues may or may not be an issue	*Childhood attachment issues create vulnerability	No evidence of childhood attachment issues	No evidence of childhood attachment issues	No evidence of childhood attachment issues
No significant functional impairment	Significant functional impairment	Functional impairment	Functional impairment	Functional impairment
Vivid dreaming may be present	Changes in EEG sleep physiology	No changes in EEG sleep physiology	No changes in EEG sleep physiology	No changes in EEG sleep physiology
No reward-related neural activity	Reward-related neural activity in nucleus accumibens in response to reminders of the deceased	No reward-related neural activity	No reward-related neural activity	No reward-related neural activity
Suicidal ideation not prominent	Elevated rates of suicidal ideation and attempts, cancer, immunological dysfunction, hypertension, cardiac events, functional impairments, hospitalizations, adverse health behaviors, reduced quality of life	Rates are not as high as CG	Rates are not as high as CG	Rates are not as high as CG
Absenteeism rates are not as high as CG	Increased absence from home and work	Absenteeism rates are not as high as CG	Absenteeism rates are not as high as CG	Absenteeism rates are not as high as CG

(*continued*)

Table 18.2. Differences Among Normal Grief, Complicated Grief (CG), Depression, PTSD, and General Anxiety Disorder (*continued*)

Normal Grief	CG	Depression	PTSD	General Anxiety Disorder
Treatment not necessary	Treatment: tricyclics alone and interpersonal psychotherapy are ineffective Focused CG therapy is efficacious	Tricyclics and SSRIs, psychotherapy efficacious	Tricyclics and SSRIs, psychotherapy efficacious	Tricyclics and SSRIs, psychotherapy efficacious

*Childhood attachment issues refer to history of childhood separation anxiety, controlling parents, parental abuse or death, close kinship relationship to deceased, insecure attachment, marital supportiveness and dependency, lack of preparation for the death.

Source: Adapted from Prigerson, H. G., Horowitz, M. J., Jacobs, S. C., Parkes, C. M., Aslan, M., Goodkin, K., Raphael, B., Marwit, S. J., Wortman, C., Neimeyer, R. A., Bonanno, G. A., Block, S. D., Kissane, D., Boelen, P., Maercker, A., Litz, B. T., Johnson, J. G., First, M. B., & Maciejewski, P. K. (2009). Prolonged grief disorder: Psychometric validation of criteria proposed for DSM-V and ICD-11. *PLOS Medicine*, *6*(8), e1000121. https://doi.org/10.1371/journal.pmed.1000121; Shear, M. K., Simon, N., Wall, M., Zisook, S., Neimeyer, R., Duan, N., Reynolds, C., Lebowitz, B., Sung, S., Ghesquiere, A., Gorscak, B., Clayton, P., Ito, M., Nakajima, S., Konishi, T., Melhem, N., Meert, K., Schiff, M., O'Connor, M. F., . . . Keshaviah, A. (2011). Complicated grief and related bereavement issues for DSM-5. *Depression and Anxiety*, *28*(2), 103–117. https://doi.org/10.1002/da.20780.

COMPLICATED GRIEF

CG is a pathological state requiring clinical intervention and has been the focus of clinical research for over 30 years. While grief is a normal response to loss, some children experience a severe and protracted course of grief that results in an increased risk of psychopathology and long-term functional impairments. Experts have long debated the necessity of including CG as a psychiatric disorder that is distinct from the normal grief response, which presents the risk of either deeming a normal grief reaction as pathologic or dismissing a pathological grief response that may be subsequently untreated. Several iterations of diagnostic criteria for CG have been proposed to formalize a clinical psychiatric diagnosis (Prigerson et al., 2009; Shear et al., 2011).

The lack of sufficient evidence supporting the biological basis and core set of CG symptoms has impeded expert consensus on its diagnostic criteria (Nakajima, 2018). The *Diagnostic and Statistical Manual of Mental Disorders* (5th ed.; *DSM-5;* American Psychiatric Association, 2013) provisionally established persistent complex grief disorder (PCGD) as a psychiatric disorder. The *DSM-5* includes PCGD as an (a) "other specific trauma- and stress-related disorder" and (b) a condition requiring future study. The 11th revision of the International Classification of Diseases (ICD-11; World Health Organization, 2018) established a new prolonged grief disorder (PGD) diagnosis for adoption in 2022. PGD differs slightly from PCGD regarding its terminology and duration of symptoms.

PROLONGED GRIEF DISORDER: DIAGNOSTIC CRITERIA

PGD requires a 6-month duration of symptoms for diagnosis rather than 12-months required with PCGD. The diagnostic criteria for PGD and PCGD include symptoms of separation distress and symptoms of reactive stress in response to the loss/death as follows:

A. Pathological grief

Persistent and pervasive grief reaction for a duration of at least 6 months

B. Separation distress

At least one of the following symptoms must be present more days than not and must result in functional impairment:

a. Persistent yearning/longing that may be expressed in play and behavior, including separation–reunion behavior with caregivers

b. Intense sorrow/emotional pain

c. Preoccupation with the deceased

d. Preoccupation with the circumstances of the death such that it may be expressed through play and behavior and worry about the possible death of others close to them

C. Reactive stress

At least six of the following symptoms must be present more days than not and must result in functional impairment:

a. Depending on the child's capacity to understand, difficulty accepting the death

b. Emotional numbness/being stunned

c. Difficulty in positive reminiscing about the deceased

d. Bitterness/anger about the loss

e. Self-blame and maladaptive cognitive self-appraisal concerning the death

f. Avoidance of thoughts and feelings regarding the deceased

g. A desire to join the deceased by death

h. Difficulty trusting others

i. Detachment from other relationships

j. Feeling life cannot be lived without the deceased

k. Diminished self-identity

l. Inability to look forward to the future

D. If the death occurred under traumatic circumstances, persistent flashbacks and magical thinking regarding the death

(Nakajima, 2018; Prigerson et al., 2009; Shear et al., 2011; WHO, 2018).

RISK FACTORS FOR PROLONGED GRIEF DISORDER

Several known risk factors have been identified that predispose a child to CG, including:

- Child history of mood disorder
- Caregiver history of mood disorder, substance abuse, or PTSD
- Traumatic death of a loved one
- Cumulative losses
- Loss associated with social stigma (e.g., HIV/AIDS, suicide, parental incarceration)
- Relationship with the deceased involved abuse, neglect, or abandonment
- Perceived lack of social support

- Surviving caregiver is disabled by their own grief
- Family history of community violence or war

(de López et al., 2020; Revet et al., 2020).

SEQUELAE OF PROLONGED GRIEF DISORDER

The sequelae of CG in childhood can be debilitating and persist throughout the life span, including:

- Decline in academic performance
- PTSD and anxiety
- Prolonged depression and social withdrawal
- Sleep disorders
- Impaired relationships and attachment issues
- Increased risk of chronic illnesses over lifetime
- Substance misuse and eating disorders
- Legal issues including truancy, delinquency, incarceration
- Increased cortisol response, toxic stress
- Family adversity
- Suicidality
- Developmental trauma disorder

(Melhem et al., 2013; Pham et al., 2018; Revet et al., 2020; Schonfeld & Demaria, 2016).

SCREENING TOOLS FOR PERSISTENT COMPLEX BEREAVEMENT-RELATED GRIEF DISORDER IN CHILDREN

1. *Inventory for Complicated Grief-Revised for Children (ICG-RC)*
2. *Complicated Grief Assessment Interview (Child Version)-Short Form, Revised (parent form also available)*

   This is a 23-item questionnaire that can be administered to children. It evaluates yearning, level of denial, trust, hopelessness, and relationships since the death. It can be obtained from the author, Dr. Holly Prigerson, at measures@twosuns.org.
3. *Prolonged Grief Disorder (PGD)-13*

   This is a 13-item questionnaire that can be administered to children as per item 2. It evaluates similar responses as the item 2 questionnaire and can also be obtained from the author, Dr. Holly Prigerson, at holly_prigerson@dfci.harvard.edu.

INVENTORY FOR COMPLICATED GRIEF-REVISED (ICG-RC) FOR CHILDREN

Each of the 28 items is scored on a 5-point Likert scale with an overall score ranging from 28 to 140:

1 = Almost never (less than once a month)

2 = Rarely (monthly)

3 = Sometimes (weekly)

4 = Often (daily)

5 = Always (several times a day)

Inventory of Complicated Grief–Revised (ICG-RC) for Children					
Item	**Almost never (less than once/month)**	**Rarely (monthly)**	**Sometimes (weekly)**	**Often (daily)**	**Always (several times/day)**
	1	**2**	**3**	**4**	**5**
1. The death feels upsetting, overwhelming or devastating	❑	❑	❑	❑	❑
2. I think about....[a] so much that it can be hard for me to do the things I normally do	❑	❑	❑	❑	❑
3. Memories of.... upset me	❑	❑	❑	❑	❑
4. I feel that I cannot accept the death[b]	❑	❑	❑	❑	❑
5. I very much miss....[b]	❑	❑	❑	❑	❑
6. I feel angry about the death	❑	❑	❑	❑	❑
7. I feel that I cannot believe the death[b]	❑	❑	❑	❑	❑
8. I feel shocked over the death[b]	❑	❑	❑	❑	❑
9. Ever since the death, it is hard for me to trust people	❑	❑	❑	❑	❑
10. Ever since the death, I feel like I don't care about other people as much and I don't feel as close to people I care about as I used to	❑	❑	❑	❑	❑
11. I avoid reminders of....	❑	❑	❑	❑	❑
12. I avoid reminders that....[a] is dead	❑	❑	❑	❑	❑
13. Sometimes people who lose a loved one feel that they cannot go back to normal life and be able to make new friends and do new activities. Do you feel that making new friends or doing new activities would be difficult for you?	❑	❑	❑	❑	❑
14. I feel that life is empty or has no meaning without....[a]	❑	❑	❑	❑	❑
15. I hear the voice of....[a] speak to me	❑	❑	❑	❑	❑
16. I feel like I have become numb (or has no feelings) since the death	❑	❑	❑	❑	❑
17. I feel that it is unfair that I should live when....[a] died	❑	❑	❑	❑	❑

(*continued*)

(*continued*)

Inventory of Complicated Grief–Revised (ICG-RC) for Children					
Item	Almost never (less than once/month)	Rarely (monthly)	Sometimes (weekly)	Often (daily)	Always (several times/day)
	1	2	3	4	5
18. I am bitter (or angry) over the death	❑	❑	❑	❑	❑
19. I feel jealous of others who have not lost someone close	❑	❑	❑	❑	❑
20. I feel like the future has no meaning or purpose without....[a]	❑	❑	❑	❑	❑
21. I feel lonely ever since the death[b]	❑	❑	❑	❑	❑
22. It is difficult for me to imagine life being satisfying without....	❑	❑	❑	❑	❑
23. I feel that a part of myself died with....[a]	❑	❑	❑	❑	❑
24. I feel that the death made me see the world differently[b]	❑	❑	❑	❑	❑
25. I don't feel safe since the death	❑	❑	❑	❑	❑
26. I feel that I don't have control over things since the death	❑	❑	❑	❑	❑
27. I am jumpy or easily startled since the death	❑	❑	❑	❑	❑
28. Since the death, my sleep has been disturbed	❑	❑	❑	❑	❑

[a]"My parent" or the relationship lost.

[b]Items constitute the ICG-RC screen.

Source: Reprinted from (Melhem, N. M., Porta, G., Walker Payne, M., & Brent, D. A. (2013). Identifying prolonged grief reactions in children: Dimensional and diagnostic approaches, *Journal of the American Academy of Child and Adolescent Psychiatry*, *52*(6), 599–607.e7, Copyright (2013), with permission from Elsevier.)

MANAGING PROLONGED GRIEF DISORDER

The previously stated strategies for facilitating normal grief can be useful in preventing CG. In addition to these methods, pediatric providers should embrace the following approach with all families who have experienced a significant loss.

- Antidepressants and other mediations may be indicated for comorbid conditions of depression, PTSD, or anxiety.
- Screen surviving caregivers for symptoms of CG.
- Support positive parenting and monitor for signs of parental distress, such as evidence of self-medication or child/abuse neglect.
- Normalize grief through open discussion and psychoeducation regarding the grief process.

- Advocate health coping skills designed to improve self-care with emphasis on stress management, healthy nutrition, regular exercise, and adequate sleep.
- Refer to a child and adolescent mental health specialist when intensive treatment is indicated for CG, especially when grief is comorbid with other mental health disorders.
- It is important to note that CG is reported across all cultures, and that while it is universal, its manifestation is also affected by the cultural mores and spiritual beliefs of the families who experience it.

COMPLICATED GRIEF THERAPY (CGT)

- Studies provide insight to the course of grief in children and suggest when and how to intervene. Pham et al. (2018) conducted a prospective, longitudinal study to evaluate the long-term mental health sequelae over the course of 7 years following the death of a parent. Compared to nonbereaved children, parentally bereaved children have higher rates of depression and PTSD in the first 2 years following the death of a parent. Children who are less than 12 years old at the time of the loss are at highest risk for developing depression, while children whose parents died by suicide or natural death are at highest risk of developing PTSD (compared to accidental death). Overall, bereaved children experience higher rates of PTSD and functional impairment across all time points following the loss of a parent.
- The focus of standard grief therapy is to facilitate the natural grief process and help to construct a continuing bond with the deceased, rather than helping the individual "let go" and move on. Cognitive behavioral therapy (CBT) as a treatment intervention has been shown to effectively reduce the symptoms of CG (Wittouck et al., 2011). (See the COPE CBT-based skills building program, and the "adolescent coping with depression course" in the Brief Interventions section.)
- Complicated grief therapy (CGT) is a short-term targeted treatment for PGD that is derived from attachment theory, interpersonal therapy, and CBT. It has been shown to be superior to psychotherapy and antidepressant medications for depression in adults, and moreover, has been shown to be effective in targeting maladaptive cognitions to help individuals accept the reality of the loss and the grief response associated with the loss (Shear & Gribbin Bloom, 2017; Skritskaya et al., 2020). CGT is delivered in a 16-session manualized protocol. Adapting CGT for developmentally appropriate use with children and adolescents may also be effective.
- The Family Bereavement Program (FBP) is a manualized, 12-session group program for parentally bereaved children (ages 8–12), adolescents (12–16), and their caregivers. The program can help increase positive caregiver-child relationships, increase positive coping, strengthen adaptive control beliefs (e.g., understanding the cause of events and making appropriate distinctions between controllable and uncontrollable events), reduce appraisals of stressful events which threatened child/youth well-being or self-esteem, and promote adaptive emotional expression (Pham et al., 2020; Sandler et al., 2013).

SPECIAL CONSIDERATIONS

Suicide

Up to 12,000 U.S. children lose a parent to suicide each year. Grief following a loss to suicide is compounded due to the social stigma, shame, and abandonment issues that are triggered by suicide. Children who lose a parent under traumatic circumstances (e.g., suicide, violence, accident, war, disaster) may suffer from traumatic grief (re-experiencing the traumatic events through intrusive memories, thoughts, and feelings that complicate the grieving process) that necessitates family support (Bergman et al., 2017). Children who lose a parent to suicide before age 18 are three times more likely to die by suicide.

When the child is orphaned by suicide, give simple, honest answers to the child's questions and use words the child is likely to understand. Do not give more information than the child asks for. Answers should be honest but sparing with details. They will likely want to know more in the future. Examples:

- "When people die by suicide their mind is not healthy, and it makes them very sad and unhappy. This is a different kind of sadness than people feel when their mind is healthy."
- "Suicide is when a person's mind is sick (depressed), and they get so sad and don't know how to get help. They think ending their life is the only way to fix it."

Children may worry that they will die by suicide too; or young children who do not understand the irreversibility of death may say that they want to die too to be with their parent. Reassure children that suicide is not something you can catch from someone and it is not inherited from your parents. Reassure children that suicide is never the answer to a problem and that there are adults who can help solve problems. Remind children than if they become very sad, they should tell a trusted adult who can help.

Military

Children of military families face special needs related to prolonged absences of the military parent. During deployment, it is essential to have regularly scheduled time to communicate with the absent parent.

When a death in the line of duty happens (military, police, fire, etc.), many children will be told that they should be proud of their dead parents for their service. This leaves the child in an untenable position to grieve the very real loss of the parent. For children of military parents, the death is only one of many significant losses that happen quite immediate to the death, and which can include moving away from military support and housing, relocating to a new school (again non-military) so that the customary family supports are stripped away at a time when they are most needed.

COVID-19 Pandemic

Public health emergencies can have both short- and long-term impacts on children and adolescent mental health. The COVID-19 pandemic necessitated strict social distancing strategies to prevent infection and contain the viral spread. These circumstances result in chronic isolation, loneliness, and persistent fears. The subsequent loss of family and friends through social distancing or COVID-related death further compounds the grief. The trauma is cumulative.

Furthermore, economic downturns are associated with increased child maltreatment and mental health problems, similar to how adult unemployment and adult mental health are affected by economic downturns (Golberstein et al., 2019). In the first 6 months of the pandemic, emergency department visits for mental health-related concerns increased for children (aged 5–11) and adolescents (aged 12–17) by approximately 24% and 31%, respectively (Leeb et al., 2020). Particularly vulnerable children include those of younger developmental age, children with special needs, children with pre-existing mental health conditions, and socioeconomically disadvantaged children.

SUMMARY

Experiencing loss in childhood is inevitable. Learning how to cope with grief through the support of loving adults helps the vast majority of children process grief effectively and grow into healthy adults. However, there is indeed a subset of adults and their children at risk for CG and for whom early identification and intervention are critical for preventing severe long-term sequelae. Screening for CG and referring for specialized care are paramount. The goal of early identification and treatment is the prevention of morbidity *and* premature mortality by promoting adaptive coping, promoting a healthy lifestyle, managing the stress response, treating CG, comorbid depression, and PTSD early in both parent and child.

CHILD-FAMILY SUPPORT RESOURCES

- **National Association of Pediatric Nurse Practitioners**

  Behavioral and Mental Health Resources

  https://www.napnap.org/behavioral-and-mental-health-resources/

  KidsHealth® Information

  https://kidshealth.org/NAPNAP/en/

  - Helping Your Child Deal with Death

    https://kidshealth.org/NAPNAP/en/parents/death.htmlm

  - Death and Grief for Teens

    https://kidshealth.org/NAPNAP/en/teens/someone-died.html?WT.ac=clk_frommob

- **Child Mind Institute—https://childmind.org**

  Helping Children Cope

  https://childmind.org/guide/helping-children-cope-grief/

  Helping Children Cope During Covid-19

  https://childmind.org/coping-during-covid-19-resources-for-parents/#loss

- **National Alliance for Grieving Children—https://childrengrieve.org**

  https://childrengrieve.org/

  NAGT Hero Toolkit (2020): Responding to Change & Loss: In support of Children & Teens

  NAGT Hero Toolkit (2019): In support of Super Heroic Grieving Children & Teens

  NAGT Hero Toolkit (2017): Supporting Grieving Children during the Season of Family

REFERENCES

American Psychiatric Association. (2013). *Diagnostic and statistical manual of mental disorders* (5th ed.). Author. https://doi.org/10.1176/appi.books.9780890425596

Bergman, A. S., Axberg, U., & Hanson, E. (2017). When a parent dies–A systematic review of the effects of support programs for parentally bereaved children and their caregivers. *BMC Palliative Care, 16*(1), 39. https://doi.org/10.1186/s12904-017-0223-y

Burns, M., Griese, B., King, S., & Talmi, A. (2020). Childhood bereavement: Understanding prevalence and related adversity in the United States. *The American Journal of Orthopsychiatry, 90*(4), 391–405. https://doi.org/10.1037/ort0000442

Centers for Disease Control and Prevention. (2019). *Preventing adverse childhood experiences: Leveraging the best available evidence*. National Center for Injury Prevention and Control, Centers for Disease Control and Prevention.

Cheung, A. H., Zuckerbrot, R. A., Jensen, P. S., Laraque, D., & Stein, R. E. K. (2018). Guidelines for adolescent depression in primary care (GLADPC): Part II. Treatment and ongoing management. *Pediatrics, 141*(3):e20174082. https://doi.org/10.1542/peds.2017-4082

de López, K. J., Søndergaard Knudsen, H., & Hansen, T. G. B. (2020). What is measured in bereavement treatment for children and adolescents? A systematic literature review. *Illness, Crisis & Loss, 4*(28), 363–387. https://doi.org/10.1177/1054137317741713

Golberstein, E., Gonzales, G., & Meara, E. (2019). How do economic downturns affect the mental health of children? Evidence from the National Health Interview Survey. *Health Economics, 28*(8), 955–970. https://doi.org/10.1002/hec.3885

Griese, B., Burns, M., & Farro, S. A. (2018). Pathfinders: Promoting healthy adjustment in bereaved children and families. *Death Studies, 42*(3), 134–142. https://doi.org/10.1080/07481187.2017.1370416

Griese, B., Burns, M. R., Farro, S. A., Silvern, L., & Talmi, A. (2017). Comprehensive grief care for children and families: Policy and practice implications. *The American Journal of Orthopsychiatry, 87*(5), 540–548. https://doi.org/10.1037/ort0000265

Haine, R. A., Ayers, T. S., Sandler, I. N., & Wolchik, S. A. (2008). Evidence-based practices for parentally bereaved children and their families. *Professional Psychology, Research and Practice*, *39*(2), 113–121. https://doi.org/10.1037/0735-7028.39.2.113

Leeb, R. T., Bitsko, R. H., Radhakrishnan, L., Martinez, P., Njai, R., & Holland, K. M. (2020). Mental health–related emergency department visits among children aged <18 years during the COVID-19 pandemic — United States, January 1–October 17, 2020. *Morbidity and Mortality Weekly Report*, *69*, 1675–1680. http://dx.doi.org/10.15585/mmwr.mm6945a3

Lundorff, M., Holmgren, H., Zachariae, R., Farver-Vestergaard, I., & O'Connor, M. (2017). Prevalence of prolonged grief disorder in adult bereavement: A systematic review and meta-analysis. *Journal of Affective Disorders*, *212*, 138–149. https://doi.org/10.1016/j.jad.2017.01.030

Lyles, M. (2004). *Navigating children's grief: How to help following a death*. Children's Grief Education Association. https://www.tiporangecounty.org/pdfs/How_to_help_chart.pdf

Melhem, N. M., Porta, G., Walker Payne, M., & Brent, D. A. (2013). Identifying prolonged grief reactions in children: Dimensional and diagnostic approaches. *Journal of the American Academy of Child and Adolescent Psychiatry*, *52*(6), 599–607, e7. https://doi.org/10.1016/j.jaac.2013.02.015

Nakajima, S. (2018). Complicated grief: Recent developments in diagnostic criteria and treatment. *Philosophical Transactions of the Royal Society of London. Series B, Biological Sciences*, *373*(1754), 20170273. https://doi.org/10.1098/rstb.2017.0273

New York Life Foundation. (2017). *New York Life's bereavement survey: Key findings*. New York Life Foundation. https://www.newyorklife.com/assets/foundation/docs/pdfs/survey_key_findings.pdf

Pham, S., Porta, G., Biernesser, C., Walker Payne, M., Iyengar, S., Melhem, N., & Brent, D. A. (2018). The burden of bereavement: Early-onset depression and impairment in youths bereaved by sudden parental death in a 7-year prospective study. *The American Journal of Psychiatry*, *175*(9), 887–896. https://doi.org/10.1176/appi.ajp.2018.17070792

Prigerson, H. G., Horowitz, M. J., Jacobs, S. C., Parkes, C. M., Aslan, M., Goodkin, K., Raphael, B., Marwit, S. J., Wortman, C., Neimeyer, R. A., Bonanno, G. A., Block, S. D., Kissane, D., Boelen, P., Maercker, A., Litz, B. T., Johnson, J. G., First, M. B., & Maciejewski, P. K. (2009). Prolonged grief disorder: Psychometric validation of criteria proposed for DSM-V and ICD-11. *PLOS Medicine*, *6*(8), e1000121. https://doi.org/10.1371/journal.pmed.1000121

Revet, A., Bui, E., Benvegnu, G., Suc, A., Mesquida, L., & Raynaud, J. P. (2020). Bereavement and reactions of grief among children and adolescents: Present data and perspectives. *L'Encephale*, *46*(5), 356–363. https://doi.org/S0013-7006(20)30092-0

Sandler, I. N., Wolchik, S. A., Ayers, T. S., Tein, J. Y., & Luecken, L. (2013). Family bereavement program (FBP): Approach to promoting resilience following the death of a parent. *Family Science*, *4*(1), 1–14. https://doi.org/10.1080/19424620.2013.821763

Schonfeld, D. J., & Demaria, T. (2016). Supporting the grieving child and family. *Pediatrics*, *138*(3), e20162147. https://doi.org/10.1542/peds.2016-2147

Shear, M. K., & Gribbin Bloom, C. (2017). Complicated grief treatment: An evidence-based approach to grief therapy. *Journal of Rational-Emotive Cognitive-Behavioral Therapy*, *35*, 6–25. https://doi.org/10.1007/s10942-016-0242-2

Shear, M. K., Simon, N., Wall, M., Zisook, S., Neimeyer, R., Duan, N., Reynolds, C., Lebowitz, B., Sung, S., Ghesquiere, A., Gorscak, B., Clayton, P., Ito, M., Nakajima, S., Konishi, T., Melhem, N., Meert, K., Schiff, M., O'Connor, M. F., . . . Keshaviah, A. (2011). Complicated grief and related bereavement issues for DSM-5. *Depression and Anxiety*, *28*(2), 103–117. https://doi.org/10.1002/da.20780

Skritskaya, N. A., Mauro, C., Garcia de la Garza, A., Meichsner, F., Lebowitz, B., Reynolds, C. F., Simon, N. M., Zisook, S., & Shear, M. K. (2020). Changes in typical beliefs in response to complicated grief treatment. *Depression and Anxiety*, *37*(1), 81–89. https://doi.org/10.1002/da.22981

Wittouck, C., Van Autreve, S., De Jaegere, E., Portzky, G., & van Heeringen K. (2011). The prevention and treatment of complicated grief: A meta-analysis. *Clinal Psychology Review*, *31*, 69–78. https://doi.org/10.1016/j.cpr.2010.09.005

World Health Organization. (2018). *International classification of diseases for mortality and morbidity statistics* (11th Revision). https://icd.who.int/browse11/l-m/en

CHAPTER 19

Tasha Childs, Candra Skrzypek, Elizabeth Mellin, Aidyn Iachini, Annahita Ball, and Dawn Anderson-Butcher

Promoting Mental Health in Schools and Universities

FAST FACTS

- Although allied healthcare professionals commonly encounter the unique mental health concerns of children and adolescents in primary care settings, estimates suggest that nearly 70% of youth who receive treatment are served in school settings (Substance Abuse and Mental Health Services Administration [SAMHSA], 2019).
- Over $247 billion are spent on youth mental health conditions each year in the United States (Torio et al., 2015).
- Despite the increased recognition of students' mental health needs only a third of students who need mental health services and supports receive them (Merikangas et al., 2010; Torio et al., 2015).
- Of the 3.2 million adolescents accessing mental health services in schools, vulnerable youth who are low-income and identify as a minority race/ethnicity are most likely to receive services in schools only (Ali et al., 2019).
- Moving beyond a focus on individual mental health disorders, mental health promotion strategies involving universal prevention, early intervention, and targeted interventions, focus on creating environments that support positive mental health and wellness.
- Allied healthcare professionals, educators, mental health practitioners, and other professionals are also increasingly recognizing the relationship between positive mental health and learning outcomes. As a result, there is a growing emphasis on mental health promotion activities in schools as they provide both an access point to initial services and continued care (Kern et al., 2017; Suldo et al., 2014).

SCHOOL MENTAL HEALTH

Mental health means more than just the absence of mental illness—it "includes our emotional, psychological, and social well-being" (U.S. Department of Health and Human Services [DHHS], 2020). As such, school mental health includes promoting positive social and emotional development, creating environments to promote wellness, enhancing protective factors, and reducing risk factors that affect mental health, as well as the prevention and intervention of mental health problems (Adelman & Taylor, 2020). Current school mental health efforts focus on health promotion/positive development strategies, universal prevention strategies aimed at entire populations of youth, selective prevention strategies focused on targeted groups, indicated prevention strategies addressing youth with significant symptoms, and treatment interventions for those with disabilities or disorders (O'Reilly et al., 2018; Weisz et al., 2005). School mental health interventions aim to provide mental health service access and use for all students, especially those who outside of school would not be able to access services (Ali et al., 2019; Kern et al., 2017).

School mental health promotion is defined as:

> "Providing a full continuum of mental health promotion programs and services in schools, including enhancing environments, broadly training and promoting social and emotional learning and life skills, preventing emotional and behavioral problems, identifying and intervening in these problems early on, and providing intervention for established problems. School mental health promotion programs should be available to all students, including those in general and special education, in diverse educational settings, and should reflect a shared agenda–with families and young people, school and community partners actively involved in building, continuously improving, and expanding them" (Weist & Murray, 2007, p. 3).

Drawing from a public health approach, school mental health promotion-related activities are often classified by the timing of the intervention (see Kutash et al., 2006). For instance:

- There are school mental health programs and activities designed **to prevent the onset of emotional or behavioral problems (Tier I)**, as well as ones that target all youth in hopes of promoting general health and well-being.
- Some school mental health programs and activities **target vulnerable youth who are at-risk and present initial signs of academic, behavioral, social, and/or emotional needs (Tier II)**. These secondary prevention programs focus on individuals and groups of young people who might benefit from early intervention to address escalating needs.
- Still others **involve extensive treatments and interventions for indicated youth (Tier III)**. These school mental health programs are implemented once a disability or disorder has been diagnosed or established.

Essentially, school mental health promotion includes all the ways in which schools allow for teachers, administrators, students, families, mental health providers, community members, and others to collaborate to promote the overall well-being and academic achievement of students (Suldo et al., 2014; see also www.schoolmentalhealth.org).

THE IMPORTANCE OF SCHOOL MENTAL HEALTH PROMOTION

Researchers have shown that well-designed school mental health promotion programs and activities impact social, emotional, and learning outcomes for youth (Durlak et al., 2011; Greenberg et al., 2003; Kutash et al., 2006, 2015; Rones & Hoagwood, 2000; Salerno, 2016; Taylor et al., 2017). In fact, in their well-cited review paper, Suldo et al. (2014) synthesized the literature demonstrating the value of school mental health interventions for increasing social and emotional outcomes, improving behaviors (such as improved engagement in learning, attendance, and academic outcomes), and decreasing externalizing behaviors and teacher stress.

Factors associated with program effectiveness include the relationship between consistent implementation, the use of multi-component, comprehensive strategies addressing the whole child, programming that focuses on changing specific behaviors and skills, and the integration of the programs seamlessly into the mainstream classroom (Rones & Hoagwood, 2000; Salerno, 2016; Taylor et al., 2017). Additionally, policies that support mental health promotion and provide funding for additional services and supports may improve access and receiving services in schools (Salerno et al., 2016; Weist et al., 2017). So far, universal mental health promotion programs and interventions have proven effective in supporting students in developing coping skills and emotional regulation, and reducing symptoms of anxiety and depression (O'Connor et al., 2018). As school and student mental health outcomes are interwoven, schools have an interest and responsibility in positive promoting mental health.

In addition to the well-recognized relationship between mental health and learning outcomes, there are several other reasons why mental health promotion activities are focused in schools:

- **Children and adolescents spend a majority of their time in schools.** Students spend over 1,000 hours in school each year (National Center for Education Statistics, 2020). From a mental health promotion framework, schools are an important environmental influence on the social and emotional well-being of young people. They also are a place where initial signs and symptoms may be identified early, allowing for intervention supports to be put in place prior to the onset of major problems and issues.
- **Schools provide unmatched access to children and adolescents for the provision of mental health services.** Nationwide, there is a lack of mental health services for youth (Cummings et al., 2013). Despite one in five youth experiencing a mental health disorder (Merikangas et al., 2010), current estimates indicate that nearly half of youth with a treatable mental health disorder do not receive mental health services (Whitney & Peterson, 2019). Schools provide increased access to services, especially for racialized students and students from low-income households who are more likely to receive mental health services in educational settings only (Ali et al., 2019). School mental health promotion provides increased access to care and offers enhanced clinical productivity for mental health providers (Flaherty et al., 1996).
- In addition to access, **schools are also a natural environment for children and adolescents** that are not connected to stigmas associated with behavioral healthcare centers. Young people and their families are often more willing to engage in mental health services that are offered in more natural settings such as schools.
- **Schools have the environment to facilitate and maximize students' social emotional learning (SEL) skills to promote positive student mental health** (Durlak et al., 2011; Jagers et al., 2019; see also the Collaborative for Academic, Social, and Emotional Learning (CASEL), https://casel.org/). Current research suggests students who master social skills are better equipped to face academic challenges and have overall more positive well-being than students without mastery (Durlak et al., 2011). Additionally, SEL programs can have a positive impact beyond the intervention for up to 6 months post-intervention (Durlak et al., 2011).
- **Many of the important adults** (e.g., teachers, school counselors, school support staff) **in the lives of children and adolescents are located in schools.** As a result, mental health promotion activities provided in schools create consistency among adults involved in the everyday lives of youth. A range of preventive services may also be offered to address early concerns or needs. Additionally, accessing services in school avoids common challenges to accessing care, such as transportation, insurance, and difficulties locating providers (Ali et al., 2019).

Common Challenges

Despite the promise of school mental health, there are common challenges that jeopardize the success of these promotion strategies. Anecdotal accounts, practice experience, and research suggest common challenges to school mental health promotion:

- **Differing Priorities:** School and mental health systems work under different mandates that may result in competing priorities. Since the No Child Left Behind Act of 2001, schools, for example, are under enormous pressure to improve academic outcomes. Although schools are now required to collect data on school climate and student engagement under the Every Student Succeeds Act (ESSA, 2015) schools still prioritize academic learning over mental health and other socio-emotional needs. School administrators may not view school mental health promotion strategies as critical to demonstrating improved academic outcomes and, as a result, they may resist efforts to address mental health in their schools.
- **Limited Knowledge and Planning:** Although there has been significant growth in school mental health promotion, there still is limited knowledge and understanding in the field

related to the best service delivery systems and strategies. Additionally, when school mental health services are in place, there still is limited awareness and knowledge among stakeholders related to the existence of these services (Weist, 1997). For instance, sometimes services and activities are not well planned for and organized, resulting in uncoordinated strategies, service duplication, and poor sustainability.

- **Role Conflict:** Teachers and other school staff are often gatekeepers to students' access of mental health supports, as teachers are frequently responsible for recognizing symptoms and initiating referrals training (Ohrt et al., 2020). Yet only 10 of 50 states have teacher mental health standards that require identification of mental health symptoms, indicating a lack of training and recognition of appropriate processes for referral may be commonplace (Ball et al., 2016; Ohrt et al., 2020). Therefore, despite the reliance on teachers in mental health promotion, their training aligns more closely with traditional priorities of academic performance and learning, rather than student well-being and positive mental health.
- **Funding:** Mental health promotion necessarily encompasses a broad range of approaches and these services require significant resources and funding. In a context of substantial cuts to federal, state, and local education and mental health budgets, the funding demands associated with school mental health promotion can create competition and tensions between schools and mental health systems that may jeopardize the work. Funding for school mental health promotion activities is also complicated by tensions between school and mental health systems around who pays for mental health services for youth who qualify for special education. The Individuals with Disabilities Education Act (IDEA, 2004) is largely viewed as an unfunded mandate by education professionals, while mental health professionals see IDEA as a requirement for schools to pay for services. Such different perspectives on IDEA often lead to disagreements about who is responsible for funding mental health promotion activities for students enrolled in special education services (Kutash et al., 2006). Additionally, Medicaid allows schools to be reimbursed for school-based health and mental health services, however, about half of states limit this funding to students with individualized education programs or 504s (Wilkinson et al., 2020).
- **School Infrastructure and Culture:** Mental health professionals, who are often unfamiliar with school infrastructure and school culture, may have trouble identifying key contacts for starting this work. In addition, mental health professionals may struggle to "fit in" in school environments where the culture is oftentimes very different. Mental health professionals, for example, often encounter more open communication about children and adolescents in schools and struggle to build relationships with teachers who do not understand the professional limits of confidentiality. Often school mental health is seen as an "add-on" program or activity that is not central to the "real work" of schools. Additionally, most public schools are understaffed and do not meet professional ratio recommendations for mental health professional (e.g., school nurses, psychologists, counselors, social workers) per student (Mann et al., 2019).
- **Privacy and Confidentiality:** The various systems involved in school mental health promotion each are mandated by law to maintain the privacy of their "clients." For instance, the Family Education and Privacy Act (FERPA, 1980) protects the privacy of student education records; whereas the Health Insurance Portability and Accountability Act of 1996 (HIPAA) protects health records. Both aim to protect privacy, but pose challenges to coordinating services and supports across different service delivery sectors. Additionally, schools also must follow the Protection of Pupil Rights Amendment (PPRA), a federal law giving parents/guardians of minor students rights in relation to surveying their children in schools. Essentially, PPRA requires schools to get written consent from parents/guardians before students are required to participate in any U.S. Department of Education–funded survey, analysis, or evaluation. This pertains to questions personal in nature asking about topics such as mental and psychological problems potentially embarrassing to the student

and his/her family, sex behavior and attitudes, illegal, anti-social, self-incriminating and demeaning behavior, and critical appraisals of other individuals with whom they have close family relationships.

- **Collaboration and Coordination of Care:** School mental health promotion activities are also challenged by interagency and interprofessional collaboration, especially when serving youth who are involved in multiple systems (e.g., healthcare, juvenile justice, child welfare). Professional turf issues, lack of trust, little support from administrators, and billing mechanisms that only reimburse for direct services represent just a few of the issues that complicate collaboration and coordination of care across systems that intersect with school mental health promotion (Mendenhall et al., 2013).

Evidence-Based Management, Including Medication Management

Conceptual Models for School Mental Health Promotion

Three conceptual models of school mental health promotion (Kutash et al., 2006) provide additional context for allied healthcare providers interested in understanding how mental health services are delivered in schools. Here we briefly introduce and review The Mental Health Spectrum, Interconnected Systems, and Multi-tiered Supports. Brief examples are offered to illustrate practical applications of each model.

- **The Mental Health Spectrum for Mental Disorders** (Mrazek & Haggerty, 1994; Weisz et al., 2005): Developed by the Institute of Medicine, the Mental Health Spectrum for Mental Disorders organizes mental health treatment on a spectrum from prevention (including universal, selective, and indicated) to treatment (including case identification, standard treatment of known disorders), and maintenance (including compliance with long-term treatment and aftercare). More recent enhancements to the model have included emphasis on evidence-based practices and the interactions among schools, families, and communities within mental health service delivery (Kutash et al., 2006, 2015).
- **Interconnected Systems** (Center for School Mental Health, University of Maryland, Weist et al., 2003; Center for Mental Health in Schools, UCLA, Adelman & Taylor, 2006): The interconnected systems framework for school mental health promotion emphasizes partnerships between school and community systems for supporting mental health among children and adolescents. Representing a person-in-environment perspective, interconnected systems seek to bridge school and community systems to support youth through the delivery of prevention, early intervention, and systems of care services. Services such as character education, graduation coaches, and trauma-focused cognitive behavior therapy are coordinated across school and community systems and braiding of resources is a common strategy for maximizing limited funding (Kutash et al., 2006, 2015).
- **Multi-tiered Supports:** Three common frameworks are used in schools to provide a continuum of care for students across multiple tiers based on their ranging mental and personal health needs. Three frameworks, Positive Behavior Intervention Supports (PBIS; Bradshaw et al., 2012), Response to Intervention (RtI; Kearney & Graczyk, 2014), and Multi-tiered Systems of Supports (MTSS; August et al., 2018), are often used interchangeably in schools to reference three levels or tiers of supports. Programs and strategies are offered at these three levels of intervention: Tier 1, universal interventions for all students (often school-wide); Tier 2, targeted interventions for students demonstrating initial signs of risk; and Tier 3, intensive (selected) interventions often involving systems of care (Horner et al., 2010; Kern et al., 2017; Mrazek & Haggerty, 1994). These school mental health promotion-related activities have shown positive effects for students in areas such as, coping, social-emotional skills, depression, and anxiety (Bates et al., 2019; O'Connor et al., 2018). Additionally, PBIS

has demonstrated effectiveness for reducing discipline referrals and suspensions as well as improving overall school climate (Bradshaw et al., 2012). Promotion across the continuum of supports requires ongoing monitoring, using screeners, assessments, and other evaluative measures (August et al., 2018).

Universal or School-Wide Mental Health Promotion

Children's overall well-being may be positively impacted by the promotion of positive mental health through a variety of programs and initiatives in schools. These may include efforts to improve children's understanding of interpersonal relationships, social skills building, health awareness, and social competence development. For instance, schools may adopt trauma informed or SEL approaches to promote student mental health through universal prevention and screening. Schools and service professionals may enhance and build upon the protective factors in children's lives that promote wellness and positive outcomes.

Children may have a variety of protective factors. Some examples include:

- Opportunities and reinforcement for involvement in prosocial activities.
- Positive school climates.
- Strong bonds, supports, and relationships with caring adults and caregivers.
- Social competencies, such as decision-making skills, conflict resolution skills, empathy, and cultural competence.
- Associations with a prosocial peer group.
- Positive self-identity.
- Strong bonds and connectedness to school, youth development groups, or extracurricular activities.
- Feelings of safety in schools, at home, and in neighborhoods.

SAMHSA outlines evidence-based universal mental health promotion strategies in their National Registry of Evidence-Based Programs and Practices (https://www.samhsa.gov/ebp-resource-center). Schools are often encouraged to use programs from the national registry or the Institute of Education Sciences' What Works Clearinghouse database (https://ies.ed.gov/ncee/wwc/). The U.S. Department of Education also identifies exemplary programs that promote overall child well-being and safety (http://www2.ed.gov/admins/lead/safety/exemplary01). These evidence-based and exemplary programs utilize a number of strategies to address mental health on the universal level. Generally, these programs may be categorized as those that are focused on school climate, classroom-based strategies, character education, social skills training, and bullying prevention. Each of these approaches relies on interprofessional collaboration among professionals in the school setting, such as teachers, administrators, school nurses, and mental health professionals.

- **School Climate:** Positive school climate is critical for students' academic success and social-emotional well-being. School climate typically refers to the general quality of school life in four distinct areas: (a) physical and emotional safety; (b) peer and adult relationships; (c) teaching and learning; and (d) school environment (Cohen, 2009; Kearney & Graczyk, 2014). Universal prevention and intervention strategies can promote students' mental health by addressing school climate in these four areas. For example, anti-violence initiatives promote student safety while school-wide community building activities promote connections to peers and adults.
- **Culturally Responsive Practices, Diversity, and Equity:** School mental health promotion activities must be culturally responsive and equitable. This is especially important given the systematic inequities and disparities present in the education system. Research shows

that most social emotional interventions in schools do not use culturally responsive practice or address the impacts of racism and oppression on development (McCallops et al., 2019). The transformative SEL framework provides equity-elaborated definitions of social and emotional competencies and emphasizes understanding one's social identity, building strong relationships across difference, critically examining inequities, and promoting empowerment through collaborative problem solving (Jagers, 2019). Additionally, the National Center for School Mental Health provides culturally responsive resources for school mental health providers (http://www.schoolmentalhealth.org/Cultural-Responsiveness--Equity/).

- **Classroom-Based Strategies:** Classroom-based strategies are commonly used to provide universal intervention related to students' mental health and wellness. Typically, classroom-based strategies include curriculum-based instruction related to safe, drug-free schools, suicide awareness, social skills and problem-solving, and alcohol, tobacco, and drug use. Classroom management strategies may also prove effective as universal interventions. These strategies are typically employed by teachers to create structured, safe learning environments for all students. The use of classroom rules, reinforcement/incentive systems, and shared practices are examples of such strategies. Specifically, behavior management techniques may be included in regular classroom activities. These techniques include redirecting students who are disrupting class or providing additional outlets for student leadership and engagement. Additionally, restorative justice and alternative discipline approaches have emerged to combat the over-representation of minority students receiving punitive discipline (i.e., office discipline referrals; Crutchfield et al., 2020).
    - One example of a successful classroom-based strategy to improve the mental health, physical health, and healthy lifestyle behaviors of diverse children and teens is the Creating Opportunities for Personal Empowerment (COPE) Programs (Melnyk, 2003). The COPE Programs are manualized 7- and 15-session evidence-based cognitive behavioral skills building programs that have been shown to decrease depression, stress, and anxiety and improve healthy lifestyle behaviors and academic performance in children, teens, and college students when delivered by teachers in classroom settings or health professionals in small group or individual format in numerous studies (Hoying & Melnyk, 2016; Hoying et al., 2016; Melnyk, 2020; Melnyk et al., 2013a, b, 2014, 2015a, b). Developmentally targeted versions of the COPE program are available for children 7 to 11 years of age, adolescents from 12 through 17 years of age, and young adults 18 to 24 years of age.
- **Character Education:** Character education programs encompass a wide variety of techniques and curricula focused on promoting values. Generally, these programs aim to impart positive qualities and strategies that children may use throughout their lives (e.g., leadership, trustworthiness, empathy). Several character education programs are supported in the research literature, such as Character Counts and Steps to Respect, and research continues to examine the ways in which structured character education may enhance students' mental health. Typically, schools utilize aspects of character education to some extent in their regular, universal school programming. However, evidence to support character education is limited and additional research is needed to better understand its use in schools (Was et al., 2006).
- **Social Skills Training:** Social skills training is another universal intervention that is provided school-wide. Oftentimes, social skills training and character education are provided in tandem, or social skills lessons are infused in other universal strategies (e.g., classroom instruction, physical education, health, and wellness programs). Increasingly evidence shows social skills are vital to students' learning success and overall well-being, as students lacking social skill mastery may struggle to maintain appropriate classroom behavior and have poor interactions with peers (Aljadeff-Abergel et al., 2012). A series of best practices (Dupper, 2006; LeCroy, 2006) are necessary to achieve the maximum benefits of social skills training:

- Present the specific social skills.
- Discuss the skills.
- Provide examples to illustrate the skills.
- Allow opportunities to practice using role play.
- Create increasingly complex practice scenarios.
- Encourage practice of skills outside of group for generalization and maintenance

In recent years educational and school mental health policy and practices have honed in on one particular type of social skills training focused on SEL (Jagers et al., 2019). The most commonly used framework comes from Collaborative to Advance of Academic, Social, and Emotional Learning (CASEL; see https://casel.org/). The CASEL framework is comprised of five key SEL skills that serve as targets of interventions in schools and community-based programming, and includes self-awareness, social awareness, self-management, relationship-management, and responsible decision-making skills. There is emergent evidence supporting social, emotional, behavioral, and academic outcomes (Graczyk et al., 2000; Ross & Tolan, 2019).

State Departments of Education are increasingly developing standards to ensure students are taught SEL skills in schools. Ohio, for example, has created K-12 standards inclusive of recognizing emotions, developing self-awareness, and exercising relationship skills (see http://education.ohio.gov/Topics/Learning-in-Ohio/Social-and-Emotional-Learning/Social-and-Emotional-Learning-Standards). There are other models of SEL emerging in research and practice. Harvard's Ecological Approaches to Social Emotional Learning (EASEL) Lab (http://exploresel.gse.harvard.edu/) is an additional resource for more information, especially if interested in comparing existing models and frameworks.

- **Bullying Prevention:** Bullying is of increasing concern for individual children, as well as concerning to schools in terms of overall school climate. Bullying is repeated aggressive behavior initiated from an individual or group toward another individual or group (Bradshaw et al., 2013). Typically, bullying involves an imbalance of power that perpetuates the cycle of aggressive and passive behaviors among children. Several best practices are suggested to prevent bullying systemically:
    - Utilize assessments to understand the extent and nature of bullying: Seek input from students, teachers, student support service professionals, and families to gain information on the frequency and intensity of bullying. Identify physical areas and times of day in which bullying may be better or worse. Use these data to guide prevention and intervention strategies.
    - Focus on school-wide prevention to create a climate that discourages bullying behavior. Everyone in the school environment, including teachers, students, parents, administrators, and school staff, should promote social norms that encourage students to interact with each other in positive, prosocial ways.
    - Train school staff in bullying prevention and establish a team or committee to oversee bullying prevention and intervention efforts at the school.
    - Encourage family involvement in bullying prevention by informing parents/guardians of school norms, strategies to address bullying, or policies and procedures related to bullying in the school. Intervene consistently to stop bullying from becoming a larger problem. Adult supervision is essential, especially in areas identified as high-bullying areas. This also includes enforcing school policies consistently and appropriately.
- **Mental Health Education:** States are increasingly requiring mental health standards to be explicitly taught in schools. For example, in 2018, New York State enacted a policy that requires mental health education to be taught as part of standard health education to students in all grade levels (NYS Education Law, 2016). Schools will teach students how

to recognize mental health signs and symptoms, develop self-care habits, and the process of identification and referral to services (MHANYS, 2017). Other states, such as Virginia, Florida, Nevada, and New Jersey, have passed similar mandates, although each policy varies in terms of the amount of mental health education required. While these policies hope to increase mental health literacy among students, teachers also need further training on student mental health and social emotional needs (Ball et al., 2016). Schools have responded to the need for further training and professional development around mental health signs, symptoms, and referral by implementing universal trainings, such as the Youth Mental Health First Aid, Gateway Provider Model, and Gatekeeper training (Splett et al., 2018). These types of universal trainings and programs allow teachers, who are gatekeepers to accessing mental health services and supports, to better understand signs of common mental health disorders and recognize signs of suicide to better support students in the classroom by differentiating instruction.

Selected/Targeted Early Intervention, Referral, and Linkage Services

Universal strategies promote overall well-being and mental health for all students. However, some children present risk factors or symptoms that are identified early in their development requiring selected/targeted intervention. In addition, children may have factors in their lives that increase their risk of negative outcomes. These risk factors can be mitigated by prevention and intervention efforts.

Examples of risk factors include:

- Poor academic performance.
- Absenteeism.
- Antisocial behavior.
- Alcohol or drug use.
- Impulsivity.
- Hyperactivity.
- Internalizing behaviors and disorders.
- Abuse and/or neglect.
- Inadequate adult supervision.
- Family or community violence.
- Association with deviant peers.
- Family and community poverty.
- Homelessness or housing insecurity.
- Food insecurity.

If children begin to demonstrate symptomology consistent with behavioral, mental, or developmental issues, then it is suggested that early, selected/targeted intervention is necessary. A variety of strategies and practices may be appropriate at the selected/targeted level of intervention.

- **Attendance monitoring** is often an initial strategy to engage children and families in school and support services. Students who are frequently absent or truant may suffer in their academic progress, school connectedness, peer relations, and overall satisfaction with their school experiences. Monitoring attendance on a regular basis and using these data to identify students with frequent absences, is an effective strategy for early identification. Schools may opt to use existing school data on attendance or implement evidence informed programs, such as Check-in Check Out, which has had positive results increasing desirable behaviors from students (Drevon et al., 2019; Hawken & Horner, 2003).

- **Assessments** are also integral in monitoring students' progress and identifying problems early. Several assessments are appropriate in school settings. Those specifically related to children's mental health are identified at the end of this chapter. Over time, school mental health professionals and other service providers may monitor students' progress to guide future interventions.
- **Differentiated instruction and classroom supports** with groups of students based on the students' academic or social-emotional skill mastery are also effective in improving student outcomes (Dombek & Connor, 2012). For instance, differentiating instruction based on students' social skills, to intentionally create student learning groups with both high and low social skills can allow students to practice and model social skills alongside their peers. These strategies may be especially useful for youth vulnerable to grade-level retention or other negative academic outcomes in order to keep students on track in their academic trajectory (Dombek & Connor, 2012).
- **Individual and family counseling** is also important to address a multitude of interpersonal and social conflicts. Students may also need medication management or consultation services, often provided by a school nurse or school-based physician.
- **Small groups in schools:** Small therapeutic and psychoeducational groups also address children's mental health needs. Topical therapeutic groups may include groups to support students experiencing grief or trauma, family stress, peer difficulties, disruptive classroom behavior, anger, anxiety, or depression. Psychoeducation also can be an effective intervention technique for children who are first identified for support services.
- **Case management** is another important strategy for selected/targeted intervention. Case management allows a single point of contact to monitor and facilitate services for children and families. This includes effective referral and linkage processes that connect children and families to needed services within the school and community, such as those that address basic needs (e.g., housing, food, clothing) and mental health services (see Ball et al., 2020 for one school-based practice framework).
- **Student support teams** are teams of professionals that are also effective in addressing students' mental health needs at the selective/targeted tier. Student support teams financed by districts are often effective at managing and coordinating services for children in need of targeted interventions. These teams are frequently multi-professional and may achieve maximum efficiency and greatest positive outcomes when interprofessional collaboration is a priority (see Mellin, 2009 for information on interprofessional collaboration in school mental health practice).

Intensive Individualized Treatment/Interventions

In addition to universal and selective/targeted interventions, intensive individualized interventions are a critical component of the three-tier prevention and intervention model. These interventions target students in need of intensive services that are offered on the individual student or family level. They may include a variety of interventions and treatments that specifically address a student's mental health needs. The mode of service delivery may differ across settings and often is dependent upon available school and community resources. Examples of common service delivery strategies and interventions at the third tier include:

- **Mental health as a special education service** is oftentimes a necessary component of a free and appropriate educational program for students with disabilities, as required under the IDEA (ESSA, 2015; IDEA, 2004). Schools are required by law to provide assessment, treatment, and education in the least restrictive education setting to students with disabilities (including emotional and behavioral disorders). As a result, education and mental health-related services are provided by special education teachers, school psychologists, and other student support personnel (i.e., school social workers) to support students' overall learning and development.

- **School-based mental health services** for intensive individualized intervention are offered by mental health providers in the school building. For example, community mental health providers may meet with students and families in the school setting. They may also consult with teachers and other school staff, as well as other health providers outside of the school. There is growing evidence of the importance of school-based services, as research demonstrates the value of this approach for increasing access to services and continuity of care (Bates et al., 2019). One model is school-based health centers (SBHCs), which are co-located at schools and provide a range of health services for students and families. Up to 30% of visits to SBHCs are mental health visits (Bains & Diallo, 2016). SBHCs have doubled over the past two decades and are now in nearly 2,000 schools nationally reducing access barriers to healthcare services, especially for low-income families and racialized youth (Love et al., 2019). Regardless of the model, school-based mental health services operate under varying governance structures. More specifically, the school or district does not necessarily employ mental health providers that offer school-based services. These providers may be district employees, but they may also be employed by local community mental health or health agencies that are partnered with the school.
- **School-linked mental health services** that are intensive and individualized are provided outside of the school setting in partnership with the school. Schools typically contract with outside providers via formalized contracts or memoranda of understanding. In turn, treatment is provided for individual students and their families at settings outside of the school. Typically, outside providers include county mental health agencies, community mental health centers, the juvenile justice system, or child welfare agencies.
- **Systems of care and wraparound** sometimes exist to support students involved in multiple systems who present co-occurring problems and needs. While the education and mental health systems have been historically divided, a school-based system of care encompasses all services necessary to meet the needs of severely emotionally disturbed children. This perspective has emphasized that schools and communities must: (a) increase access to services; (b) provide individualized services in the least restrictive setting; (c) engage parents and families for service planning and delivery; and (d) coordinate and integrate services across agencies, including schools (Leaf et al., 2003).
- **School-based mental health teams** do not provide direct service to individual students; instead, they are multidisciplinary groups that focus on coordinating services for students in need of intensive interventions. These teams are typically composed of multiple professionals, including teachers, social workers, psychologists, administrators, nurses, counselors, and other student support personnel (e.g., occupational therapists, speech pathologists). Parents and students also may serve on these teams. School-based mental health teams provide case management, triage, and referral, as well.
- **Medication management services in schools** are typically led by school nurses and include the storage, administration, and tracking of medications. This service is critical to many children and adolescents, especially those with chronic healthcare needs and disabilities, who rely on medications to help manage mental health symptoms. Students receive a variety of different types of medication in schools, though medication for ADHD and asthma are the most common. Older children and adolescents are more likely to receive psychiatric medication in schools than younger children (Maughan et al., 2018). While not all schools have registered nurses present each day, the National Association of School Nurses [NASN] advocates for school nurses to be responsible for the development and leadership of

medication management policies and procedures in schools to reduce medication errors, improve safety, and coordinate care among students, parents, providers, and schools (NASN, 2017).

- **Telehealth services** where students and families access healthcare providers remotely while on-site at a school campus have become increasingly popular, especially within rural communities (Love et al., 2019). As schools continue to promote mental health, the COVID-19 pandemic has pushed schools to increasingly rely on telehealth services. For instance, in one state, about 33 % of school districts provided tele-mental health and telehealth services on their websites (Iachini & Childs, 2021).

Overall, a number of practices and intervention strategies are supported in the existing research on school mental health. Collectively, services that are provided across the intervention continuum maximize schools' and allied health professionals' ability to address student mental health needs.

Comprehensive Approaches

The complex needs of children, families, and schools oftentimes require more comprehensive approaches to promoting children's mental health and well-being. These approaches are multi-faceted and dynamic, often including multiple disciplinary perspectives and practitioners.

- **Coordinated school health programs** (CSHP) involve the interaction of multiple components all centered on promoting student well-being (Centers for Disease Control and Prevention [CDC], 2007). The key CSHP components span health education and physical education, health services and nutrition services, counseling and psychological services, healthy school environment, and family/community involvement (CDC, 2007). CSHP promotes the coordination of policies, activities, and services that address these components and, ultimately, provide for the health of school students and staff while strengthening schools to be "critical facilities" for service provision and coordination (CDC, 2007, n.d.). School-based health centers (described later in this chapter) are one way that the CSHP has been implemented in practice.
- An **interconnected systems framework (ISF)** for meeting the needs of all students is another comprehensive approach to address student needs across all three tiers of supports (Splett et al., 2017). In this framework, Adelman and Taylor (1999, 2006, 2020) advocate for the maximization and alignment of community and school resources and services across the learning support continuum. This work requires collaboration among jurisdictions, school districts, community agencies, and the public and private sectors across systems of prevention, early intervention, and care. Common core standards for comprehensive systems of learning supports addressing whole child development are currently in development (Adelman & Taylor, 2012). Additionally, implementation relies on ongoing data collection to support informed decision-making on universal mental health promotion and evidence-informed intervention selection (Splett et al., 2017).
- **Full-service and community schools** (FSCS; Dryfoos, 1994; Lubell, 2011) models have grown in use over the last 20 years. These models view the school as the "hub" of community support, co-locating education, health, positive youth development, mental health, workforce development, and social services together at schools. These models exist across the country but vary widely as some schools have a vast array of services whereas others may have only one or two service sectors represented (Dryfoos, 1994). One example of the FSCS approach is the *Communities in Schools* initiative which utilizes community partnerships to support school improvement and priority areas based on each school's individual needs (see https://www.communitiesinschools.org/our-model/). There is emergent research

to demonstrate the value of the community schools approach for promoting student- and school-level outcomes (Anderson-Butcher et al., 2017; Johnston et al., 2020).

- **Trauma-informed schools** aim to minimize the impact of trauma on students' performance and experience in school (Maynard et al., 2019; Wiest-Stevenson & Lee, 2016). As up to 60 % of students have experienced a traumatic event, schools are beginning to implement trauma-informed practices (Wiest-Stevenson & Lee, 2016). These practices may include universal prevention and evidence-informed targeted interventions, such as Cognitive Behavioral Intervention for Trauma in Schools (CBITS; see https://cbitsprogram.org/). CBITS has been used in schools to reduce symptoms of trauma and/or post-traumatic stress disorder (PTSD) in students through individual or group sessions and has strong evidence of effectiveness with students (Chafouleas et al., 2019; Jaycox et al., 2012). Additionally, CBITS screens for current symptoms of PTSD, then identified students participate in the program, which mainly focuses on providing psychoeducation and management of symptoms related to anxiety and depression.
- **Whole school, whole child, whole community** (WSCC; Lewallen et al., 2015) is a framework with 10 components, including the eight from CSHP, and provides a holistic approach to student health and education. This framework aims to promote wellness across all stakeholders, such as families, teachers, and students. Additionally, WSCC emphasizes the reliant roles of education and health in students' lives across their lifetime in terms of financial and emotional well-being.
- The **community collaboration model for school improvement** (CCMSI) also provides an example of new models of school improvement focused on students' nonacademic barriers to learning, including mental health issues (Anderson-Butcher et al., 2008, 2010). This model addresses the need for schools and educators to gain influence over students' out-of-school time and on the need for schools to further utilize existing family and community resources to optimize student learning and healthy development using systematic organization of numerous improvement components. Focused on building system capacity for improvement, the CCMSI involves continuous planning and improvement processes that are evaluation-driven and anchored in "milestones" that mark developmental progress for school leaders. Five content areas guide the CCMSI expanded school improvement initiative – academic learning, youth development, parent/family engagement and support, health and social services, and community partnerships.

Oftentimes, these comprehensive approaches are rooted in more traditional school improvement processes, such as standards-based accountability and curriculum realignment. As such, local, state, and federal policy are integral in the development, implementation, and sustainability of these approaches. More specifically, several federal policy initiatives guide the promotion of mental health in schools.

Federal Policies

Current federal policy initiatives emphasize including mental health services within existing school improvement frameworks, while others promote the development and strengthening of existing mental health services in partnership with schools.

- **ESSA** (also formerly known as the **Elementary and Secondary Education Act** or the **No Child Left Behind Act**) is the federal law that funds public education, providing equal access to high quality education for all youth (Solomon et al., 2020). The law focuses on raising student achievement and addressing disproportionality and disparities through standards-based reforms and accountabilities. Title I is a key component of this policy, and provides additional learning supports and resources for students from disadvantaged circumstances. The 2015 revision of ESSA requires schools to collect a fifth accountability measure, school quality or student success, which may include student engagement, post-secondary readiness, and school climate and safety (Solomon et al., 2020; ESSA, 2015).

- **IDEA** is the long-standing federal policy to protect and provide intervention services for children with disabilities. Students with disabilities (physical, emotional, and learning) have the right to formalized school support services that are data-based and -driven. States are provided with partial funding to implement service strategies and systems that address students' learning needs within special education. In addition, states that receive federal funds under IDEA are required to provide a free and public education in the least restrictive setting for all students. This is implemented via ongoing assessment, individualized education plans (IEP), appropriate accommodations and related services, and impartial hearings.
- **Section 504 of the Rehabilitation Act of 1973** prohibits discrimination based upon disability. Similar to the provisions of IDEA, Section 504 requires that students with disabilities receive a free and appropriate education and are entitled to appropriate accommodations and related services. Written plans, termed 504 plans, are developed and enacted to specify these accommodations. 504 plans are different from IEPs, however, because any child with a disability may have a 504 plan. Only students eligible for special education services may have an IEP.
- **The McKinney-Vento Homeless Assistant Act** (Title IX, Part A of ESSA) provides educational protections for students experiencing homelessness and aims to reduce barriers to a high-quality education for these youth. For example, under this Act, homeless students can remain in their school of origin if it is in their best interest and must have access to all eligible programs and services. Under the provisions of McKinney-Vento, each local education agency must designate a liaison who is responsible for the identification and enrollment of homeless youth and removing barriers that may hinder their attendance and educational success. McKinney-Vento local educational agency subgrant funds may be used for the provision of mental health services.
- **School-based health centers** remain a policy priority as recent federal initiatives provide states considerable funds to establish school-based health centers. Based on the CDC's Coordinated School Health model, school-based health centers provide a myriad of health services within schools. These may include primary healthcare, mental health and behavioral healthcare, health and mental health education and promotion, case management, and crisis intervention. Additionally, in response to COVID-19 the Coronavirus Aid, Relief and Economic Security (CARES) Act allotted states additional funding to support students with disabilities, internet access, food distribution, personnel protective equipment, and other emerging needs (U.S. Department of Education, n.d.).

Screening and Assessment Tools for School Mental Health Promotion

As part of school mental health promotion efforts, many schools utilize a wide variety of screening and assessment tools. Some screening and assessment tools are designed to assess the health and well-being of individual students, and some are designed to assess the overall school system. Examples of key constructs assessed at the individual level include depression and suicide, bullying, alcohol and other drug use, as well as other specific social-emotional barriers to learning. School-wide assessment tools examine the overall system, specifically in relationship to improvement processes that support student learning and development.

Prior to providing examples of these individual-level and system-wide screening and assessment tools, it is important to note that schools already collect academic and behavioral data as part of normal educational practices. For example, schools not only track grades, but also track attendance and behavioral data such as suspensions and expulsions. Many schools also collect rapid assessment academic data on individual students in order to track students' trajectories over time, known as "value-added" data.

Individual-Level Screening and Assessment Tools.

Individual-level screening and assessment tools allow practitioners to identify and understand the nature of problems children and adolescents might be experiencing. They also help identify related assets and strengths. Using these tools is important in practice, particularly as it ensures students are identified, referred, and provided with the best services and supports to meet their needs.

The U.S. Preventive Services Task Force (USPSTF) makes recommendations regarding preventive screening and other prevention services for the primary care setting (http://www.uspreventiveservicestaskforce.org/). While the focus of this chapter is on screening and assessment in the school setting, these recommendations are still important for nurses to consider in their practice and are presented next. Relevant Task Force recommendations for screening are overviewed here.

- Some key areas for screening and assessment in the school setting include depression, suicide, and alcohol, tobacco, and other drug (ATOD) use. With regard to depression, the USPSTF (2016) recommends screening adolescents between 12 and 18 years of age for major depressive disorder if services and supports are available for identified students. For children (ages younger than 11 years old), the USPSTF (2016) suggests there is inconclusive evidence to make a recommendation. The USPSTF (2014; 2020b) also suggests there is inconclusive evidence regarding screening for suicidal risk and ATOD use in children and adolescents. The American Academy of Pediatrics (AAP, 2020), however, suggests that adolescents should be screened for alcohol, tobacco, and other drug use with psychometrically validated measures.
- Another resource for screening and assessment, for middle and high school students, is the Youth Risk Behavior Surveillance System (YRBSS). The YRBSS survey is conducted by the Centers for Disease Control and Prevention (CDC) and freely accessible in the public domain (see https://www.cdc.gov/healthyyouth/data/yrbs/index.htm). The YRBSS asks questions regarding youths' behaviors with alcohol, tobacco, and other drug use, dietary, physical activity, and sexual activity. Additionally, the YRBSS is available in a Spanish version (https://www.cdc.gov/healthyyouth/data/yrbs/pdf/2021/2021_YRBS_National_HS_Questionnaire-Spanish.pdf).

In addition, a variety of tools exist to screen and assess these three key areas (depression, suicide, and ATOD use), including:

- Some commonly used assessment tools for depression include the **Patient Health Questionnaire for Teens** (PHQ-9 for Teens; Kroenke et al., 2001), the **Reynold's Children or Adolescent Depression Scale** (Reynolds, 1994), and the **Beck's Depression Inventory-II** (BDI-II: Beck et al., 1996). These tools have demonstrated psychometric properties. Following are the websites where these tools can be purchased or freely used with author permission.
  - PHQ-9 for Teens: https://www.aap.org/en-us/professional-resources/quality-improvement/Project-RedDE/Pages/Depression.aspx
  - Reynold's Child Depression Scale-2nd edition: http://www4.parinc.com/Products/Product.aspx?ProductID=RCDS-2
  - Reynold's Adolescent Depression Scale-2nd edition: http://www4.parinc.com/Products/Product.aspx?ProductID=RADS-2
  - BDI-II: https://www.pearsonassessments.com/store/usassessments/en/Store/Professional-Assessments/Personality-%26-Biopsychosocial/Beck-Depression-Inventory-II/p/100000159.html

- One widely adopted screening tool for suicide is the **Suicidal Ideation Questionnaire–Junior** (SIQ-JR)
  - SIQ-Jr: http://www4.parinc.com/Products/Product.aspx?ProductID=SIQ
- AAP (2020) recommends using the **CRAFFT, GAIN,** or **AUDIT** as a screening measure for ATOD use, substance use disorders, and mental health disorders. Additional screeners and assessment tools recommended by AAP can be found here: https://www.aap.org/en-us/advocacy-and-policy/aap-health-initiatives/Pages/Substance-Use-Screening.aspx

Another key area for assessment in the school setting is bullying. In 2011, the CDC developed a compendium of assessment tools to assess bullying. Some of these tools are available in the public domain, but others are not.

- One commonly used tool presented in this compendium with good psychometric properties is the **Olweus Bullying Questionnaire** (OBQ; Solberg & Olweus, 2003). This tool must be purchased for use.
  - OBQ: https://www.hazelden.org/store/item/14432

In addition to measures of specific mental and behavioral health concerns, there also are other more global tools that exist. These tools assess a wide range of constructs that are of interest to school mental health promotion. Examples of these tools are presented next. All of these need to be purchased for use in the school settings. The websites to purchase these tools are listed after each description of the tool.

- The **Behavior Assessment System for Children, 3rd Edition (BASC-3;** Reynolds & Kamphaus, 2015) is a commonly used tool that can be completed by teachers, parents, or students. Depending on version, the BASC-3 assesses constructs such as anxiety, depression, social skills, self-esteem, and attention problems. Additionally, the Behavioral and Emotional Screening System (BESS) is a subsection of the BASC-3 that may be used to screen student's ages 3 to 18 years old (Reynolds & Kamphaus, 2015).
  - BASC-3: https://www.pearsonassessments.com/store/usassessments/en/Store/Professional-Assessments/Behavior/Comprehensive/Behavior-Assessment-System-for-Children-%7C-Third-Edition-/p/100001402.html
  - BASC-3 BESS: https://www.pearsonassessments.com/store/usassessments/en/Store/Professional-Assessments/Behavior/Comprehensive/BASC-3-Behavioral-and-Emotional-Screening-System/p/100001482.html
- Another commonly used tool is the **Child Behavior Checklist** (CBCL). The CBCL also can be completed by teachers, parents, or students. The tool assesses constructs such as social relationship competence, school competence, and youths' emotional and behavioral problems.
  - CBCL: https://aseba.org/school-age/
- The **Developmental Assets Profile** (DAP; Search Institute, 2004) is another available tool that assesses the extent to which youth experience a range of assets across a variety of contexts, including at home, in school, and in the community.
  - DAP: https://www.search-institute.org/surveys/choosing-a-survey/dap/
- The **Social, Academic, and Emotional Behaviors Risk Screener (SAEBRS;** Kilgus et al., 2016) is a 19-item tool completed by teachers through an online platform to universally screen students for risk factors, including social skills, and internalizing and externalizing behaviors.
  - SAEBRS: https://www.fastbridge.org/saebrs/

- The **Direct Behavior Rating scale (DBR;** Chafouleas et al., 2010, 2013) has been used to screen elementary, middle, and high school students for academic, disruptive, and respectful behaviors in the classroom. The measure is completed by teachers and includes questions, such as "How well did the student pay attention today?."
    - DBR: https://www.fastbridge.org/product-seb/
- **The Student Strengths Assessment (DESSA;** LeBuffe et al., 2018) has two main versions, DESSA (72 items) and DESSA-mini (8 items) which are used to assess, plan, and monitor behaviors relating to students, social-emotional well-being during both in- and out-of-school time. This tool aligns items with the CASEL SEL dimensions, including self-awareness and relationship skills. Measures are completed by teachers, program staff, and/or parents at one or multiple time points.
    - DESSA: https://apertureed.com/products-solutions/dessa-system-2/dessa-overview/

School mental health promotion also involves ensuring students have their basic needs met (Adelman & Taylor, 2020). Other measures have been developed to assess students' access to basic needs, such as safety, food insecurity, homelessness, and internet access. Screeners are presented in the following that measure food insecurity.

- The U.S. Department of Agriculture (USDA, 2020) **Self-Administered Food Security Survey Module** (Connell et al., 2004) is a 9-item survey, which asks students to recall answers to questions around their food access in the past month. The survey is appropriate for youth 12 years and older.
    - Youth Self-Administered Food Security Survey Module: https://www.ers.usda.gov/media/8283/youth2006.pdf
- The **Child Food Security Assessment** is a 9-item survey that asks children to report how many times they have experienced instances of food insecurity in the last year. For instance, statements include, "I worry about not having enough to eat" and "I try not to eat a lot so that there is enough food for everyone to eat" (Fram et al., 2013, 2015). This tool is appropriate for children older than 6 years old and is available in English and Spanish versions.

Other global tools have been developed that are available for free in the public domain. The Safe and Supportive Schools Technical Assistance Center School Climate Survey Compendium provides a host of assessment tools. The Compendium can be found here: https://safesupportivelearning.ed.gov/topic-research/school-climate-measurement/school-climate-survey-compendium

- One tool found in the Center Compendium is the **Community and Youth Collaborative Institute (CAYCI) School Experience Surveys** (CAYCI-SES; Anderson-Butcher & Amorose, 2012; Anderson-Butcher et al., 2013, 2020), which assess student well-being and school climate. For instance, the surveys include measures of internalizing behaviors, such as feeling anxious and worried, and externalizing behaviors such as fighting and bullying. The CAYCI-SES surveys also assess a range of other constructs including academic motivation, school connectedness, academic stress, parent involvement/support, teacher/student relationships, and community and learning supports. All of these surveys are in English and Spanish, and there are elementary and secondary youth, parent, and teacher versions of these tools. Surveys are in the public domain and may be used with permission of the author (see http://cayci.osu.edu/surveys/overview-and-development/). Schools can also explore the data collected from students, teachers, and parents together for common themes and priorities, and identify targets for system-wide improvements. Technical support is available related to data collection, analyses, and report generation (with normed data) for a nominal charge (http://cayci.osu.edu/surveys/overview-and-development/getting-started-with-ses/).

System-Level Assessment Tools

Several school-wide assessment tools also have been developed to assess system-level factors across school mental health promotion efforts. Although schools have their own system of accountability for reporting student performance measures, schools also use existing data from office discipline referrals, attendance, and other ratings to approximate student experiences. These tools are meant to identify priority areas for school-wide planning efforts, and therefore do not have validated psychometric properties.

- One relevant tool for school mental health promotion is the **School Mental Health Quality Assessment Questionnaire** (SMH-QAQ; Weist, 2006). The SMH-QAQ assesses the extent to which a school has in place a variety of SMH best practice principles, including (a) access to care, (b) funding, (c) needs assessment, (d) addressing needs and strengths, (e) evidence-based practice, (f) stakeholder involvement and feedback, (g) quality assessment and improvement, (h) continuum of care, (i) referral process, (j) clinician training, support, and service delivery, (k) competently addressing developmental, cultural, and personal differences, (l) interdisciplinary collaboration and communication, and (m) community coordination (http://www.theshapesystem.com/).
- Another relevant planning tool is the CDC's **School Health Index** (SHI). The SHI assesses the eight key dimensions of the coordinated school health model. These dimensions include (a) school health and safety policies/environment, (b) health education, (c) physical education and other physical activity programs, (d) nutrition services, (e) health services, (f) counseling, psychological, and social services, (g) health promotion for staff, and (h) family and community involvement (http://www.cdc.gov/healthyyouth/shi/).
- The guidelines for school mental health, developed by the **Center for Mental Health in Schools at UCLA** (2001), also are important to consider for school-wide assessments (http://www.smhp.psych.ucla.edu/). Specifically, six overarching guidelines are shared related to (a) domains of intervention, (b) barriers to student learning, (c) types of services/support provided, (d) timing of interventions, (e) quality of interventions, and (f) accountability mechanisms. Examining this list and identifying the extent to which a school mental health program meets these guidelines may be a helpful step in planning efforts.
- The National Center for School Mental Health (NCSMH) at the University of Maryland School of Medicine, in partnership with the field, developed **The School Health Assessment and Performance Evaluation System (SHAPE System**; https://www.theshapesystem.com/) to increase the quality, accountability, and sustainability of school mental health systems in schools. The SHAPE system is an interactive tool which allows school communities to assess their overall approach to school mental health services and supports. Districts use the SHAPE system to look at areas where their schools can improve in relation to best practices and impact. Please note there also are ample school mental health resources available on the SHAPE website.

Resources Available, Including Excellent Websites on the Topic

- Caring Across Communities: http://healthinschools.org/caring-across-communities/#sthash.KlgjTXxR.dpbs
- Center for Health and Health Care in Schools: www.healthinschools.com
- Center for Resilient Children: https://centerforresilientchildren.org/

- Center on School Mental Health: www.csmh.umaryland.edu
- Communities in Schools: https://www.communitiesinschools.org/
- Community and Youth Collaborative Institute at The Ohio State University: https://cayci.osu.edu/
- Creating Opportunities for Personal Empowerment Programs for Children, Teens and Young Adults: www.cope2thrive.com
- Georgetown University Center for Child and Human Development: http://gucchd.georgetown.edu/
- Harvard Family Research Project: www.hfrp.org
- Mental Health First-Aid Training: https://www.mentalhealthfirstaid.org/take-a-course/
- Mental Health-Education Integration Grant Programs: https://www2.ed.gov/programs/mentalhealth/index.html
- National Assembly on School-Based Health Care: https://www.sbh4all.org/school-health-care/national-census-of-school-based-health-centers/
- National Center on Safe Supportive Learning Environments: https://safesupportivelearning.ed.gov/promoting-mental-health
- National Center for School Mental Health: http://www.schoolmentalhealth.org/
- School Mental Health Playbook: https://www.azahcccs.gov/AHCCCS/Downloads/Initiatives/BehavioralHealthServices/Helios/Tucson_09252019/ToolkitResource/School-Mental-Health-Screening-Playbook.pdf
- National Child Traumatic Stress Network: https://www.nctsn.org/
- National Dissemination Center for Children with Disabilities: http://nichcy.org/
- National Technical Assistance Center for Children's Mental Health: https://www.samhsa.gov/nttac
- National Technical Assistance Center on Positive Behavior and Intervention Supports: http://www.pbis.org/
- Panorama Education: https://www.panoramaed.com/
- Research and Training Center for Children's Mental Health at USF's Louis de la Parte Florida Mental Health Institute: http://rtckids.fmhi.usf.edu/default.cfm
- Safe Schools/Healthy Students: https://healthysafechildren.org/grantee/safe-schools-healthy-students
- SAMHSA National Registry of Evidence-Based Programs and Practices: https://www.samhsa.gov/ebp-resource-center
- School-Based Behavioral Health: http://www.sbbh.pitt.edu/
- School Mental Health Training Center: https://www.mentalhealthednys.org/mh-education-readiness/
- School Social Work.Net: https://schoolsocialwork.net/
- Technical Assistance Center on Social Emotional Intervention for Young Children: http://www.challengingbehavior.org/
- UCLA School Mental Health Clearinghouse: http://smhp.psych.ucla.edu/clearing.htm
- USDOE Exemplary Programs: http://www2.ed.gov/admins/lead/safety/exemplary01
- U.S. Department of Education, Laws & Guidance: https://www2.ed.gov/policy/landing.jhtml?src=pn

Appropriate Handouts With Important and Age-Appropriate Information

Presented next is a list of forms oftentimes helpful within school mental health promotion efforts. Each form is briefly described and a link to a template form is provided.

- **Release of Information:** This form allows parents/guardians to determine with whom professionals can share private and confidential information about their child and/or family. Until a release is signed, information should not be shared with professionals from other agencies. A template release of information can be found in the Appendix of the School Linkage Protocol (Anderson-Butcher et al., 2011) at the following website: http://cayci.osu.edu/wp-content/uploads/2015/03/2-10-10SchoolLinkageProtocol_ForPrint.pdf
- **Telehealth Consent Form:** This form is a free resource provided by the National Association of Social Workers (NASW) in response to a shift to alternative methods of services, such as online and over the phone, due to COVID-19 closures (n.d.). The form can be used as a basis for developing informed consent forms for your schools' specific needs and service delivery. A telehealth consent form shoud be used.
- **Memorandum of Understanding (MOU):** An MOU, also oftentimes referred to as a Memo of Agreement (MOA), is a form that ensures that all parties entering a collaborative partnership are aware of their roles and responsibilities. In addition, an MOU outlines the timeframe for the agreement. A template MOU can be found in the Appendix of the School Linkage Protocol (Anderson-Butcher et al., 2012) at the following website: http://cayci.osu.edu/wp-content/uploads/2015/03/2-10-10SchoolLinkageProtocol_ForPrint.pdf
- **Medication Management Checklist:** The Center for Health and Health Care in Schools has developed a brief checklist for parents to assess whether their child's school has policies in place to ensure students receive the appropriate medications at the appropriate times. This checklist can be found at http://healthinschools.org/issue-areas/other-school-health-issues/school-health-services/medication-management/state-policies-on-administration-of-medication-in-schools/#sthash.OWyhDkzj.dpbs

REFERENCES

Adelman, H. S., & Taylor, L. (1999). Mental health in schools and system restructuring. *Clinical Psychology Review, 19*(2), 137–165. https://doi.org/10.1016/s0272-7358(98)00071-3

Adelman, H. S., & Taylor, L. (2006). *The school leader's guide to student learning and supports: New directions for addressing barriers to learning*. Corwin Press.

Adelman, H. S., & Taylor, L. (2012). *Common core standards and learning supports*. http://smhp.psych.ucla.edu/pdfdocs/comcorannounce.pdf.

Adelman, H. S., & Taylor, L. (2020). *Addressing barriers to learning: In the classroom and schoolwide*. http://smhp.psych.ucla.edu/pdfdocs/barriersbook.pdf

Ali, M. M., West, K., Teich, J. L., Lynch, S., Mutter, R., & Dubenitz, J. (2019). Utilization of mental health services in educational setting by adolescents in the united states. *The Journal of School Health, 89*(5), 393–401. https://doi.org/10.1111/josh.12753

Aljadeff-Abergel, E., Ayvazo, S., & Eldar, E. (2012). Social skills training in natural play settings: Educating through the physical theory to practice. *Intervention in School and Clinic, 48*(2), 76–86. https://doi.org/10.1177/1053451212449737

Anderson-Butcher, D., & Amorose, A. J. (2012). *Community and Youth Collaborative Initiative School Community Surveys technical reports*. College of Social Work, The Ohio State University.

Anderson-Butcher, D., Amorose, A., Bates, S., Iachini, A., Ball, A., & Henderson, T. (2020). Driving school improvement planning with community and youth collaborative institute school experience surveys. *Children & Schools, 42*(1), 7–17. https://doi.org/10.1093/cs/cdz028

Anderson-Butcher, D., Amorose, A., Iachini, A., & Ball, A. (2012). The development of the perceived school experiences scale. *Research on Social Work Practice, 22*(2), 186–194. https://doi.org/10.1177/1049731511419866

Anderson-Butcher, D., Amorose, A. J., Iachini, A., & Ball, A. (2013). *Community and youth collaborative institute school experience surveys*. College of Social Work, The Ohio State University.

Anderson-Butcher, D., Lawson, H. A., Bean, J., Flaspohler, P., Boone, Barbara, & Kwiatkowski, A. (2008). Community collaboration to improve schools: Introducing a new model from Ohio. *Children & Schools, 30*(3), 161–172. https://psycnet.apa.org/doi/10.1093/cs/30.3.161s

Anderson-Butcher, D., Lawson, H. A., Iachini, A., Bean, J., Flaspohler, P., & Zullig, K. (2010). Capacity-related innovations resulting from pilot school and district implementation of a community collaboration model for school improvement. *Journal of Educational and Psychological Consultation, 20*(4), 257–287. https://doi.org/10.1080/10474412.2010.500512

Anderson-Butcher, D., Paluta, L., Sterling, K., & Anderson, C. (2017). Ensuring healthy youth development through community schools: A case study. *Children & Schools, 1*(1), 7–16.

August, G. J., Piehler, T. F., & Miller, F. G. (2018). Getting "smart" about implementing multi-tiered systems of support to promote school mental health. *Journal of School Psychology, 66*, 85–96. https://doi.org/10.1016/j.jsp.2017.10.001

Bains, R. M., & Diallo, A. F. (2016). Mental health services in school-based health centers: Systematic review. *The Journal of School Nursing, 32*(1), 8–19. https://doi.org/10.1177%2F1059840515590607

Ball, A., Iachini, A. L., Bohnenkamp, J. H., Togno, N. M., Brown, E. L., Hoffman, J. A., & George, M. W. (2016). School mental health content in state in-service K-12 teaching standards in the United States. *Teaching and Teacher Education, 60*, 312–320. https://doi.org/10.1016/j.tate.2016.08.020

Ball, A., Skrzypek, C., & Lynch, M. (2020). The family engagement practice framework: A comprehensive framework developed from the voices of school-based practitioners. *Family Relations*. Advance online publication. https://doi.org/10.1111/fare.12513

Bates, S., Mellin, E., Paluta, L., Anderson-Butcher, D., Vogeler, M., & Sterling, K. (2019). Examining the influence of interprofessional team collaboration on student-level outcomes through school-community partnerships. *Children & Schools, 41*(2), 119–122.

Beck, A. T., Steer, R. A., & Brown, G. K. (1996). *Beck depression inventory – II manual*. Psychological Corporation.

Bradshaw, C. P. (2013). Preventing bullying through positive behavioral interventions and supports (PBIS): A multitiered approach to prevention and integration. *Theory into Practice, 52*(4), 288–295. https://doi.org/10.1080/00405841.2013.829732

Bradshaw, C. P., Pas, E. T., Bloom, J., Barrett, S., Hershfeldt, P., Alexander, A., McKenna, M., Chafin, A. E., & Leaf, P. J. (2012). A state-wide partnership to promote safe and supportive schools: the PBIS Maryland Initiative. *Administration and Policy in Mental Health and Mental Health Services Research, 39*(4), 225–237. https://doi.org/10.1007/s10488-011-0384-6

Centers for Disease Control. (2007). *Coordinated school health program*. http://www.cdc.gov/HealthyYouth/CSHP/.

Center for Disease Control and Prevention. (n.d.). *Mental health*. https://www.cdc.gov/mentalhealth/index.htm

Centers for Disease Control and Prevention. (2012). *School health index*. http://www.cdc.gov/healthyyouth/shi/

Centers for Disease Control and Prevention. (2020). *Youth risk behavior surveillance system*. https://www.cdc.gov/healthyyouth/data/yrbs/index.htm

Center for Mental Health in Schools at UCLA. (2001). *Mental health in schools: Guidelines, models, resources, & policy considerations*. Policy Leadership Cadre for Mental Health in Schools.

Chafouleas, S. M., Briesch, A. M., Riley-Tillman, T. C., Christ, T. J., Black, A. C., & Kilgus, S. P. (2010). An investigation of the generalizability and dependability of direct behavior rating single item scales (DBR-SIS) to measure academic engagement and disruptive behavior of middle school students. *Journal of School Psychology, 48*, 219–246. https://doi.org/10.1016/j.jsp.2010.02.001

Chafouleas, S. M., Kilgus, S. P., Jaffery, R., Riley-Tillman, T. C., Welsh, M., & Christ, T. J. (2013). Direct behavior rating as a school-based behavior screener for elementary and middle grades. *Journal of School Psychology, 5*, 367–385. https://doi.org/10.1016/j.jsp.2013.04.002

Chafouleas, S. M., Koriakin, T. A., Roundfield, K. D., & Overstreet, S. (2019). Addressing childhood trauma in school settings: A framework for evidence-based practice. *School Mental Health: A Multidisciplinary Research and Practice Journal, 11*(1), 40–53. https://doi.org/10.1007/s12310-018-9256-5

Cohen, J. (2009). Transforming school climate: educational and psychoanalytic perspectives: Introduction. *Schools: Studies in Education, 6*(1), 99–103. https://doi.org/10.1086/597659

Connell, C. L., Nord, M., Lofton, K. L., & Yadrick, K. (2004). Food security of older children can be assessed using a standardized survey instrument. *The Journal of Nutrition, 134*(10), 2566. https://doi.org/10.1093/jn/134.10.2566

Crutchfield, J., Phillippo, K. L., & Frey, A. (2020). Structural racism in schools: A view through the lens of the national school social work practice model. *Children & Schools, 42*(3), 187–193.

Cummings, J. R., Wen, H., & Druss, B. G. (2013). Improving access to mental health services for youth in the United States. *JAMA, 309*(6), 553–554. https://doi.org/10.1001/jama.2013.437

Dombek, J. L., & Connor, C. M. D. (2012). Preventing retention: first grade classroom instruction and student characteristics. *Psychology in the Schools, 49*(6), 568–588. https://doi.org/10.1002/pits.21618

Drevon, D. D., Hixson, M. D., Wyse, R. D., & Rigney, A. M. (2019). A meta-analytic review of the evidence for check-in check-out. *Psychology in the Schools, 56*(3), 393–412. https://doi.org/10.1002/pits.22195

Dryfoos, J. (1994). *Full-Service Community schools: A revolution in Health and Social Services for Children, Youth and Families*. Jossey-Bass.

Dupper, D. (2006). Design and utility of life schools groups in schools. In C. Franklin, M. B. Harris, & P. Allen-Meares (Eds.), *The school services sourcebook: A guide for school-based professionals*. Oxford University Press.

Durlak, J. A., Weissberg, R. P., Dymnicki, A. B., Taylor, A. D., & Schellinger, K. B. (2011). The impact of enhancing students' social and emotional learning: A meta-analysis of school-based universal interventions. *Child Development, 82*(1), 405–432. https://doi.org/10.1111/j.1467-8624.2010.01564.x

Every Student Succeeds Act. (2015). *Public law 114-95: Reauthorization of the elementary and secondary education act of 1965–Every student succeeds act*. https://www.congress.gov/bill/114th-congress/senate-bill/1177

Family Educational Rights and Privacy Act. (1980). 20 U.S.C. § 1232g; 34 CFR Part 99. https://www.govinfo.gov/content/pkg/USCODE-2017-title20/pdf/USCODE-2017-title20-chap31-subchapIII-part4-sec1232g.pdf

Flaherty, L. T., Weist, M. D., & Warner, B. S. (1996). School-based mental health services in the United States: History, current models, and needs. *Community Mental Health Journal, 32*(4), 341–52. https://doi.org/10.1007/bf02249452

Fram, M. S., Frongillo, E. A., Draper, C. L., & Fishbein, E. M. (2013). Development and validation of a child report assessment of child food insecurity and comparison to parent report assessment. *Journal of Hunger & Environmental Nutrition, 8*(2), 128–145. https://doi.org/10.1080/19320248.2013.790775

Fram, M. S., Ritchie, L. D., Rosen, N., & Frongillo, E. A. (2015). Child experience of food insecurity is associated with child diet and physical activity. *Journal of Nutrition, 145*(3), 499–504. https://doi.org/10.3945/jn.114.194365

Graczyk, P., Matjasko, J., Weissberg, R., Greenberg, M., Elias, M., & Zins, J. (2000). The role of the Collaborative to Advance Social and Emotional Learning (CASEL) in supporting the implementation of quality school-based prevention programs. *Journal of Educational and Psychological Consultation, 11*(1), 3–6.

Greenberg, M. T., Weissberg, R. P., O'Briend, M. E., Zins, J. E., Fredericks, L., Resnick, H., et al. (2003). Enhancing school-based prevention and youth development through coordinated social, emotional, and academic learning. *American Psychologist, 58*, 466–474.

Hawken, L. S., & Horner, R. H. (2003). Evaluation of a targeted intervention within a schoolwide system of behavior support. *Journal of Behavioral Education, 12*(3), 225–240.

Herrenkohl, T. I. (2019). Cross-system collaboration and engagement of the public health model to promote the well-being of children and families. *Journal of the Society for Social Work and Research, 10*(3), 319–332. https://doi.org/10.1086/704958

Horner, R. H., Sugai, G., & Anderson, C. M. (2010). Examining the evidence base for school-wide positive behavior support. *Focus on Exceptional Children, 42*(8), 1–14. https://doi.org/10.17161/foec.v42i8.6906

Hoying, J., & Melnyk, B. M. (2016). COPE: A pilot study with urban-dwelling minority sixth-grade youth to improve physical activity and mental health outcomes. *The Journal of School Nursing, 32*(5), 347–356. https://doi.org/10.1177/1059840516635713

Hoying, J., Melnyk, B. M., Arcoleo, K. (2016). Effects of the COPE cognitive behavioral skills building TEEN program on the healthy lifestyle behaviors and mental health of Appalachian early adolescents, *Journal of Pediatric Health Care, 30*(1), 65–72. https://doi.org/10.1016/j.pedhc.2015.02.005

Iachini, A. L. & Childs, T. M. (2021). Resources for families during COVID-19: A content analysis of information provided on school district websites. *Children & Schools*, cdab001. https://doi.org/10.1093/cs/cdab001

Individuals with Disabilities Education Act. (2004). *Public law 114-95: Chapter 33—Education of individuals with disabilities*. https://www.govinfo.gov/content/pkg/USCODE-2011-title20/pdf/USCODE-2011-title20-chap33.pdf

Jagers, R. J., Rivas-Drake, D., & Williams, B. (2019). Transformative social and emotional learning (SEL): Toward SEL in service of educational equity and excellence. *Educational Psychologist, 54*(3), 162–184. https://doi.org/10.1080/00461520.2019.1623032

Jaycox, L. H., Kataoka, S. H., Stein, B. D., Langley, A. K., & Wong, M. (2012). Cognitive behavioral intervention for trauma in schools. *Journal of Applied School Psychology, 28*(3), 239–255.

Johnston, W. R., Engberg, J., Opper, I. M., Sontag-Padilla, L., & Xenakis, L. (2020). *What is the impact of the New York City community schools initiative?* Rand Corporation.

Kearney, C. A., & Graczyk, P. (2014). A response to intervention model to promote school attendance and decrease school absenteeism. *Child Youth Care Forum, 43*, 1–25. https://doi.org/10.1007/s10566-013-9222-1

Kern, L., Mathur, S. R., Albrecht, S. F., Poland, S., Rozalski, M., & Skiba, R. J. (2017). The need for school-based mental health services and recommendations for implementation. *School Mental Health: A Multidisciplinary Research and Practice Journal*, *9*(3), 205–217. https://doi.org/10.1007/s12310-017-9216-5

Kilgus, S. P., Eklund, K., von der E. N. P., Taylor, C. N., & Sims, W. A. (2016). Psychometric defensibility of the social, academic, and emotional behavior risk screener (saebrs) teacher rating scale and multiple gating procedure within elementary and middle school samples. *Journal of School Psychology*, *58*, 21–39. https://doi.org/10.1016/j.jsp.2016.07.001

Kroenke, K., Spitzer, R. L., & Williams, J. B. W. (2001). The phq-9: Validity of a brief depression severity measure. *Journal of General Internal Medicine*, *16*(9), 606–613. https://doi.org/10.1046/j.1525-1497.2001.016009606.x

Kutash, K., Duchnowski, A. J., & Green, A. L. (2015). Meeting the mental health needs of youth with emotional and behavioral disorders. *Beyond Behavior*, *24*(2), 4–13. https://doi.org/10.1177%2F107429561502400202

Kutash, K., Duchnowski, A. J., & Lynn, N. (2006). *School-based mental health: An empirical guide for decision makers*. The Research & Training Center for Children's Mental Health, Louis de la Parte Florida Mental Health Institute, University of South Florida.

Leaf, P. J., Schultz, D., Kiser, L. J., Pruitt, D. B. (2003). School mental health in systems of care. In M. D. Weist, S. W. Evans, & N. A. Lever (Eds.), *Handbook of school mental health: Advancing practice and research*. Springer Publishing Company.

LeBuffe, P. A., Shapiro, V. B., & Robitaille, J. L. (2018). The Devereux student strengths assessment (DESSA) comprehensive system: Screening, assessing, planning, and monitoring. *Journal of Applied Developmental Psychology*, *55*, 62–70. https://doi.org/10.1016/j.appdev.2017.05.002

LeCroy, C. W. (2006). Designing and facilitating groups with children. In C. Franklin, M. B. Harris, & P. Allen-Meares (Eds.), *The school services sourcebook: A guide for school-based professionals*. Oxford University Press.

Lewallen, T. C., Hunt, H., Potts-Datema, W., Zaza, S., & Giles, W. (2015). The whole school, whole community, whole child model: A new approach for improving educational attainment and healthy development for students. *The Journal of School Health*, *85*(11), 729–39. https://doi.org/10.1111/josh.12310

Love, H. E., Schlitt, J., Soleimanpour, S., Panchal, N., & Behr, C. (2019). Twenty years of school-based health care growth and expansion. *Health Affairs*, *38*(5), 755–764. https://doi.org/10.1377/hlthaff.2018.05472

Lubell, E. (2011). *Building community schools: A guide for action*. Children's Aid Society.

Mann, A., Whitaker, A., Torres-Gullien, S., Morton, M., Jordan, H., Coyle, S., & Sun, W. L. (2019). *Cops & no counselors: How the lack of school mental health staff is harming students*. American Civil Liberties Union. https://www.aclu.org/report/cops-and-no-counselors

Maughan, E. D., McCarthy, A. M., Hein, M., Perkhounkova, Y., & Kelly, M. W. (2018). Medication management in schools: 2015 survey results. *The Journal of School Nursing*, *34*(6), 468–479. https://doi.org/10.1177/1059840517729739

Maynard, B. R., Farina, A., Dell, N. A., & Kelly, M. S. (2019). Effects of trauma-informed approaches in schools: A systematic review. *Campbell Systematic Reviews*, *15*(1), 1–18. https://doi.org/10.1002/cl2.1018

McCallops, K., Barnes, T. N., Berte, I., Fenniman, J., Jones, I., Navon, R., & Nelson, M. (2019). Incorporating culturally responsive pedagogy within social-emotional learning interventions in urban schools: An international systematic review. *International Journal of Educational Research*, *94*, 11–28. https://doi.org/10.1016/j.ijer.2019.02.007

Mellin, E. A. (2009). Unpacking interdisciplinary collaboration in expanded school mental health service utilization for children and adolescents. *Advances in School Mental Health Promotion*, *2*, 5–15. https://doi.org/10.1080/1754730X.2009.9715706

Melnyk, B. M. (2003). *Creating opportunities for personal empowerment (COPE) programs for children, adolescents and college students/young adults*. COPE2Thrive, LLC.

Melnyk, B. M. (2020). Reducing healthcare costs for mental health hospitalizations with the evidence-based COPE program for child and adolescent depression and anxiety: A cost analysis. *Journal of Pediatric Health Care*, *34*(2), 117–121. https://doi.org/10.1016/j.pedhc.2019.08.002

Melnyk, B. M., Amaya, M., Szalacha, L. A., Hoying, J., Taylor, T. & Bowersox, K. (2015a). Feasibility, acceptability and preliminary effects of the COPE on-line cognitive-behavioral skills building program on mental health outcomes and academic performance in freshmen college students: A randomized controlled pilot study. *Journal of Child and Adolescent Psychiatric Nursing*, *28*(3), 147–154. https://doi.org/10.1111/jcap.12119

Melnyk, B. M., Jacobson, D., Kelly, S. A., Belyea, M. J., Shaibi, G. Q., Small, L., O'Haver, J. A., & Marsiglia, F. F. (2015b). Twelve-month effects of the COPE healthy lifestyles TEEN program on overweight and depression in high school adolescents. *Journal of School Health*, *85*(12), 861–870.

Melnyk, B. M., Jacobson, D., Kelly, S., Belyea, M., Shaibi, G., Small, L., O'Haver, J., & Marsiglia, Fx. F. (2013b). Promoting healthy lifestyles in high school adolescents: A randomized controlled trial. *American Journal of Preventive Medicine*, *45*(4), 407–415.

Melnyk, B. M., Kelly, S., Jacobson, D., Arcoleo, K., & Shaibi, G. (2013a). Improving physical activity, mental health outcomes and academic retention of college students with freshman 5 to thrive: COPE/healthy lifestyles. *Journal of the American Academy of Nurse Practitioner*, *26*(6), 314–322.

Melnyk, B. M., Kelly, S., & Lusk, P. (2014). Outcomes and feasibility of a manualized cognitive-behavioral skills building intervention: Group COPE for depressed and anxious adolescents in school settings. *Journal of Child and Adolescent Psychiatric Nursing*, *27*(1), 3–13. [Epub ahead of print]. https://doi.org/10.1111/jcap.12058

Mendenhall, A. N., Iachini, A., & Anderson-Butcher, D. (2013). Exploring facilitators and barriers to implementation of an expanded school improvement model. *Children & Schools*, *4*, 225–234.

Mental Health Association in New York State, Inc. (2017). *Mental health education in New York Schools—A review of legislative history, intent, and vision for implementation.* https://mhanys.org/wp-content/uploads/2015/04/MHANYS-2017-Mental-Health-Education-in-Schools-White-Paper-FINAL-3.pdf

MentalHealth.gov. (2020). What is mental health? https://www.mentalhealth.gov/basics/what-is-mental-health

Merikangas, K. R., He, J. P., Burstein, M., Swanson, S. A., Cui, L., Avenevoli, S., Cui, L., Benjet, C., Georgiades, K., & Swendsen, J. (2010). Lifetime prevalence of mental disorders in U.S. adolescents: Results from the national comorbidity survey replication-adolescent supplement (NCS-A). *Journal of the American Academy of Child and Adolescent Psychiatry*, *49*(10), 980–989. https://doi.org/10.1016/j.jaac.2010.05.017

Mrazek, P. J., & Haggerty, R. J. (1994). *Reducing risks for mental disorders: Frontiers for preventive intervention research.* National Academy Press.

National Association of School Nurses. (2017). *Medication administration in schools (Position Statement).* https://www.nasn.org/advocacy/professional-practice-documents/position-statements/ps-medication

National Association of Social Workers. (n.d.). *Tele-mental health: Legal considerations for social workers.* https://www.socialworkers.org/About/Legal/HIPAA-Help-For-Social-Workers/Telemental-Health

National Center for Education Statistics. (2020). *Education commission of the states, 50 state comparison: Instructional time policies.* https://nces.ed.gov/programs/statereform/tab5_14.asp

New York State Education Law, § 804 – Health Education Regarding Alcohol, Drugs, Tobacco Abuse and the Prevention and Detection of Certain Cancers. (2016). https://newyork.public.law/laws/n.y._education_law_section_804

O'Connor, C. A., Dyson, J., Cowdell, F., & Watson, R. (2018). Do universal school-based mental health promotion programmes improve the mental health and emotional wellbeing of young people? A literature review. *Journal of Clinical Nursing*, *27*(3–4), 426. https://doi.org/10.1111/jocn.14078

Ohrt, J. H., Deaton, J. D., Linich, K., Guest, J. D., Wymer, B., & Sandonato, B. (2020). Teacher training in k-12 student mental health: a systematic review. *Psychology in the Schools*, *57*(5), 833–846. https://doi.org/10.1002/pits.22356

O'Reilly, M., Svirydzenka, N., Adams, S., & Dogra, N. (2018). Review of mental health promotion interventions in schools. *Social Psychiatry and Psychiatric Epidemiology: The International Journal for Research in Social and Genetic Epidemiology and Mental Health Services*, *53*(7), 647–662. https://doi.org/10.1007/s00127-018-1530-1

Reynolds, C. R., & Kamphaus, R. W. (2015). *BASC-3: Behavior assessment system for children, third edition manual.* Pearson.

Reynolds, W. M. (1994). Assessment of depression in children and adolescents by self-report questionnaires. In W. M. Reynolds & H. F. Johnston (Eds.), *Handbook of depression in children and adolescents* (pp. 209–234). Plenum.

Rones, M., & Hoagwood, K. (2000). School-based mental health services: A research review. *Clinical Child and Family Psychology Review*, *3*(4), 223–241.

Ross, K. M., & Tolan, P. (2018). Social and emotional learning in adolescence: Testing the CASEL model in a normative sample. *Journal of Early Adolescence*, *38*(8), 1170–1199.

Salerno, J. P. (2016). Effectiveness of universal school-based mental health awareness programs among youth in the United States: A systematic review. *Journal of School Health*, *86*(12), 922–931. https://doi.org/10.1111/josh.12461

Solberg, M. E., & Olweus, D. (2003). aPrevalence estimation of school bullying with the Olweus Bully/Victim Questionnaire. *Aggressive Behavior*, *29*(3), 239–268. https://doi.org/10.1002/ab.10047

Solomon, B. J., Sun, S., & Temkin, D. (2020). *When providing school climate data, researchers and districts should also provide supports for data-informed decision making*. Child Trends. https://www.childtrends.org/publications/when-providing-school-climate-data-researchers-and-districts-should-also-provide-supports-for-data-informed-decision-making

Splett, J. W., Garzona, M., Gibson, N., Wojtalewicz, D., Raborn, A., & Reinke, W. M. (2018). Teacher recognition, concern, and referral of children's internalizing and externalizing behavior problems. *School Mental Health*, *11*(2), 228–239. https://doi.org/10.1007/s12310-018-09303-z

Splett, J. W., Perales, K., Halliday-Boykins, C. A., Gilchrest, C. E., Gibson, N., & Weist, M. D. (2017). Best practices for teaming and collaboration in the interconnected systems framework. *Journal of Applied School Psychology, 33*(4), 347–368. https://doi.org/10.1080/15377903.2017.1328625

Substance Abuse and Mental Health Services Administration. (2019). *Ready, set, go, review: Screening for behavioral health risk in schools.* Office of the Chief Medical Officer, Substance Abuse and Mental Health Services Administration.

Suldo, S., Gormley, M., DuPaul, G., & Anderson-Butcher, D. (2014). Connecting school mental health to students' and schools' academic outcomes. *School Mental Health, 6*(2), 84–98.

Taylor, R. D., Oberle, E., Durlak, J. A., & Weissberg, R. P. (2017). Promoting positive youth development through school-based social and emotional learning interventions: A meta-analysis of follow-up effects. *Child Development, 88*(4), 1156–1171. https://doi.org/10.1111/cdev.12864

Torio, C. M., Encinosa, W., Berdahl, T., McCormick, M. C., & Simpson, L. A. (2015). Annual report on health care for children and youth in the United States: National estimates of cost, utilization and expenditures for children with mental health conditions. *Academic Pediatrics, 15*(1), 19–35. https://doi.org/10.1016/j.acap.2014.07.007

The Search Institute. (2004). *Developmental assets profile.* Search Institute.

United States Department of Agriculture. (2020). *Food security in the U.S.* https://www.ers.usda.gov/topics/food-nutrition-assistance/food-security-in-the-us/survey-tools/

United States Department of Education. (n.d.). *CARES act education stabilization fund.* https://covid-relief-data.ed.gov/?utm_content=&utm_medium=email&utm_name=&utm_source=govdelivery&utm_term=

United States Department of Health and Human Services. (1999). *Mental health: A report of the surgeon general.* U.S. Department of Health and Human Services, Substance Abuse and Mental Health Services Administration, Center for Mental Health Services, National Institutes of Health, National Institutes of Mental Health.

United States Department of Health and Human Services. (2020). What is mental health? https://www.mentalhealth.gov/basics/what-is-mental-health

United States Preventive Services Task Force. (2014). *Screening for suicide risk in adolescents, adults, and older adults in primary care: U.S. preventive services task force recommendation statement.* http://www.uspreventiveservicestaskforce.org/3rduspstf/suicide/suiciderr.htm

United States Preventive Services Task Force. (2016). *Screening for depression in children and adolescents: U.S. preventive services task force recommendation statement.* https://www.uspreventiveservicestaskforce.org/uspstf/recommendation/depression-in-children-and-adolescents-screening

United States Preventive Services Task Force. (2020a). *Primary care–based interventions to prevent illicit drug use in children, adolescents, and young adults: US preventive services task force recommendation statement.* https://www.uspreventiveservicestaskforce.org/uspstf/recommendation/drug-use-illicit-primary-care-interventions-for-children-and-adolescents

United States Preventive Services Task Force. (2020b). *Screening and behavioral counseling interventions to reduce unhealthy alcohol use in adolescents and adults: US preventive services task force recommendation statement.* https://www.uspreventiveservicestaskforce.org/uspstf/recommendation/unhealthy-alcohol-use-in-adolescents-and-adults-screening-and-behavioral-counseling-interventions

Was, C. A., Woltz, D. J., & Drew, C. (2006). Evaluating character education programs and missing the target: a critique of existing research. *Educational Research Review, 1*(2), 148–156. https://doi.org/10.1016/j.edurev.2006.08.001

Weist, M. D. (1997). Expanded school mental health services: A national movement in progress. *Advances in Clinical Child Psychology, 19*, 319–352. https://doi.org/10.1007/978-1-4757-9035-1_9

Weist, M. D., Bruns, E. J., Whitaker, K., Wei, Y., Kutcher, S., Larsen, T., Holsen, I., Cooper, J. L., Geroski, A., & Short, K. H. (2017). School mental health promotion and intervention: Experiences from four nations. *School Psychology International, 38*(4), 343–362. https://doi.org/10.1177%2F0143034317695379

Weist, M. D., Goldstein, A., Morris, L., & Bryant, T. (2003). Integrating expanded school mental health programs and school-based health centers. *Psychology in the Schools, 40*(3), 297–308. https://doi.org/10.1002/pits.10089

Weist, M. D., & Murray, M. (2007). Advancing school mental health promotion globally. *Advances in School Mental Health Promotion, 1*, 2–12. https://doi.org/10.1080/1754730X.2008.9715740

Weist, M., Stephan, S., Lever, N., Moore, E. &, Lewis, K. (2006). *School Mental Health Quality Assessment Questionnaire (SMHQAQ).* http://www.schoolmentalhealth.org/Resources/Clin/QAIRsrc/QAI

Weisz, H., Sandler, I., Durlak, J., & Anton, B. (2005). Promoting and protecting youth mental health through evidence-based prevention and treatment. *American Psychologist, 60*(6), 628–648. https://doi.org/10.1037/0003-066x.60.6.628

Whitney, D. G., & Peterson, M. D. (2019). US national and state-level prevalence of mental health disorders and disparities of mental health care use in children. *JAMA Pediatrics, 173*(4), 389–391. https://doi/10.1001/jamapediatrics.2018.5399

Wiest-Stevenson, C., & Lee, C. (2016). Trauma-informed schools. *Journal of Evidence-Informed Social Work, 13*(5), 498–503. https://doi.org/10.1080/23761407.2016.1166855

Wilkinson, A., Gabriel, A., Stratford, B., Carter, M., Rodriguez, Y., Okogbue, O., Somers, S., Young, D., & Harper, K. (2020). *Early evidence of Medicaid's important role in school-based health services*. Child Trends. https://www.childtrends.org/publications/early-evidence-medicaid-role-school-based-heath-services

CHAPTER 20

Bernadette Mazurek Melnyk, Kate Gawlik, and Alice M. Teall

Self-Care for Clinicians Who Care for Children and Adolescents With Mental Health Problems

FAST FACTS

- Rates of depression, burnout, suicidal intent, and chronic health conditions tend to be higher in nurses than in the general population.
- A significant number of pediatric nurses report moderate to high levels of emotional exhaustion and depersonalization, and low levels of personal accomplishment.
- The onset of the COVID-19 pandemic was overwhelming for an already overwhelmed system and healthcare workforce.
- Pediatric clinicians face unique challenges when delivering patient care due to the complexity of the family dynamics and the special needs of caring for an ill child.
- Children, especially young children, often do not understand how and why they are ill and why they must comply with necessary treatments, painful procedures, therapy, and/or hospitalizations. This inability to understand and rationalize can cause an additional layer of stress and moral distress for pediatric providers.
- Burnout in pediatric clinicians is multifactorial. Commonly cited reasons for burnout include: prostration (mental and physical exhaustion); chaotic work environments; the demanding roles and hours expected and maintained; lack of confidence in job achievement; lack of time to achieve organized and priority-setting schedules; poor/ineffective leadership; low nurse to high patient ratios; and dealing with stressed parents, critically ill children, death and dying, and other emotionally difficult events.
- Good self-care by pediatric clinicians and systems that support clinician wellness are imperative to prevent burnout, compassion fatigue, and other mental health disorders.

INTRODUCTION: THE IMPORTANCE OF CLINICIAN HEALTH AND WELL-BEING

The prevalence of depression, burnout, suicidal intent, and chronic health conditions (e.g., hypertension, diabetes) tends to be higher in healthcare clinicians than in the general population (Melnyk & Orsolini et al., 2018). Burnout consists of emotional exhaustion, no longer finding work meaningful,

Special thanks to Springer Publishing for permission to adapt this chapter from Melnyk et al. (2021). Evidence-based assessment of personal health and well-being for clinicians with key strategies to achieve optimal wellness. In *Evidence-Based Physical Examination: Best Practices for Health and Well-Being Assessment*. Springer Publishing Company.

feeling ineffective, and a tendency to view patients, students, and colleagues as objects rather than as human beings (Fred & Scheid, 2018). Conditions associated with burnout include headaches, tension, insomnia, fatigue, anger, impaired memory, decreased attention, thoughts of quitting work, drug and alcohol use, and suicide. Burnout not only has adverse effects on clinician population health and healthcare quality and safety, but it contributes to high turnover and substantial financial losses (Willard-Grace et al., 2019). For every physician who leaves a practice, it is estimated that $500,000 to $1,000,000 in revenue is lost (Fred & Scheid, 2018). For every newly licensed registered nurse who is lost in the first year of practice, it costs the organization up to three times the nurse's annual salary when taking into consideration the cost of recruitment, training, and orientation (Unruh & Zhang, 2014). Burnout currently affects more than 50% of health professionals (Shanafelt et al., 2015) and impacts the quality and safety of healthcare. Depression and burnout in clinicians have been linked to reductions in healthcare quality, increased medical errors, patient dissatisfaction, reduced productivity, and very costly staff turnover (Hall et al., 2016; Melnyk & Orsolini et al., 2018). Because burnout can lead to adverse consequences for clinicians and patients, urgent attention must be given to this public health epidemic. Preventable medical errors are the third leading cause of death in America (Makary, 2016). In a national study of nearly 1,900 nurses from 19 healthcare systems throughout the United States, greater than 50% of them reported poor physical and mental health. Approximately one-third of the nurses reported depression, which was the leading cause of medical errors (Melnyk & Orsolini et al., 2018).

Clinicians typically do a wonderful job of caring for their patients and family members, but they often do not prioritize their own self-care. Coupled with healthcare system challenges, including documentation requirements of electronic health records that results in clinicians spending less time with patients, maintenance of certification, loss of autonomy, unhealthy workplace cultures, and heavy workloads, these issues are a prescription for an unhealthy population and unsafe provision of care.

The onset of the COVID-19 pandemic was overwhelming for an already overwhelmed system and healthcare workforce. The exceptional response of clinicians to meet the demands of the COVID-19 pandemic has been significant and inspiring. Unfortunately, courageousness and selflessness can take an emotional toll on clinician health and well-being. The impact of the pandemic includes exacerbation of the anxiety, burnout, fatigue, and distress that were already being experienced in ever greater numbers (Jun et al., 2020; Melnyk, 2020; Muller et al., 2020). Consequently, calls to support clinician well-being have become even more urgent.

THE NATIONAL ACADEMY OF MEDICINE'S ACTION COLLABORATIVE ON CLINICIAN WELL-BEING AND RESILIENCE

Because of the high prevalence of clinician burnout, depression, and suicide, the National Academy of Medicine (NAM) launched an *Action Collaborative on Clinician Well-being and Resilience* in 2017 in order to enhance visibility on this issue and to develop evidence-based solutions to tackle this public health epidemic and improve clinician health (Dzau et al., 2018). The NAM collaborative identified both external and individual factors that affect clinician well-being and resistance. See Figure 20.1.

The NAM also emphasized the urgent need for healthcare systems to implement system interventions to combat this problem, including prioritizing the hiring of Chief Wellness Officers (CWOs) whose responsibility is to lead a culture of well-being and implement strategies to create a healthier workforce (Kishore et al., 2018). CWOs should have a role within the executive suite to elevate the importance of the position and be equipped with the needed resources to effectively build cultures of well-being and implement evidence-based interventions to enhance well-being in clinicians. A knowledge hub with best practices has been developed by the NAM collaborative and can be accessed at nam.edu/clinicianwellbeing/. This hub provides numerous resources and solutions for trying to

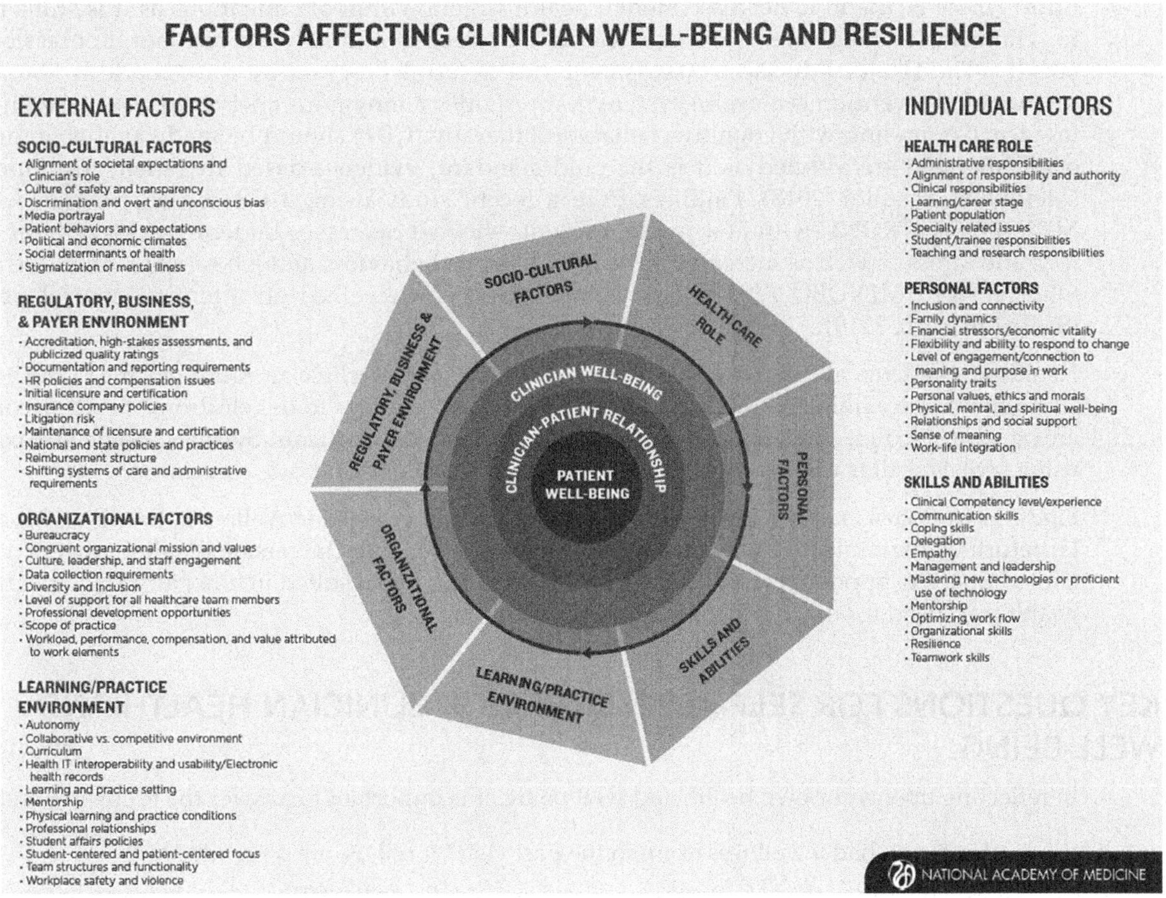

FACTORS AFFECTING CLINICIAN WELL-BEING AND RESILIENCE

EXTERNAL FACTORS

SOCIO-CULTURAL FACTORS
- Alignment of societal expectations and clinician's role
- Culture of safety and transparency
- Discrimination and overt and unconscious bias
- Media portrayal
- Patient behaviors and expectations
- Political and economic climates
- Social determinants of health
- Stigmatization of mental illness

REGULATORY, BUSINESS, & PAYER ENVIRONMENT
- Accreditation, high-stakes assessments, and publicized quality ratings
- Documentation and reporting requirements
- HR policies and compensation issues
- Initial licensure and certification
- Insurance company policies
- Litigation risk
- Maintenance of licensure and certification
- National and state policies and practices
- Reimbursement structure
- Shifting systems of care and administrative requirements

ORGANIZATIONAL FACTORS
- Bureaucracy
- Congruent organizational mission and values
- Culture, leadership, and staff engagement
- Data collection requirements
- Diversity and Inclusion
- Level of support for all healthcare team members
- Professional development opportunities
- Scope of practice
- Workload, performance, compensation, and value attributed to work elements

LEARNING/PRACTICE ENVIRONMENT
- Autonomy
- Collaborative vs. competitive environment
- Curriculum
- Health IT interoperability and usability/Electronic health records
- Learning and practice setting
- Mentorship
- Physical learning and practice conditions
- Professional relationships
- Student affairs policies
- Student-centered and patient-centered focus
- Team structures and functionality
- Workplace safety and violence

SOCIO-CULTURAL FACTORS
HEALTH CARE ROLE
PERSONAL FACTORS
SKILLS AND ABILITIES
LEARNING/PRACTICE ENVIRONMENT
ORGANIZATIONAL FACTORS
REGULATORY, BUSINESS & PAYER ENVIRONMENT
CLINICIAN WELL-BEING
CLINICIAN-PATIENT RELATIONSHIP
PATIENT WELL-BEING

INDIVIDUAL FACTORS

HEALTH CARE ROLE
- Administrative responsibilities
- Alignment of responsibility and authority
- Clinical responsibilities
- Learning/career stage
- Patient population
- Specialty related issues
- Student/trainee responsibilities
- Teaching and research responsibilities

PERSONAL FACTORS
- Inclusion and connectivity
- Family dynamics
- Financial stressors/economic vitality
- Flexibility and ability to respond to change
- Level of engagement/connection to meaning and purpose in work
- Personality traits
- Personal values, ethics and morals
- Physical, mental, and spiritual well-being
- Relationships and social support
- Sense of meaning
- Work-life integration

SKILLS AND ABILITIES
- Clinical Competency level/experience
- Communication skills
- Coping skills
- Delegation
- Empathy
- Management and leadership
- Mastering new technologies or proficient use of technology
- Mentorship
- Optimizing work flow
- Organizational skills
- Resilience
- Teamwork skills

NATIONAL ACADEMY OF MEDICINE

Figure 20.1. Factors affecting clinician burn-out

Source: Reproduced with permission from the National Academy of Sciences. https://nam.edu/wp-content/uploads/2018/01/Conceptual_Model_Paper_Figure_1_FINAL.png

combat clinician burn-out, compassion fatigue, depression, and anxiety symptoms at both the individual and organizational levels.

HEALTHCARE SYSTEM INTERVENTIONS

Healthcare organizations should implement a comprehensive, multi-component wellness strategy that targets evidence-based interventions to individual clinicians, the family and social network, the workplace culture and environment, and organizational policies that are built on a clear vision and mission (Melnyk, Gascon, et al., 2018). Central to this strategy is the building of a culture of well-being that makes healthy choices the easy choices for clinicians to make (Melnyk, Szalacha, et al., 2018). Leaders as well as supervisors and managers must role model and provide support for wellness; if not, it is unlikely that their clinicians will engage in healthy lifestyle behaviors (Melnyk, 2019).

It should be made clear to all clinicians that their well-being is a high priority for the organization, and they should be made aware of wellness resources within the institution that are available to them. It is critical to have a "menu of options" for wellness as not all clinicians will benefit from the same interventions (Melnyk, 2019). Grassroots tactics, such as wellness champions are an effective and low-cost strategy in creating a wellness culture throughout the organization (Amaya et al., 2017).

Efforts must be made to decrease mental health stigma within organizations as it is still a barrier for clinicians seeking care. Clinicians should be screened annually for burnout, depression, and anxiety. The Healer Education Assessment and Referral Program by the American Foundation for Suicide Prevention is a useful system that provides anonymous encrypted risk screening for a low fee. Counseling with cognitive behavioral therapy (CBT) should be made available for those clinicians who are affected as it is the gold standard, evidence-based treatment for depression (Melnyk & Orsolini, 2018). Findings from a recent study using a CBT-based program entitled MINDBODYSTRONG with new nurse residents showed decreases in depressive symptoms, anxiety, and stress as well as increases in healthy lifestyle behaviors and job satisfaction in the nurses who received MINDBODYSTRONG versus those who received an attention control program (Sampson et al., 2019).

Healthcare systems also must address staffing where patient–clinician ratios are high, and 12-hour shifts should be eliminated (Melnyk, 2019). In addition, changes to the electronic health record also are necessary so that clinicians can spend more time with their patients. Systems should also consider using scribes as they can decrease the data entry workload of healthcare clinicians.

Findings from cost analyses indicate that, for every dollar invested in wellness, there is a $3 to $6 dollar return on investment (Baiker et al., 2010). At The Ohio State University, the first university in the United States to appoint a CWO, investment in wellness has resulted in a negative faculty and staff healthcare spend for the fourth year in a row.

KEY QUESTIONS FOR SELF-ASSESSMENT OF CLINICIAN HEALTH AND WELL-BEING

In reflecting upon your own health and well-being, it is important to answer the following questions:

1. Have you had a wellness exam in the past year? If not, is one scheduled?
2. Do you follow the U.S. Preventive Services Task Force (USPTSF) recommendations for **your own** preventive health screenings that apply to your age, sex, and smoking status? The USPTSF has an online calculator that can be used to determine applicable and individualized screenings and preventive measures. Visit epss.ahrq.gov/ePSS/search.jsp to access it and determine what screenings apply to you.
3. How high is your current level of stress according to the Perceived Stress Scale-10 (PSS-10)? Please answer the 10-question PSS-10 scale (Exhibit 20.1) and total your score.
4. Are you currently experiencing depressive symptoms according to the nine-item Patient Health Questionnaire (PHQ-9)? Please answer the nine-question PHQ-9 (Exhibit 20.2) and total your score.
5. Are you currently experiencing anxiety symptoms according to the seven-item Generalized Anxiety Disorder Questionnaire (GAD-7)? Please answer the GAD-7 scale (Exhibit 20.3) and total your score.
6. Are you currently experiencing burnout? Complete the Assessment of Burnout (Exhibit 20.4) and total your score.

Exhibit 20.1 10-Item Perceived Stress Scale

	Never	Almost never	Sometimes	Fairly often	Very often
1. In the last month, how often have you been upset because of something that happened unexpectedly?	0	1	2	3	4
2. In the last month, how often have you felt that you were unable to control the important things in your life?	0	1	2	3	4
3. In the last month, how often have you felt nervous and stressed?	0	1	2	3	4
4. In the last month, how often have you felt confident about your ability to handle your personal problems?	4	3	2	1	0
5. In the last month, how often have you felt that things were going your way?	4	3	2	1	0
6. In the last month, how often have you found that you could not cope with all the things that you had to do?	0	1	2	3	4
7. In the last month, how often have you been able to control irritations in your life?	4	3	2	1	0
8. In the last month, how often have you felt that you were on top of things?	4	3	2	1	0
9. In the last month, how often have you been angered because of things that happened that were outside of your control?	0	1	2	3	4
10. In the last month, how often have you felt difficulties were piling up so high that you could not overcome them?	0	1	2	3	4
Column Totals					
Sum of Columns (total score)					

(*continued*)

Exhibit 20.1 10-Item Perceived Stress Scale (*Continued*)

Scoring of the PSS	
Total Score	Perceived Stress Severity
0–13	Low perceived stress
14–26	Moderate perceived stress
27–40	High perceived stress

Source: Reproduced with permission from Cohen, S., Kamarch, T., & Mermelstein, R. (1983). A global measure of perceived stress. *Journal of Health and Social Behavior, 24*, 385–396. https://doi.org/10.2307/2136404

Exhibit 20.2 Nine-Item Patient Health Questionnaire (PHQ-9)

Over the last 2 weeks, how often have you been bothered by any of the following problems?	**Not at all**	**Several days**	**More than half the days**	**Nearly every day**
1. Little interest or pleasure in doing things	0	1	2	3
2. Feeling down, depressed, or hopeless	0	1	2	3
3. Trouble falling or staying asleep, or sleeping too much	0	1	2	3
4. Feeling tired or having little energy	0	1	2	3
5. Poor appetite or overeating	0	1	2	3
6. Feeling bad about yourself or that you are a failure or have let yourself or your family down	0	1	2	3
7. Trouble concentrating on things, such as reading the newspaper or watching television	0	1	2	3
8. Moving or speaking so slowly that other people have noticed. Or the opposite—being so fidgety or restless that you have been moving around a lot more than usual	0	1	2	3
9. Thoughts that you would be better off dead, or of hurting yourself	0	1	2	3
Column Totals	0			
Sum of Columns (total score)				

Scoring

Sum of all items to create a total score

(continued)

Exhibit 20.2 Nine-Item Patient Health Questionnaire (PHQ-9) *(Continued)*

Interpretation of Total Score

Total Score	Depression Severity
1–4	Minimal depression
5–9	Mild depression
10–14	Moderate depression
15–19	Moderately severe depression
20–27	Severe depression

Note: Developed by Drs. Robert L. Spitzer, Janet B.W. Williams, Kurt Kroenke, and colleagues, with an educational grant from Pfizer, Inc.

Source: Kroenke, K., Spitzer, R. L., & Williams, J. B. (2001). The PHQ-9: Validity of a brief depression severity measure. *Journal of General Internal Medicine, 16*(9), 606–613. https://doi.org/10.1046/j.1525-1497.2001.016009606.x

Exhibit 20.3 Seven-Item Generalized Anxiety Disorder Screener (GAD-7)

Over the last 2 weeks, how often have you been bothered by the following problems?	Not at all	Several days	More than half the days	Nearly every day
1. Feeling nervous, anxious, or on edge	0	1	2	3
2. Not being able to stop or control worrying	0	1	2	3
3. Worrying too much about different things	0	1	2	3
4. Trouble relaxing	0	1	2	3
5. Being so restless that it is hard to sit still	0	1	2	3
6. Becoming easily annoyed or irritated	0	1	2	3
7. Feeling afraid as if something awful might happen	0	1	2	3
Column Totals	0			
Sum of Columns (total score)				

Scoring and Interpretation

GAD-7 Score	Provisional Diagnosis
0–7	None
8+	Probable anxiety disorder

Note: Developed by Drs. Robert L. Spitzer, Janet B.W. Williams, Kurt Kroenke, and colleagues, with an educational grant from Pfizer, Inc.

Source: Reproduced with permission from Spitzer, R. L., Kroenke, K., Williams, J. B., & Lowe, B. (2006). A brief measure for assessing generalized anxiety disorder: The GAD-7. *Archives of Internal Medicine, 166*(10), 1092–1097. https://doi.org/10.1001/archinte.166.10.1092

Exhibit 20.4 Assessment of Burnout

Overall, based on your definition of burnout, how would you rate your level of burnout?

Response	Score
I enjoy my work. I have no symptoms of burnout.	1
Occasionally I am under stress, and I don't always have as much energy as I once did, but I don't feel burned out.	2
I am definitely burning out and have one or more symptoms of burnout, such as physical and emotional exhaustion.	3
The symptoms of burnout that I'm experiencing won't go away. I think about frustration at work a lot.	4
I feel completely burned out and often wonder if I can go on. I am at the point where I may need some changes or may need to seek some sort of help.	5

Scoring:

≤2 : No symptoms of burnout.

≥3 : One or more symptoms of burnout.

If you are currently experiencing elevated symptoms of stress, depressive symptoms, anxiety, or burnout according to your scores on the above scales, are they interfering with your ability to concentrate or function? If yes, it is time to seek assistance. Do not let stigma interfere with you seeking help for your symptoms. Everyone has difficulty coping or functioning at certain times in their lives. For the sake of your own health and the people who love you as well as for the patients for whom you care, *seek help now!*

If you ever have thoughts of suicide, immediately seek help or call the national suicide prevention hot-line at 1-800-273-8255.

The Suicide Lifeline provides 24/7, free and confidential support for people in distress. It also provides prevention and crisis resources for you or your loved ones, in addition to best practice resources for clinicians.

Source: Reproduced with permission from Dolan, E. D., Mohr, D., Lempa, M., Joos, S., Fihn, S. D., Nelson, K. M., & Helfrichm, C. D. (2014). Using a single item to measure burnout in primary care staff: A psychometric evaluation. *Journal of General Internal Medicine, 30*(5), 582–587. https://doi.org/10.1007/s11606-014-3112-6

KEY STRATEGIES FOR OPTIMIZING YOUR OWN PERSONAL HEALTH AND WELL-BEING IN THE NINE DIMENSIONS OF WELL-BEING

When we board an airplane and hear safety messaging, we are told by a flight attendant to place the oxygen mask on ourselves first before placing it on your child or loved one. Remember, you cannot take good care of your family and/or your patients unless you practice good self-care. As briefly discussed in Chapter 1 of this text, good self-care should encompass the nine dimensions of wellness. These dimension of wellness are physical, emotional, financial, social, intellectual, career, creative, environmental, and spiritual. Each of these are discussed in the subsequent sections.

Physical Wellness

Chronic disease affects one in two Americans, yet approximately 80% of chronic disease can be prevented with just a few healthy lifestyle behaviors. Although cardiovascular disease remains the number one killer of Americans, if all causes of death and disease are taken into consideration, it is really our behaviors that are the number one killer, including physical in activity, unhealthy eating, drug abuse, and smoking. In order to substantially reduce your risk of chronic disease, make a commitment to achieve the following, including:

- 30 minutes of moderate intensity physical activity 5 days per week.
- Five servings of fruits and vegetables per day.
- Do not smoke.
- If you drink alcohol, limit it to no more than one drink a day if you are a woman and two a day if you are a man (Ford et al., 2011).

> Engage in some physical activity each day; even small amounts can increase your energy and decrease fatigue.

Aim for at least 7 hours of sleep per night, sit less, and practice regular stress reduction for even more preventive benefits (Melnyk & Neale, 2018). For a person who is inactive, even small increases in moderate intensity physical activity (e.g., 11 minutes a day) has health benefits (Physical Activity Guidelines Advisory Committee, 2018). There is no threshold that has to be exceeded before benefits occur. For more energy, it also is important to sit less and stand more. Several chronic diseases and conditions result from prolonged sitting. One recent study found that prolonged sitting (i.e., 6 or more hours a day versus less than 3 hours per day) was related to a higher risk of mortality from all causes, including cardiovascular disease, cancer, diabetes, kidney disease, suicide, chronic obstructive pulmonary disease, pneumonitis due to solids and liquids, liver disease, peptic ulcer and other digestive diseases, Parkinson disease, Alzheimer disease, nervous disorders, and musculoskeletal disorders (Patel et al., 2018). Try having standing meetings instead of sitting meetings. In addition to being good for your cardiovascular health, you will get through your meetings more quickly! Instead of waiting until January 1st to set a new healthy lifestyle behavior goal, consider today your January 1st. Remember, it takes 30 to 60 days to make or break a new health habit. It is important to write down your new healthy lifestyle behavior goal and place that goal where you can see it every day (e.g., by where you brush your teeth or at your computer). If you do fall off track, just start again the following day. Habits take consistent practice to make or break.

In addition, know your own numbers, including total cholesterol, low density lipoproteins, high density lipoproteins, body mass index, hemoglobin A1c, and waist circumference. The 2017 American College of Cardiology (ACC)/American Heart Association (AHA) guideline defines normal blood pressure (BP) as less than 120/80 Hg, and recommends BP checks at every healthcare clinician visit, or at least once every 2 years if your BP is normal. (Whelton & Carey, 2018).

It also is important to engage in strength training at least twice a week as it provides several benefits, including increased muscle mass, increased bone strength, better stability, and lower blood pressure. Resistance bands are an ideal convenient way to build strength as you can keep them at your desk and place one in your suitcase when you travel. Many websites contain resistance band workouts, such as greatist.com/fitness/resistance-band-exercises.

It also is important to limit your sodium intake to less than 1,500 mg/day and drink plenty of water as even mild dehydration can make you feel fatigued. The recommended amount is approximately 15.5 cups for men and 11.5 cups a day for women.

Emotional Wellness

Emotional wellness is the ability to identify, express, and manage the full range of your feelings. It includes practicing techniques to deal with stress, depression, and anxiety, and seeking help when your feelings become overwhelming or interfere with everyday functioning.

There is a wise saying: change your thinking, change your life! CBT or skills building is the gold standard recommended first-line treatment for mild to moderate depression and anxiety, yet so few people suffering with these symptoms receive it due to the inadequate numbers of mental health professionals throughout the United States. In CBT, people are taught that how they think is related to how they feel and how they behave. The ABCs are taught in CBT. The letter "A" stands for an activating event that triggers a negative Belief or thought. The Consequence of the negative belief is feeling stressed, anxious or depressed or acting in unhealthy ways. In CBT, individuals are taught how to monitor for activating events and stop negative beliefs when they occur. The consequence is feeling emotionally better and behaving in healthier ways. The next time that you feel stressed, anxious, angry, or depressed, ask yourself "What was I just thinking?" Chances are it was a negative thought. Monitoring for these activating events and turning negative thought patterns around is key to experiencing less negative moods. A recent randomized controlled trial testing a CBT-based program entitled MINDSTRONG, originally created by Bernadette Melnyk, with new nurse residents in a large academic medical center in the Midwest revealed that those who received the MINDSTRONG program versus those who received an attention control program had less stress, anxiety and depression as well as healthier behaviors and job satisfaction (Sampson et al., 2019). For more information on this MINDSTRONG program, contact Dr. Melnyk at Melnyk.15@osu.edu.

Try monitoring your thoughts for the next 30 days or keeping a journal of negative thoughts patterns and the emotions that come with them. Write down how you will respond to the stressor the next time. With time and practice, you can actually change your thinking in response to the stressors in your life, and that will change how you feel (Melnyk & Neal, 2018). Other tactics that can enhance your emotional well-being include:

- Engage in some physical activity each day; even small amounts can increase your energy and decrease fatigue.
- Keep a journal of what causes your stress and strategies that help to reduce it.
- Get at least 7 hours of sleep a night to avoid excess cortisol from being released.
- Practice mindfulness—the ability to stay in the present moment. Mindfulness decreases worry about the future and guilt about the past, which are two wasted emotions.
- Manage your energy by taking short recovery breaks throughout the day (even 5 minutes of activity every hour can increase your level of energy).
- Read 5 minutes in a positive thinking book of your choice every morning to elevate your mood and protect yourself against negativity that can arise each day.
- When stressed, take just five slow deep breaths in and out—deep breathing works to decrease stress and lower blood pressure. As you breathe in, say "I am calm." As you breathe out, say "I am blowing out all of my stress."
- Help others and be kind; compassion for others helps you to feel good.
- Talk to someone you trust about how you feel.
- Resolve to keep your workplace positive.
- Practice a daily attitude of gratitude. Naming or writing down three people or things you are grateful for every morning and evening can boost your mood.

If symptoms of anxiety, stress, or depression persist for more than 2 weeks and interfere with your daily functioning, do not wait; seek help from a qualified therapist or your healthcare clinician. Emotional wellness includes seeking help when needed (Melnyk & Neale, 2018).

Financial Wellness

Financial well-being includes being fully aware of your financial state and budget, and managing your finances to achieve your goals. Detailed analysis and planning is important so that you can make decisions regarding how you will spend and save your income. According to a study conducted by the American Psychological Association (APA) (2015), approximately three in four Americans experience financial stress, which typically affects physical and emotional well-being. According to the APA, high levels of financial stress are associated with an increased risk for ulcers, migraines, heart attacks, depression, anxiety, and sleep disturbance, and may lead to unhealthy coping mechanisms, such as binge drinking, smoking, and overeating. By analyzing, planning, and managing your spending, you can improve your financial well-being. The following are helpful strategies.

- **Evaluate your finances**. Analyze the amount of monthly income that you make and how you are currently spending it. Three months' worth of credit card and bank statements will give you a clear picture of your income and expenses. Identify your fixed expenses, such as the mortgage, car payments, student loans, and utility bills, and your variable expenses, such as money spent on food, clothing, vacations, emergencies, and health.
- **Prioritize**. Decide what you want to spend your income on every month and draw up a realistic budget. Online resources like Quicken, YNAB, and Moneydance can help.
- **Save rather than borrow**. Paying cash for things is best. If you use a credit card to obtain airline miles or other benefits, be sure to pay it off at the end of the month. It is much better to save to pay for something rather than borrow it. If you are thinking about a big purchase, sit on it overnight and see if you feel the same sense of urgency to buy it as you did when you saw it.
- **Protect yourself from unexpected expenses**. Reduce worry about financial emergencies by saving at least 6 months of pay.
- **Seek help**. A certified financial planner (CFP) can help you evaluate your current situation and show you ways to pay off debt and invest in your future. Look for fee-based CFPs, who charge a one-time fee rather than taking a percentage of your investments' earnings.
- **Find healthy outlets for your stress that are free.** Physical activity and stress reduction practices can reduce your overall stress, which will help you to think more clearly and get a better handle on your finances (Melnyk & Neale, 2018).

Social Wellness

> Take time to connect to people and activities that bring you joy.

Social wellness can be defined as our ability to effectively interact with people around us and to create a support system that includes family and friends (Melnyk & Neale, 2018). Findings from studies indicate that social connections help people to deal with stress and keep us healthy. It is important to build positive relationships at home and at work and to learn to have crucial conversations. It is fine to disagree with co-workers or loved ones as long as the disagreements are handled respectfully. Disconnecting from emails and technology to connect with the important people in your life on a regular basis will improve your mood. If you are feeling frustrated with how little time you have to connect with the people in your life who are important, consider saying "no" more to opportunities that create work overload in your life. Studies on the impact of loneliness on physical and mental health are alarming. Loneliness has been found to cause inflammation and raise stress hormone levels, which can increase the risk of heart disease, arthritis, type 2 diabetes, depression, pain, fatigue, and dementia (Jaremka et al., 2014). Jaremka et al. (2014) also found that people who are lonely may have suppressed immune systems, brought on by stress. Bottom line: Prioritize taking time to connect to people and activities that bring you joy.

Intellectual Wellness

When a person is intellectually healthy, he or she appreciates lifelong learning, fosters critical thinking, develops moral reasoning, expands worldviews, and engages in education for the pursuit of knowledge. Any time that you learn a new skill or concept and attempt to understand a different viewpoint or exercise your mind with puzzles and games, you are building intellectual well-being. Studies show that intellectual exercise may improve the physical structure of your brain to help prevent cognitive decline (Melnyk & Neale, 2018). Research supports that physical and mental exercise support the growth of new neurons, while stress and depression can hinder it (Barry, 2011). Challenging your brain also helps existing neurons form new connections. Combining intellectual growth with mindfulness can enhance your brain's health and prevent the cognitive decline that often occurs with aging.

Strategies that can help with intellectual well-being include: reading 5 to 10 minutes in a positive thinking book every day, which can also elevate your mood; giving your brain a rest with at least a few minutes of quiet time every few hours; not multi-tasking as it is the enemy of full engagement; disrupting your typical routines; and engaging in life-long learning.

Career Wellness

If you are engaged in work that you are truly passionate about throughout your career, you will never feel like you work a day in your life. It is important to answer the following question.

What will you do in the next 5 to 10 years if you know that you cannot fail?

Then, write the answer down to this question, put a date on it and place it where you can see it every day. So many people get immersed in day-to-day living and "to do's" or grinding chores or work that they lose their ability to dream. "Nothing happens without first a dream" is a famous saying by Carl Sandburg. When your work is aligned with your dreams and passions, you will wake up every day with energy and enthusiasm. If you are experiencing chronic stress, dissatisfaction, and burnout at work, it should prompt you to do an evaluation of your career wellness. People who are the happiest in their careers are those who have purpose, passion, and pride (Buettner, 2017).

Even if you cannot change where you work right now, you can change your approach to the stressors and challenges you face at work. Several strategies can help you re-evaluate your career, cope with change and stress, and re-energize your work life.

- Practice mindfulness at select times during the day at work. Research supports that mindfulness can increase on-the-job resiliency and improve effectiveness and safety.
- Cultivate a positive mindset. By staying positive, you will feel emotionally better and be more productive.
- Do not multi-task. Multi-tasking can drain your energy.

- Evaluate your work hours, including time you spend commuting. If you cannot cut your commuting time, try making use of drive time to listen to audiobooks or positive music. Use your vacation hours to disconnect and get away at regular intervals.

Creative Wellness

Creativity has long been a part of well-being. A review of more than 100 studies of the benefits of the arts (music, visual arts, dance, and writing) found that creative expression has a powerful impact on health and well-being among various populations (Jacobs, 2015). Findings from studies indicate that participating in the arts decreases depressive symptoms, increases positive emotions, reduces stress, and, in some cases, improves immune system functioning. Creative wellness means valuing and participating in a diverse range of arts and cultural experiences to understand and appreciate your surrounding world (Melnyk & Neale, 2018). If you do not consider yourself creative, attempt doodling in a blank journal to relieve stress, or try a free doodling app like Doodle Buddy and You Doodle. Freewriting, journaling, and writing poetry and stories can be stress reducing and healing. Creativity can include cooking, gardening, redecorating your home or office, and more. Research shows that creative pursuits also boost intellectual wellness and may delay cognitive decline in older people.

> Participating in the arts decreases depressive symptoms, increases positive emotions, reduces stress, and can improve immune system functioning.

Environmental Wellness

Environmental wellness means recognizing the responsibility to preserve, protect, and improve the environment, and to appreciate your connection to nature (Melnyk & Neale, 2018). Environmental wellness intersects with social wellness when you work to conserve the environment for future generations and improve conditions for others around the world. Studies have shown that green space, such as parks, forests, and river corridors, are good for our physical and mental health (World Health Organization, 2016). Your environment includes everything that surrounds you— your home, your car, your workplace, the food you eat, and the people with whom you interact.

Paying attention to environment is especially important at work, where our surroundings can have a profound effect on how we feel and function. We tend to thrive better when we are surrounded by people who support our goals and provide support to help us to succeed. We cannot usually choose the people with whom we work, but we can support an environment of workplace civility, and choose to spend more time with those who support and uplift us. Also, we can contribute to making our physical surroundings healthier, from recycling to creating a culture of respect and gratitude (Melnyk & Neale, 2018).

You can improve your environment by taking steps to be conscious about how you use natural resources, such as recycling, turning off water or electric appliances and lights when not in use, saving gas by walking, biking, or taking public transportation instead of driving, and supporting your colleagues' efforts to recycle at the office. When you show respect for the natural environment, you show respect for others and for future generations.

Spiritual Wellness

Spiritual wellness is largely about your purpose, not religion. Dossey (2015) contends that our spirituality involves a sense of connection outside ourselves and includes our values, meaning, and purpose. Your spiritual well-being is about what inspires you, what gives you hope, and what you feel strongly about (Melnyk & Neale, 2018). Your spirit is the seat of your deepest values and character.

Although religion and spirituality can be connected, they are different. A faith community can give you an outlet for your spirituality, but religion is not spirituality's only expression. Hope, purpose, job, love, meaning, connection, appreciation of beauty, and caring and compassion for others are associated with spiritual well-being.

Our purpose is at the foundation of our spiritual nature. If you are feeling disconnected from your values and purpose, try the following strategies.

- Set aside some quiet time to think about your purpose and whether you are fulfilling it. Identify what you need to do to adjust. Ask yourself what you would do in the next 5 to 10 years if you knew you could not fail.
- Retain a positive outlook. Actively seek ways to increase positivity, such as keeping a gratitude journal, celebrating your strengths, and recognizing and practicing small acts of kindness daily.
- Adopt a meditative practice. Traditional forms of meditation can include prayer or sitting in stillness with a quiet mind. Some people prefer physical action that incorporates meditation, such as yoga, tai chi, or walking. Find out what you like best and do what works for you.

> Forms of meditation include prayer, sitting in stillness with a quiet mind, and physical activities such as yoga, tai chi, or walking.

TAKE ACTION TO IMPROVE YOUR HEALTH AND WELL-BEING NOW: BERN'S STORY

Do not procrastinate taking good self-care. Your life and others' lives depend on it.

Now that you have nearly completed this chapter and reviewed evidence-based strategies that can assist you in achieving optimal health and well-being, evaluate your strengths and needs in each of the nine dimensions of well-being. Choose one dimension that you will focus on in the next 30 to 60 days. If you are finding it difficult to prioritize your own self-care, think about all of the people who love you and want you to be around for a long time. The first author of this chapter (Bernadette [Bern] Melnyk) lost her mom suddenly at the age of 15 years. After a wonderful breakfast interchange when they were home alone, Bern's mom sneezed, suffered a stroke and died. The sad part of this story is that Bern's mother had a history of headaches for over a year. She finally visited her physician for an evaluation a week before she died, was diagnosed with high blood pressure, and given a prescription for a blood pressure medication. However, she never filled the prescription; Bern's father found it in her mom's purse after she died. Due to this traumatic event, Bern suffered with post-traumatic stress disorder for a few years. Unfortunately, there was no help or counseling for her in the small town of Republic, Pennsylvania, where she grew up. In the next 4 years, Bern also lost a cousin after a motor vehicle accident, the only grandparent she ever knew and loved, and her father suffered a major heart attack. However, what does not break us only makes us stronger. As a result of these adversities, Bern developed a passion and purpose to become a nurse, a pediatric nurse practitioner and psychiatric nurse practitioner, and obtain a PhD so that she could develop and test evidence-based programs to improve mental health outcomes in children, teens, college students, and parents. These programs are now bringing her evidence-based Creating Opportunities for Personal Empowerment (COPE) cognitive-behavioral skills building intervention programs to thousands of children and youth with depression and anxiety across the United States and five other countries. We tell this story to encourage you because often we do not understand why we are experiencing life's challenges when they are happening, but as a result of these types of experiences, we grow stronger and pursue our purpose to make a positive impact in the world.

If it is difficult for you to prioritize your own self-care, think about doing it for the people who love you—who want you to be around for a very long time. Bern lost her mom suddenly when she was 15 years old due to a stroke that may have been able to be prevented if she had filled her prescription and started taking the medication. She did not have a mother to see her graduate from high school, become a nurse, and go on to have her three beautiful daughters. When she lacks the energy to exercise or the motivation to make healthy food choices, Bern thinks about her husband, three daughters, and two small grandsons who provide the motivation for her to continue to make healthy lifestyle choices. Who is the person/people in your life that will serve as the motivator(s) for you to make healthy choices and take better self-care?

ACT NOW: Take one step today and commit to improving one wellness dimension that can lead you on a better path to optimal health and well-being. If you do not take the time for good self-care today, you will need to take the time to deal with chronic illness in the future. We believe in you; you can do it!

REFERENCES

Amaya, M., Melnyk, B. M., Buffington, B., & Battista, L. (2017). Workplace wellness champions: lessons learned and implications for future programming. *Building Healthy Academic Communities Journal, 1*(1), 59–67. https://doi.org/10.18061/bhac.v1i1.5744.

American Psychological Association. (2015). *Paying with our health.* https://www.apa.org/news/press/releases/stress/2014/stress-report.pdf

Baicker, K., Cutler, D., & Song, Z. (2010). Workplace wellness programs can generate savings. *Health Affairs, 29*(2), 304–311. https://doi.org.10.1377/hlthaff.2009.0626

Barry, S. R. (2011). How to grow new neurons in your brain. *Psychology Today.* https://www.psychologytoday.com/us/blog/eyes-the-brain/201101/how-grow-new-neurons-in-your-brain

Buettner, D. (2017). *The blue zones of happiness: Lessons from the world's happiest people.* National Geographic Partners.

Cohen, S., Kamarch, T., & Mermelstein, R. (1983). A global measure of perceived stress. *Journal of Health and Social Behavior, 24,* 385–396. https://doi.org/10.2307/2136404

Dolan, E. D., Mohr, D., Lempa, M., Joos, S., Fihn, S. D., Nelson, K. M., & Helfrich, C. D. (2014). Using a single item to measure burnout in primary care staff: A psychometric evaluation. *Journal of General Internal Medicine, 30*(5), 582–587. https://doi.org/10.1007/s11606-014-3112-6

Dossey, B. M. (2015). Integrative health and wellness assessment. In B. M. Dossey, S. Luck, & B. S. Schaub (Eds.), *Nurse coaching: Integrative approaches for health and well – being* (pp. 109–121). International Nurse Coach Association.

Dzau, V. J., Kirch, D. G., & Nasca, T. J. (2018). To care is human—collectively confronting the clinician-burnout crisis. *New England Journal of Medicine, 378*(4), 312–314. https://doi.org/10.1056/NEJMp1715127.

Ford, E. S., Zhao, G, Tsai, J., & Li, C. (2011). Low-risk lifestyle behaviors and all-cause mortality: Findings from the national health and nutrition examination survey III mortality study. *American Journal of Public Health, 101,* 1922–1929. https://doi.org/10.2105/AJPH.2011.300167.

Fred, H. L., & Scheid, M. S. (2018). Physician burnout: Causes, consequences, and (?) cures. *Texas Heart Institute Journal, 45*(4), 198–202. http://doi.org.10.14503/THIJ-18-6842

Hall, L. H., Johnson, J., Watt, I., Tsipa, A., & O'Connor, D. B. (2016). Healthcare staff wellbeing, burnout, and patient safety: A systematic review. *PLOS One, 11*(7), e0159015. https://doi.org/10.1371/journal.pone.0159015.

Jacobs, T. (2015, April 8). Making art tied to fewer cognitive problems in old age. *Pacific Standard.* Retrieved from https://psmag.com/social-justice/making-art-tied-to-fewer-cognitive-problems-in-old-age

Jaremka, L. M., Andridge, R. R., Fagundes, C. P., Alfano, C. M., Povoski, S. P., Lipari, A. M., Agnese, D. M., Arnold, M. W., Farrar, W. B., Yee, L. D., Carson, W. E., Bekaii-Saab, T., Martin, E. W., Schmidt, C. R., & Kiecolt-Glaser, J. K. (2013). Pain, depression, and fatigue: Loneliness as a longitudinal risk factor. *Health Psychology, 33*(9), 948–957. https://doi.org/10.1037/a0034012.

Jaremka, L. M., Fagundes, C. P., Peng, J., Bennett, J. M., Glaser, R., Malarkey, W. B., & Kiecolt-Glaser, J. K. (2014). Loneliness promotes inflammation during acute stress. *Psychology Science, 24*(7), 1089–1097. https://doi.org/10.1177/0956797612464059

Jun, J., Tucker, S., & Melnyk, B. M. (2020). Clinician mental health and well-being during global healthcare crises: Evidence learned from prior epidemics for COVID-19 pandemic. *Worldviews on Evidence-Based Nursing, 17*(3), 182–184. https://doi.org/10.1111/wvn.12439

Kishore, S., Ripp, J., Shanafelt, T., Melnyk, B. M., Roger, D., Brigham, T., Busis, N., Charney, D., Cipriano, P., Minor, L., Rothman, P., Spisso, J., Kirch, D. G., Nasca, T., & Dzau, V. (2018). Making the case for the chief wellness officer in America's health systems: A call to action. *Health Affairs*. Blog website. healthaffairs.org/do/10.1377/hblog20181025.308059/full. Published October 26, 2018. Accessed November 1, 2018.

Kroenke, K., Spitzer, R. L., & Williams, J. B. (2001). The PHQ-9: Validity of a brief depression severity measure. *Journal of General Internal Medicine*, *16*(9), 606–613. https://doi.org/10.1046/j.1525-1497.2001.016009606.x

Makary, M. A. (2016). Medical error-the third leading cause of death in the US. *BMJ*, *353*, i2139 https://doi.org/10.1136/bmj.i2139

Melnyk, B. M. (2019). Making an evidence-based case for urgent action to address clinician burnout. *American Journal of Accountable Care*, *7*(2), 12–14.

Melnyk, B. M. (2020). Burnout, depression and suicide in nurses/clinicians and learners: An urgent call for action to enhance professional well-being and healthcare safety. *Worldviews on Evidence-Based Nursing*, *17*(1), 2–5. https://doi.org/10.1111/wvn.12416

Melnyk, B. M., Gascon, G. M., Amaya, M., & Mehta, L. S. (2018). A comprehensive approach to university wellness emphasizing million hearts demonstrates improvement in population cardiovascular risk. *Building Healthy Academic Communities Journal*, *2*(2), 6–11. https://doi.org/10.18061/bhac.v2i2.6555.

Melnyk, B. M., Gawlik, K., & Teall, A. M. (2021). Evidence-based assessment of personal health and wellbeing for clinicians: Key strategies to achieve optimal wellness. In (Chapter 28, p. 723–736). In Gawlik, K., Melnyk, B. M., & Teall, A. M. *Evidence-Based Physical Examination: Best Practices for Health & Well-Being Assessment*. Springer Publishing Company.

Melnyk, B. M., & Neale, S. (2018). *9 dimensions of wellness. Evidence-based tactics for optimizing your health and well-being*. The Ohio State University.

Melnyk, B. M., Orsolini, L., Tan, A., Arslanian-Engoren, C., Melkus, G., Dunbar-Jacobs, J., Rice, V., Millian, A., Dunbar, S., Braun, L., Wilber, J., Chyun, D., Gawlik, K., & Lewis, L. (2017). A national study links nurses' physical and mental health to medical errors and perceived worksite wellness. *Journal of Occupational Medicine*, *60*(2), 126–131. https://doi.org. 10.1097/JOM.0000000000001198

Melnyk B. M., Szalacha, L. A., & Amaya, M. (2018). Psychometric properties of the perceived wellness culture and environment scale. *American Journal of Health Promotion*, *32*(4), 1021–1027. https://doi.org/10.1177/0890117117737676.

Muller, A. E., Hafstad, E. V., Himmels, J. P. W., Smedslund, G., Flottorp, S., Stensland, S., & Vist, G. E. (2020). The mental health impact of the covid-19 pandemic on healthcare workers, and interventions to help them: A rapid systematic review. *MedRxiv*, *293*, 113441. https://doi.org/10.1101/2020.07.03.20145607

Patel, A. V., Maliniak, M. L., Rees-Punia, E., Matthews, C. E., & Gapstur, S. M. (2018). Prolonged leisure time spent sitting in relation to cause-specific mortality in a large US cohort. *American Journal of Epidemiology*, *187*(10), 2151–2158. https://doi.org/10.1093/aje/kwy125

Physical Activity Guidelines Advisory Committee. (2018). *2018 physical activity guidelines advisory committee*. U.S. Department of Health and Human Services.

Sampson, M., Melnyk, B. M., & Hoying, J. (2019). Intervention effects of the MINDBODYSTRONG© cognitive behavioral skills-building program on newly licensed registered nurses' mental health, healthy lifestyle behaviors and job satisfaction. *JONA: The Journal of Nursing Administration*, *49*(10), 487–495. https://doi.org.10.1097/NNA.0000000000000792.

Shanafelt, T. D., Hasan, O., Dyrbye, L. N., Sinsky, C., Satele, D., Sloan, J., & West, C. P. (2015). Changes in burnout and satisfaction with work-life balance in physicians and the general US working population between 2011 and 2014. *Mayo Clinic Proceeding*, *90*, 1600–1613. https://doi.org/10.1016/j.mayocp.2015.08.023

Spitzer, R. L., Kroenke, K., Williams, J. B., & Lowe, B. (2006). A brief measure for assessing generalized anxiety disorder: the GAD-7. *Archives of Internal Medicine*, *166*(10), 1092–1097. https://doi.org/10.1001/archinte.166.10.1092

Unruh, L. Y., & Zhang, N. J. (2014). Newly licensed registered nurse job turnover and turnover intent. *Journal of Nurses in Professional Development*, *30*(5), 220–230. https://doi.org/10.1097/NND.0000000000000079.

Whelton, P. K., & Carey, R. M. (2018). The 2017 American College of Cardiology/American Heart Association clinical practice guideline for high blood pressure in adults. *JAMA Cardiology*, *3*(4), 352–353. https://doi.org.10.1001/jamacardio.2018.0005

Willard-Grace, R., Knox, M., Huang, B., Hammer, H., Kivlahan, C., & Grumbach, K. (2019). Burnout and health care workforce turnover. *Annals of Family Medicine*, *17*(1), 36–41. https://doi.org/10.1370/afm.2338.

World Health Organization. (2016). *Urban green spaces and health: A review of evidence*. http://www.euro.who.int/__data/assets/pdf_file/0005/321971/Urban-green-spaces-and-health-review-evidence.pdf?ua=1

Index